50% OFF Online HESI A2 Prep Course!

Dear Customer,

We consider it an honor and a privilege that you chose our HESI A2 Study Guide. As a way of showing our appreciation and to help us better serve you, we have partnered with Mometrix Test Preparation to offer **50% off our online HESI A2 Prep Course.** Many HESI A2 courses are needlessly expensive and don't deliver enough value. With their course, you get access to the best HESI A2 prep material, and you only pay half price.

Mometrix has structured their online course to perfectly complement your printed study guide. The HESI A2 Prep Course contains **in-depth lessons** that cover all the most important topics, **150+ video reviews** that explain difficult concepts, **over 2,500 practice questions** to ensure you feel prepared, and **300 digital flashcards** so you can fit some studying in while you're on the go.

Online HESI A2 Prep Course

Topics Covered:

- English Language
  - Main Ideas, Supporting Details, and Context
  - Vocabulary and General Knowledge
  - Agreement and Sentence Structure
- Math
  - Operations
  - Factoring
  - Proportions and Ratios
- Science
  - Biology
  - Chemistry
  - Anatomy and Physiology

Course Features:

- HESI A2 Study Guide
  - Get content that complements our best-selling study guide.
- 7 Full-Length Practice Tests
  - With over 2,500 practice questions, you can test yourself again and again.
- Mobile Friendly
  - If you need to study on-the-go, the course is easily accessible from your mobile device.
- HESI A2 Flashcards
  - The course includes a flashcard mode consisting of over 300 content cards to help you study.

To receive this discount, simply head to their website: mometrix.com/university/hesi or simply scan this QR code with your smartphone. At the checkout page, enter the discount code: **TPBHESI50**

If you have any questions or concerns, please don't hesitate to contact Mometrix at universityhelp@mometrix.com.

Sincerely,

 in partnership with

FREE Test Taking Tips Video/DVD Offer

To better serve you, we created videos covering test taking tips that we want to give you for FREE. **These videos cover world-class tips that will help you succeed on your test.**

We just ask that you send us feedback about this product. Please let us know what you thought about it—whether good, bad, or indifferent.

To get your **FREE videos**, you can use the QR code below or email freevideos@studyguideteam.com with "Free Videos" in the subject line and the following information in the body of the email:

    a. The title of your product

    b. Your product rating on a scale of 1-5, with 5 being the highest

    c. Your feedback about the product

If you have any questions or concerns, please don't hesitate to contact us at info@studyguideteam.com.

Thank you!

HESI A2 Study Guide 2022-2023

1,000+ Practice Questions and HESI Admission Assessment Exam Review Book [9th Edition]

Joshua Rueda

Written and edited by TPB Publishing.

TPB Publishing is not associated with or endorsed by any official testing organization. TPB Publishing is a publisher of unofficial educational products. All test and organization names are trademarks of their respective owners. Content in this book is included for utilitarian purposes only and does not constitute an endorsement by TPB Publishing of any particular point of view.

Interested in buying more than 10 copies of our product? Contact us about bulk discounts: bulkorders@studyguideteam.com

ISBN 13: 9781637754016
ISBN 10: 1637754019

Table of Contents

//Test Prep Books///

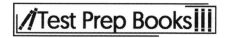

Quick Overview

As you draw closer to taking your exam, effective preparation becomes more and more important. Thankfully, you have this study guide to help you get ready. Use this guide to help keep your studying on track and refer to it often.

This study guide contains several key sections that will help you be successful on your exam. The guide contains tips for what you should do the night before and the day of the test. Also included are test-taking tips. Knowing the right information is not always enough. Many well-prepared test takers struggle with exams. These tips will help equip you to accurately read, assess, and answer test questions.

A large part of the guide is devoted to showing you what content to expect on the exam and to helping you better understand that content. In this guide are practice test questions so that you can see how well you have grasped the content. Then, answer explanations are provided so that you can understand why you missed certain questions.

Don't try to cram the night before you take your exam. This is not a wise strategy for a few reasons. First, your retention of the information will be low. Your time would be better used by reviewing information you already know rather than trying to learn a lot of new information. Second, you will likely become stressed as you try to gain a large amount of knowledge in a short amount of time. Third, you will be depriving yourself of sleep. So be sure to go to bed at a reasonable time the night before. Being well-rested helps you focus and remain calm.

Be sure to eat a substantial breakfast the morning of the exam. If you are taking the exam in the afternoon, be sure to have a good lunch as well. Being hungry is distracting and can make it difficult to focus. You have hopefully spent lots of time preparing for the exam. Don't let an empty stomach get in the way of success!

When travelling to the testing center, leave earlier than needed. That way, you have a buffer in case you experience any delays. This will help you remain calm and will keep you from missing your appointment time at the testing center.

Be sure to pace yourself during the exam. Don't try to rush through the exam. There is no need to risk performing poorly on the exam just so you can leave the testing center early. Allow yourself to use all of the allotted time if needed.

Remain positive while taking the exam even if you feel like you are performing poorly. Thinking about the content you should have mastered will not help you perform better on the exam.

Once the exam is complete, take some time to relax. Even if you feel that you need to take the exam again, you will be well served by some down time before you begin studying again. It's often easier to convince yourself to study if you know that it will come with a reward!

Test-Taking Strategies

1. Predicting the Answer

When you feel confident in your preparation for a multiple-choice test, try predicting the answer before reading the answer choices. This is especially useful on questions that test objective factual knowledge. By predicting the answer before reading the available choices, you eliminate the possibility that you will be distracted or led astray by an incorrect answer choice. You will feel more confident in your selection if you read the question, predict the answer, and then find your prediction among the answer choices. After using this strategy, be sure to still read all of the answer choices carefully and completely. If you feel unprepared, you should not attempt to predict the answers. This would be a waste of time and an opportunity for your mind to wander in the wrong direction.

2. Reading the Whole Question

Too often, test takers scan a multiple-choice question, recognize a few familiar words, and immediately jump to the answer choices. Test authors are aware of this common impatience, and they will sometimes prey upon it. For instance, a test author might subtly turn the question into a negative, or he or she might redirect the focus of the question right at the end. The only way to avoid falling into these traps is to read the entirety of the question carefully before reading the answer choices.

3. Looking for Wrong Answers

Long and complicated multiple-choice questions can be intimidating. One way to simplify a difficult multiple-choice question is to eliminate all of the answer choices that are clearly wrong. In most sets of answers, there will be at least one selection that can be dismissed right away. If the test is administered on paper, the test taker could draw a line through it to indicate that it may be ignored; otherwise, the test taker will have to perform this operation mentally or on scratch paper. In either case, once the obviously incorrect answers have been eliminated, the remaining choices may be considered. Sometimes identifying the clearly wrong answers will give the test taker some information about the correct answer. For instance, if one of the remaining answer choices is a direct opposite of one of the eliminated answer choices, it may well be the correct answer. The opposite of obviously wrong is obviously right! Of course, this is not always the case. Some answers are obviously incorrect simply because they are irrelevant to the question being asked. Still, identifying and eliminating some incorrect answer choices is a good way to simplify a multiple-choice question.

4. Don't Overanalyze

Anxious test takers often overanalyze questions. When you are nervous, your brain will often run wild, causing you to make associations and discover clues that don't actually exist. If you feel that this may be a problem for you, do whatever you can to slow down during the test. Try taking a deep breath or counting to ten. As you read and consider the question, restrict yourself to the particular words used by the author. Avoid thought tangents about what the author *really* meant, or what he or she was *trying* to say. The only things that matter on a multiple-choice test are the words that are actually in the question. You must avoid reading too much into a multiple-choice question, or supposing that the writer meant something other than what he or she wrote.

2

5. No Need for Panic

It is wise to learn as many strategies as possible before taking a multiple-choice test, but it is likely that you will come across a few questions for which you simply don't know the answer. In this situation, avoid panicking. Because most multiple-choice tests include dozens of questions, the relative value of a single wrong answer is small. As much as possible, you should compartmentalize each question on a multiple-choice test. In other words, you should not allow your feelings about one question to affect your success on the others. When you find a question that you either don't understand or don't know how to answer, just take a deep breath and do your best. Read the entire question slowly and carefully. Try rephrasing the question a couple of different ways. Then, read all of the answer choices carefully. After eliminating obviously wrong answers, make a selection and move on to the next question.

6. Confusing Answer Choices

When working on a difficult multiple-choice question, there may be a tendency to focus on the answer choices that are the easiest to understand. Many people, whether consciously or not, gravitate to the answer choices that require the least concentration, knowledge, and memory. This is a mistake. When you come across an answer choice that is confusing, you should give it extra attention. A question might be confusing because you do not know the subject matter to which it refers. If this is the case, don't eliminate the answer before you have affirmatively settled on another. When you come across an answer choice of this type, set it aside as you look at the remaining choices. If you can confidently assert that one of the other choices is correct, you can leave the confusing answer aside. Otherwise, you will need to take a moment to try to better understand the confusing answer choice. Rephrasing is one way to tease out the sense of a confusing answer choice.

7. Your First Instinct

Many people struggle with multiple-choice tests because they overthink the questions. If you have studied sufficiently for the test, you should be prepared to trust your first instinct once you have carefully and completely read the question and all of the answer choices. There is a great deal of research suggesting that the mind can come to the correct conclusion very quickly once it has obtained all of the relevant information. At times, it may seem to you as if your intuition is working faster even than your reasoning mind. This may in fact be true. The knowledge you obtain while studying may be retrieved from your subconscious before you have a chance to work out the associations that support it. Verify your instinct by working out the reasons that it should be trusted.

8. Key Words

Many test takers struggle with multiple-choice questions because they have poor reading comprehension skills. Quickly reading and understanding a multiple-choice question requires a mixture of skill and experience. To help with this, try jotting down a few key words and phrases on a piece of scrap paper. Doing this concentrates the process of reading and forces the mind to weigh the relative importance of the question's parts. In selecting words and phrases to write down, the test taker thinks about the question more deeply and carefully. This is especially true for multiple-choice questions that are preceded by a long prompt.

9. Subtle Negatives

One of the oldest tricks in the multiple-choice test writer's book is to subtly reverse the meaning of a question with a word like *not* or *except*. If you are not paying attention to each word in the question, you can easily be led astray by this trick. For instance, a common question format is, "Which of the following is…?" Obviously, if the question instead is, "Which of the following is not…?," then the answer will be quite different. Even worse, the test makers are aware of the potential for this mistake and will include one answer choice that would be correct if the question were not negated or reversed. A test taker who misses the reversal will find what he or she believes to be a correct answer and will be so confident that he or she will fail to reread the question and discover the original error. The only way to avoid this is to practice a wide variety of multiple-choice questions and to pay close attention to each and every word.

10. Reading Every Answer Choice

It may seem obvious, but you should always read every one of the answer choices! Too many test takers fall into the habit of scanning the question and assuming that they understand the question because they recognize a few key words. From there, they pick the first answer choice that answers the question they believe they have read. Test takers who read all of the answer choices might discover that one of the latter answer choices is actually *more* correct. Moreover, reading all of the answer choices can remind you of facts related to the question that can help you arrive at the correct answer. Sometimes, a misstatement or incorrect detail in one of the latter answer choices will trigger your memory of the subject and will enable you to find the right answer. Failing to read all of the answer choices is like not reading all of the items on a restaurant menu: you might miss out on the perfect choice.

11. Spot the Hedges

One of the keys to success on multiple-choice tests is paying close attention to every word. This is never truer than with words like almost, most, some, and sometimes. These words are called "hedges" because they indicate that a statement is not totally true or not true in every place and time. An absolute statement will contain no hedges, but in many subjects, the answers are not always straightforward or absolute. There are always exceptions to the rules in these subjects. For this reason, you should favor those multiple-choice questions that contain hedging language. The presence of qualifying words indicates that the author is taking special care with their words, which is certainly important when composing the right answer. After all, there are many ways to be wrong, but there is only one way to be right! For this reason, it is wise to avoid answers that are absolute when taking a multiple-choice test. An absolute answer is one that says things are either all one way or all another. They often include words like *every*, *always*, *best*, and *never*. If you are taking a multiple-choice test in a subject that doesn't lend itself to absolute answers, be on your guard if you see any of these words.

12. Long Answers

In many subject areas, the answers are not simple. As already mentioned, the right answer often requires hedges. Another common feature of the answers to a complex or subjective question are qualifying clauses, which are groups of words that subtly modify the meaning of the sentence. If the question or answer choice describes a rule to which there are exceptions or the subject matter is complicated, ambiguous, or confusing, the correct answer will require many words in order to be expressed clearly and accurately. In essence, you should not be deterred by answer choices that seem excessively long. Oftentimes, the author of the text will not be able to write the correct answer without offering some qualifications and modifications. Your job is to read the answer choices thoroughly and completely and to select the one that most accurately and precisely answers the question.

13. Restating to Understand

Sometimes, a question on a multiple-choice test is difficult not because of what it asks but because of how it is written. If this is the case, restate the question or answer choice in different words. This process serves a couple of important purposes. First, it forces you to concentrate on the core of the question. In order to rephrase the question accurately, you have to understand it well. Rephrasing the question will concentrate your mind on the key words and ideas. Second, it will present the information to your mind in a fresh way. This process may trigger your memory and render some useful scrap of information picked up while studying.

14. True Statements

Sometimes an answer choice will be true in itself, but it does not answer the question. This is one of the main reasons why it is essential to read the question carefully and completely before proceeding to the answer choices. Too often, test takers skip ahead to the answer choices and look for true statements. Having found one of these, they are content to select it without reference to the question above. Obviously, this provides an easy way for test makers to play tricks. The savvy test taker will always read the entire question before turning to the answer choices. Then, having settled on a correct answer choice, he or she will refer to the original question and ensure that the selected answer is relevant. The mistake of choosing a correct-but-irrelevant answer choice is especially common on questions related to specific pieces of objective knowledge. A prepared test taker will have a wealth of factual knowledge at their disposal, and should not be careless in its application.

15. No Patterns

One of the more dangerous ideas that circulates about multiple-choice tests is that the correct answers tend to fall into patterns. These erroneous ideas range from a belief that B and C are the most common right answers, to the idea that an unprepared test-taker should answer "A-B-A-C-A-D-A-B-A." It cannot be emphasized enough that pattern-seeking of this type is exactly the WRONG way to approach a multiple-choice test. To begin with, it is highly unlikely that the test maker will plot the correct answers according to some predetermined pattern. The questions are scrambled and delivered in a random order. Furthermore, even if the test maker was following a pattern in the assignation of correct answers, there is no reason why the test taker would know which pattern he or she was using. Any attempt to discern a pattern in the answer choices is a waste of time and a distraction from the real work of taking the test. A test taker would be much better served by extra preparation before the test than by reliance on a pattern in the answers.

FREE Videos/DVD OFFER

Doing well on your exam requires both knowing the test content and understanding how to use that knowledge to do well on the test. We offer completely FREE test taking tip videos. **These videos cover world-class tips that you can use to succeed on your test.**

To get your **FREE videos**, you can use the QR code below or email freevideos@studyguideteam.com with "Free Videos" in the subject line and the following information in the body of the email:

    a. The title of your product

    b. Your product rating on a scale of 1-5, with 5 being the highest

    c. Your feedback about the product

If you have any questions or concerns, please don't hesitate to contact us at info@studyguideteam.com.

Thanks again!

Introduction to the HESI Admission Assessment

Function of the Test

The Health Education Systems, Inc. (HESI) Admission Assessment (A2) Exam is an entrance exam intended for high school graduates seeking admission to post-secondary health programs such as nursing schools. Test-takers have typically not received any training in specific medical subjects. The test is offered nationwide by the colleges and universities that require it as part of an applicant's admission package.

Test Administration

Many of the specifics of the process of HESI administration are determined at the discretion of the testing institution. For instance, each school may choose to administer the entire HESI exam or any portion thereof. Accordingly, there is no set process or schedule for taking the exam; instead, the schedule is determined on a case-by-case basis by the institution administering the exam. Likewise, the cost of the HESI is set by the administering institution. The typical cost is usually around $40-$70.

Find out ahead of time which sections you will be required to take so that you can focus your studying on those areas.

Retesting is generally permitted by HESI, but individual schools may have their own rules on the subject. Likewise, individual schools may set their own policies on whether section scores from different sessions of the HESI can be combined to get one score, or whether a score must come from one coherent session. Students with disabilities may seek accommodations from the schools administering the exam.

Test Format

The exam can include up to eight academic sections with the following distribution of questions:

Section	# of Questions
Mathematics	55
Reading Comprehension	55
Vocabulary	55
Grammar	55
Biology	30
Chemistry	30
Anatomy & Physiology	30
Physics	30

Each academic section contains five unscored pilot questions that are only used to gather data on their effectiveness before potentially including them as scored questions on future exams. Additionally, there is a Personality Profile and Learning Style Assessment that may be included. Like the academic sections, schools can pick and choose whether to include one, both, or neither of these assessments. Each takes about 15 minutes, and you do not need to study for them.

Scoring

Prospective students and their educational institutions both receive detailed score reports after a prospective applicant completes the exam. Individual student reports include scoring explanations and breakdowns by topic for incorrect answers. The test taker's results can also include study tips based on the individual's Learning Style assessment and identification of the test taker's dominant personality type, strengths, weaknesses, and suggested learning techniques, based on the Personality Profile.

There is no set passing score for the HESI. Instead, individual schools set their own requirements and processes for incorporating scores into admissions decisions. However, HESI recommends that RN and HP programs require a 75% score to pass, and that LPN/LVN programs require a 70% score to pass

Study Prep Plan for the HESI Admission Assessment

1 **Schedule** - Develop a study schedule based on the sections of the exam that you will be taking.

2 **Relax** - Test anxiety can hurt event the best students. There are many ways to reduce stress. Find the one that works best for you.

3 **Execute** - Once you have a good plan in place, be sure to stick to it

Sample Study Plans

One Week Study Schedule

Day 1	_____
Day 2	_____
Day 3	_____
Day 4	_____
Day 5	_____
Day 6	_____
Day 7	Take Your Exam!

Two Week Study Schedule

Day 1	_____	Day 8	_____
Day 2	_____	Day 9	_____
Day 3	_____	Day 10	_____
Day 4	_____	Day 11	_____
Day 5	_____	Day 12	_____
Day 6	_____	Day 13	_____
Day 7	_____	Day 14	Take Your Exam!

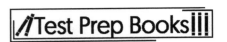
One Month Study Schedule

Day 1 _____	Day 11 _____	Day 21 _____
Day 2 _____	Day 12 _____	Day 22 _____
Day 3 _____	Day 13 _____	Day 23 _____
Day 4 _____	Day 14 _____	Day 24 _____
Day 5 _____	Day 15 _____	Day 25 _____
Day 6 _____	Day 16 _____	Day 26 _____
Day 7 _____	Day 17 _____	Day 27 _____
Day 8 _____	Day 18 _____	Day 28 _____
Day 9 _____	Day 19 _____	Day 29 _____
Day 10 _____	Day 20 _____	Day 30 Take Your Exam!

Mathematics

Numbers usually serve as an adjective representing a quantity of objects. They function as placeholders for a value. Numbers can be better understood by their type and related characteristics.

Definitions

A few definitions:

Whole numbers: describes a set of numbers that does not contain any fractions or decimals. The set of whole numbers includes zero.

> Example: 0, 1, 2, 3, 4, 189, 293 are all whole numbers.

Integers: describes whole numbers and their negative counterparts. (Zero does not have a negative counterpart here. Instead, zero is its own negative.)

> Example: -1, -2, -3, -4, -5, 0, 1, 2, 3, 4, 5 are all integers.

-1, -2, -3, -4, -5 are considered negative integers, and 1, 2, 3, 4, 5 are considered positive integers.

Absolute value: describes the value of a number regardless of its sign. The symbol for absolute value is $| |$.

> Example: The absolute value of 24 is 24 or $|24|=24$.

The absolute value of -693 is 693 or $|-693|=693$.

Even numbers: describes any number that can be divided by 2 evenly, meaning the answer has no decimal or remainder portion.

> Example: 2, 4, 9082, -2, -16, -504 are all considered even numbers, because they can be divided by 2, without leaving a remainder or forming a decimal. It does not matter whether the number is positive or negative.

Odd numbers: describes any number that does not divide evenly by 2.

> Example: 1, 21, 541, 3003, -9, -63, -1257 are all considered odd numbers, because they cannot be divided by 2 without a remainder or a decimal.

Prime numbers: describes a number that is only evenly divisible, resulting in no remainder or decimal, by 1 and itself.

> Example: 2, 3, 7, 13, 113 are all considered prime numbers because each can only be evenly divided by 1 and itself.

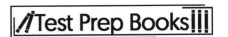

Composite numbers: describes a positive integer that is formed by multiplying two smaller integers together. Composite numbers can be divided evenly by numbers other than 1 or itself.

Example: 9, 24, 66, 2348, 10002 are all considered composite numbers because they are the result of multiplying two smaller integers together. In particular, these are all divisible by 2.

Decimals: designated by a decimal point which indicates that what follows the point is a value that is less than 1 and is added to the integer number preceding the decimal point. The digit immediately following the decimal point is in the tenths place, the digit following the tenths place is in the hundredths place, and so on.

For example, the decimal number 1.735 has a value greater than 1 but less than 2. The 7 represents seven tenths of the unit 1 (0.7 or $\frac{7}{10}$); the 3 represents three hundredths of 1 (0.03 or $\frac{3}{100}$); and the 5 represents five thousandths of 1 (0.005 or $\frac{5}{1000}$).

Real numbers: describes rational numbers and irrational numbers.

Rational numbers: describes any number that can be expressed as a fraction, with a non-zero denominator. Since any integer can be written with 1 in the denominator without changing its value, all integers are considered rational numbers. Every rational number has a decimal expression that terminates or repeats. That is, any rational number either will have a countable number of nonzero digits or will end with an ellipsis or a bar (3.6666... or 3.$\overline{6}$) to depict repeating decimal digits. Some examples of rational numbers include 12, -3.54, 110.$\overline{256}$, $\frac{-35}{10}$, and 4.$\overline{7}$.

Irrational numbers: describes numbers that cannot be written as a finite decimal. Pi (π) is considered to be an irrational number because its decimal portion is unending or a non-repeating decimal. The most common irrational number is π, which has an endless and non-repeating decimal, but there are other well-known irrational numbers like e and $\sqrt{2}$.

Basic Addition and Subtraction

Addition
Addition is the combination of two numbers so their quantities are added together cumulatively. The sign for an addition operation is the+symbol. For example, $9 + 6 = 15$. The 9 and 6 combine to achieve a cumulative value, called a **sum**.

Addition holds the **commutative property**, which means that the order of the numbers numbers in an addition equation can be switched without altering the result. The formula for the commutative property is $a + b = b + a$. Let's look at a few examples to see how the commutative property works:

$$7 = 3 + 4 = 4 + 3 = 7$$

$$20 = 12 + 8 = 8 + 12 = 20$$

Addition also holds the **associative property**, which means that the grouping of numbers doesn't matter in an addition problem. In other words, the presence or absence of parentheses is irrelevant. The formula for the associative property is $(a + b) + c = a + (b + c)$. Here are some examples of the associative property at work:

$$30 = (6 + 14) + 10 = 6 + (14 + 10) = 30$$

$$35 = 8 + (2 + 25) = (8 + 2) + 25 = 35$$

There are set columns for addition: ones, tens, hundreds, thousands, ten-thousands, hundred-thousands, millions, and so on. To add how many units there are total, each column needs to be combined, starting from the right, or the ones column.

THOUSANDS	HUNDREDS	TENS	ONES

Every 10 units in the ones column equals one in the tens column, and every 10 units in the tens column equals one in the hundreds column, and so on.

Example: The number 5432 has 2 ones, 3 tens, 4 hundreds, and 5 thousands. The number 371 has 3 hundreds, 7 tens and 1 one. To combine, or add, these two numbers, simply add up how many units of each column exist. The best way to do this is by lining up the columns:

$$
\begin{array}{r}
5\ 4\ 3\ 2 \\
+\quad 3\ 7\ 1 \\
\hline
\end{array}
$$

The ones column adds $2 + 1$ for a total (sum) of 3.

The tens column adds $3 + 7$ for a total of 10; since 10 of that unit was collected, add 1 to the hundreds column to denote the total in the next column:

$$
\begin{array}{r}
1 \\
5\ 4\ 3\ 2 \\
+\quad 3\ 7\ 1 \\
\hline
0\ 3 \\
\end{array}
$$

When adding the hundreds column, this extra 1 needs to be combined, so it would be the sum of 4, 3, and 1.

$$4 + 3 + 1 = 8$$

The last, or thousands, column listed would be the sum of 5. Since there are no other numbers in this column, that is the final total.

The answer would look as follows:

$$
\begin{array}{r}
5\ 4\ 3\ 2 \\
+\quad 3\ 7\ 1 \\
\hline
5\ 8\ 0\ 3 \\
\end{array}
$$

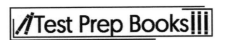

Example
Find the sum of 9,734 and 895.

Set up the problem:

$$
\begin{array}{r}
9\ 7\ 3\ 4 \\
+\ \ \ 8\ 9\ 5 \\
\hline
\end{array}
$$

Total the columns:

$$
\begin{array}{r}
9\ 7\ 3\ 4 \\
+\ \ \ 8\ 9\ 5 \\
\hline
1\ 0\ 6\ 2\ 9
\end{array}
$$

In this example, another column (ten-thousands) is added to the left of the thousands column, to denote a carryover of 10 units in the thousands column. The final sum is 10,629.

When adding using all negative integers, the total is negative. The integers are simply added together and the negative symbol is tacked on.

$$(-12) + (-435) = -447$$

Subtraction
Subtraction is taking away one number from another, so their quantities are reduced. The sign designating a subtraction operation is the $-$ symbol, and the result is called the **difference**. For example, $9 - 6 = 3$. The number 6 detracts from the number 9 to reach the difference 3.

Unlike addition, subtraction follows neither the commutative nor associative properties. The order and grouping in subtraction impact the result.

$$15 = 22 - 7 \neq 7 - 22 = -15$$

$$3 = (10 - 5) - 2 \neq 10 - (5 - 2) = 7$$

When working through subtraction problems involving larger numbers, it's necessary to regroup the numbers. Let's work through a practice problem using regrouping:

$$
\begin{array}{r}
3\ 2\ 5 \\
-\ \ 7\ 7 \\
\hline
\end{array}
$$

Here, it is clear that the ones and tens columns for 77 are greater than the ones and tens columns for 325. To subtract this number, borrow from the tens and hundreds columns. When borrowing from a column, subtracting 1 from the lender column will add 10 to the borrower column:

$$
\begin{array}{ccc}
3\text{-}1 & 10+2\text{-}1 & 10+5 \\
 & 7 & 7 \\
\hline
\end{array}
=
\begin{array}{ccc}
2 & 11 & 15 \\
 & 7 & 7 \\
\hline
2 & 4 & 8
\end{array}
$$

After ensuring that each digit in the top row is greater than the digit in the corresponding bottom row, subtraction can proceed as normal, and the answer is found to be 248.

Addition and Subtraction with Negative Integers

When adding mixed-sign integers, determine which integer has the larger absolute value. Absolute value is the distance of a number from zero on the number line. Absolute value is indicated by these symbols: ||.

Take this equation for example:

$$12 + (-435)$$

The absolute value of each of the numbers is as follows:

$$|12| = 12$$

$$|-435| = 435$$

Since -435 is the larger integer, the final number will have its sign. In this case, that sign is negative. Now, subtract the smaller integer from the larger one. If you work out the equation, it will look like this:

$$12 + (-435) = -423$$

Mathematically, the equation looks like the one above, but practically speaking you will be doing it like this:

$$435 - 12 = 423$$

(then add the negative sign)

When using subtraction with negative integers, every unmarked integer is assumed to have a positive sign unless it is clearly marked as a negative integer. Subtracting an integer is the same as adding a negative integer.

Example:
$$-3 - 4$$
$$-3 + (-4)$$
$$-3 + (-4) = -7$$

Subtracting a negative integer is the same as adding a positive integer.

Example
$$-3 - (-4)$$
$$-3 + 4$$
$$-3 + 4 = 1$$

Multiplication of Whole Numbers

Multiplication involves adding together multiple copies of a number. It is indicated by an $\times$ symbol or a number immediately outside of a parenthesis. For example:

$$5(8 - 2)$$

The two numbers being multiplied together are called **factors**, and their result is called a **product**. For example, $9 \times 6 = 54$. This can be shown alternatively by expansion of either the 9 or the 6:

$$9 \times 6 = 9 + 9 + 9 + 9 + 9 + 9 = 54$$

$$9 \times 6 = 6 + 6 + 6 + 6 + 6 + 6 + 6 + 6 + 6 = 54$$

Like addition, multiplication holds the commutative and associative properties:

$$115 = 23 \times 5 = 5 \times 23 = 115$$

$$84 = 3 \times (7 \times 4) = (3 \times 7) \times 4 = 84$$

Multiplication also follows the **distributive property**, which allows the multiplication to be distributed through parentheses. The formula for distribution is $a \times (b + c) = ab + ac$. This is clear after the examples:

$$45 = 5 \times 9 = 5(3 + 6) = (5 \times 3) + (5 \times 6) = 15 + 30 = 45$$

$$20 = 4 \times 5 = 4(10 - 5) = (4 \times 10) - (4 \times 5) = 40 - 20 = 20$$

For larger-number multiplication, how the numbers are lined up can ease the process. It is simplest to put the number with the most digits on top and the number with fewer digits on the bottom. If they have the same number of digits, select one for the top and one for the bottom. Line up the problem, and begin by multiplying the far-right column on the top and the far-right column on the bottom. If the answer to a column is more than 9, the ones place digit will be written below that column and the tens place digit will carry to the top of the next column to be added after those digits are multiplied. Write the answer below that column. Move to the next column to the left on the top, and multiply it by the same far-right column on the bottom. Keep moving to the left one column at a time on the top number until the end.

Example
Multiply 37×8

Line up the numbers, placing the one with the most digits on top.

$$
\begin{array}{r}
3\ 7 \\
\times\ \ \ 8 \\
\hline
\end{array}
$$

Multiply the far-right column on the top with the far-right column on the bottom (7×8). Write the answer, 56, as below: The ones value, 6, gets recorded, the tens value, 5, is carried.

$$
\begin{array}{r}
{\scriptstyle +5} \\
3\ 7 \\
\times\ \ \ 8 \\
\hline
6
\end{array}
$$

Move to the next column left on the top number and multiply with the far-right bottom (3×8). Remember to add any carry over after multiplying: $3 \times 8 = 24$, $24 + 5 = 29$. Since there are no more digits on top, write the entire number below.

$$
\begin{array}{r}
{\scriptstyle +5} \\
3\ 7 \\
\times\ \ \ 8 \\
\hline
2\ 9\ 6
\end{array}
$$

The solution is 296.

If there is more than one column to the bottom number, move to the row below the first strand of answers, mark a zero in the far-right column, and then begin the multiplication process again with the far-right column on top and the second column from the right on the bottom. For each digit in the bottom number, there will be a row of answers, each padded with the respective number of zeros on the right. Finally, add up all of the answer rows for one total number.

Example: Multiply 512×36.

Line up the numbers (the one with the most digits on top) to multiply.

Begin with the right column on top and the right column on bottom (2×6).

$$
\begin{array}{r}
5\ 1\ 2 \\
\times\ \ \ 3\ 6 \\
\hline
\end{array}
$$

17

Move one column left on top and multiply by the far-right column on the bottom (1×6). Add the carry over after multiplying: $1 \times 6 = 6, 6 + 1 = 7$.

```
        +1
     5  1  2
  x     3  6
  ─────────────
        7  2
```

Move one column left on top and multiply by the far-right column on the bottom (5×6). Since this is the last digit on top, write the whole answer below.

```
     5  1  2
  X     3  6
  ─────────────
  3  0  7  2
```

Now move on to the second column on the bottom number. Starting on the far-right column on the top, repeat this pattern for the next number left on the bottom (2×3). Write the answers below the first line of answers; remember to begin with a zero placeholder on the far right.

```
     5  1  2
  X     3  6
  ─────────────
  3  0  7  2
        6  0
```

Continue the pattern (1×3).

```
     5  1  2
  X     3  6
  ─────────────
  3  0  7  2
     3  6  0
```

Since this is the last digit on top, write the whole answer below.

```
     5  1  2
  x     3  6
  ─────────────
  3  0  7  2
  1  5  3  6  0
```

Now add the answer rows together. Pay attention to ensure they are aligned correctly.

```
     5  1  2
  x     3  6
  ─────────────
  3  0  7  2
  1  5  3  6  0
  ─────────────
  1  8  4  3  2
```

The solution is 18,432.

18

Division of Whole Numbers

Division and multiplication are inverses of each other in the same way that addition and subtraction are opposites. The signs designating a division operation are the ÷ and / symbols. In division, the second number divides into the first.

The number before the division sign is called the **dividend** or, if expressed as a fraction, the **numerator**. For example, in $a \div b$, a is the dividend, while in $\frac{a}{b}$, a is the numerator.

The number after the division sign is called the **divisor** or, if expressed as a fraction, the **denominator**. For example, in $a \div b$, b is the divisor, while in $\frac{a}{b}$, b is the denominator.

Like subtraction, division doesn't follow the commutative property, as it matters which number comes before the division sign, and division doesn't follow the associative or distributive properties for the same reason. For example:

$$\frac{3}{2} = 9 \div 6 \neq 6 \div 9 = \frac{2}{3}$$

$$2 = 10 \div 5 = (30 \div 3) \div 5 \neq 30 \div (3 \div 5) = 30 \div \frac{3}{5} = 50$$

$$25 = 20 + 5 = (40 \div 2) + (40 \div 8) \neq 40 \div (2 + 8) = 40 \div 10 = 4$$

The answer to a division problem is called the **quotient**. If a divisor doesn't divide into a dividend an integer number of times, whatever is left over is termed the **remainder**. The remainder can be further divided out into decimal form by using long division; however, this doesn't always give a quotient with a finite number of decimal places, so the remainder can also be expressed as a fraction over the original divisor.

Example
Divide $\frac{1,050}{42}$ or $1,050 \div 42$.

Set up the problem with the denominator being divided into the numerator.

$$4\,2\overline{)1\,0\,5\,0}$$

Check for divisibility into the first unit of the numerator, 1.

42 cannot go into 1, so add on the next unit in the denominator, 0.

42 cannot go into 10, so add on the next unit in the denominator, 5.

19

42 can be divided into 105 two times. Write the 2 over the 5 in 105 and multiply 42 x 2. Write the 84 under 105 for subtraction and note the remainder, 21 is less than 42.

$$
\begin{array}{r}
2 \\
42\overline{)1\,0\,5\,0} \\
-8\,4 \\
\hline
2\,1
\end{array}
$$

Drop the next digit in the numerator down to the remainder (making 21 into 210) to create a number 42 can divide into. 42 divides into 210 five times. Write the 5 over the 0 and multiply 42×5.

$$
\begin{array}{r}
2\,5 \\
42\overline{)1\,0\,5\,0} \\
-8\,4 \\
\hline
2\,1\,0
\end{array}
$$

Write the 210 under 210 for subtraction. The remainder is 0.

$$
\begin{array}{r}
2\,5 \\
42\overline{)1\,0\,5\,0} \\
-8\,4 \\
\hline
2\,1\,0 \\
-2\,1\,0 \\
\hline
0
\end{array}
$$

The solution is 25.

Example
Divide 375/4 or 375 ÷ 4.

Set up the problem.

$$
4\overline{)3\,7\,5}
$$

4 cannot divide into 3, so add the next unit from the numerator, 7. 4 divides into 37 nine times, so write the 9 above the 7. Multiply $4 \times 9 = 36$. Write the 36 under the 37 for subtraction. The remainder is 1 (1 is less than 4).

$$
\begin{array}{r}
9 \\
4\overline{)3\,7\,5} \\
-3\,6 \\
\hline
1
\end{array}
$$

20

Drop the next digit in the numerator, 5, making the remainder 15. 4 divides into 15, three times, so write the 3 above the 5. Multiply 4 × 3. Write the 12 under the 15 for subtraction, remainder is 3 (3 is less than 4).

$$\begin{array}{r} 9\ 3 \\ 4\overline{)3\ 7\ 5} \\ -\ 3\ 6 \\ \hline 1\ 5 \\ -\ 1\ 2 \\ \hline 3 \end{array}$$

The solution is 93 remainder 3 or 93 ¾ (the remainder can be written over the original denominator).

Decimals

Decimals mark the division between the whole portion and the fractional (or decimal) portion of a number. For example, 3.15 has 3 in the whole portion and 15 in the fractional or decimal portion. A number such as 645 is all whole, but there is still a decimal place. The decimal place in 645 is to the right of the 5, but usually not written, since there is no fractional or decimal portion to this number. The same number can be written as 645.0 or 645.00 or 645.000, etc. The position of the decimal place can change the entire value of a number, and impact a calculation. In the United States, the decimal place is used when representing money. You'll often be asked to round to a certain decimal place. Here is a review of some basic decimal **place value** names:

thousands	hundreds	tens	ones	tenths	hundredths	thousandths

Decimal

The number 12,302.2 would be read as "twelve thousand, three hundred two and two-tenths."

In the United States, a period denotes the decimal place; however, some countries use a comma. The comma is used in the United States to separate thousands, millions, and so on.

To round to the nearest whole number (eliminating the decimal portion), the example would become 12,302. For rounding, go to the number that is one place to the right of what you are rounding to. If the number is 0 through 4, there will be no change. For numbers 5 through 9, round up to the next whole number.

Example
Round 6,423.7 to the ones place.

Since the tenths place is the position to the right of the ones place, we use that number to determine if we round up or not. In this case, the 3 is in the ones place and the 7 is in the tenths place. (6,42<u>3</u>.7)

The 7 in the tenths place means we round the 3 up, so the final number will be 6,424.0

Example
Round 542.88 to the nearest tens

Since the ones place is the position to the right of the tens, we use that number to determine if we round up or not. In this case, the 4 is in the tens place and the 2 is in the ones place (5<u>4</u>2.88).

The 2 in the ones place means we do not round the 4 up, so the final number will be 540.00

Note: Everything to the right of the rounded position goes to 0 as a placeholder.

Example: Say you wanted to post an advertisement to sell a used vehicle for $2000.00. However, when typing the price, you accidentally moved the decimal over one place to the left. Now the asking price appears as $200.00. This difference of a factor of 10 is dramatic. As numbers get bigger or smaller, the impact of this mistake becomes more pronounced. If you were looking to sell a condo for $1,000,000.00, but made an error and moved the decimal place to the left one position, the price posts at $100,000.00. A mistake of a factor of 10 cost $900,000.00.

In dividing by 10, you move the decimal one position to the left, making a smaller number than the original. If multiplying by 10, move the decimal one position to the right, making a larger number than the original.

<u>Example</u>
Divide 100 by 10 or $100 \div 10$.

Move the decimal one place to the left, so the result is a smaller number than the original.

$$100 \div 10 = 10$$

<u>Example</u>
Divide 1.0 by 10 or $1.0 \div 10$.

Move the decimal one place to the left, so the result is a smaller number than the original.

$$1.0 \div 10 = 0.1$$

<u>Example</u>
Multiply 100 by 10 or 100×10.

Move the decimal one place to the right, so the result is a larger number than the original.

$$100 \times 10 = 1,000$$

<u>Example</u>
Multiply 0.1 by 10 or 0.1×10.

Move the decimal one place to the right, so the result is a larger number than the original.

$$0.1 \times 10 = 1.0$$

Prefixes

Moving the decimal place to the left or to the right illustrates multiplying or dividing by factors of 10. The metric system of units for measurement utilizes factors of 10 as displayed in the following table:

kilo	1000 units
hecto	100 units
deca	10 units
base unit	
deci	0.1 units
centi	0.01 units
milli	0.001 units

It is important to have the ability to quickly manipulate by 10 according to prefixes for units.

Example: How many milliliters are in 5 liters of saline solution?

There are 1,000 milliliters for every 1 liter. If we have 5 liters, it would be $5 \times 1,000 = 5,000$ mL

You may also count the zeros and which side of the decimal place they are on: 1000 has three zeroes to the left of the decimal, so insert three zeroes between the 5 and the decimal, or move the decimal place over three places to the right, for your answer of 5000 mL.

Example
How many kilograms are in 4.8 grams?

There is 1 gram for every 0.001 kilograms. Since there is one-thousandth of a kilogram for each gram, that means divide by 1,000, or move the decimal to the left by 3 places – 1 place for each 0. So, the result would be 0.0048 kg.

For quick conversions, move the decimal place the set number of spaces left or right to match the column/slot, as depicted below.

To convert from one prefix to another to the left or right of the base unit (follow the arrow to the left or right), move the decimal place the number of columns/slots as counted.

mega			kilo	hecto	deca	base	deci	centi	milli			micro
1,000,000	100,000	10,000	1,000	100	10	unit	.1	.01	.001	.0001	.00001	.000001

move decimal to the left   move decimal to the right

Example
How many centiliters are in 4.7 kiloliters?

To convert a number with a unit prefixed as kilo into a unit prefixed as centi, move across five columns to the right, meaning move the decimal place five places to the right.

$$4.7 \text{ kL} = 470,000 \text{ cL}$$

23

<u>Example</u>
How many liters are in 30 microliters?

Start with the unit marked micro and count the columns moving to the left until you reach the base unit for liters. Be sure to count the blank columns, as they are important placeholders. There are six columns from micro to the base unit moving to the left, so move the decimal place six places to the left.

$$30 \text{ mL} = 0.000030 \text{ L}$$

Decimal Addition

Addition with decimals is done the same way as regular addition. All numbers could have decimals, but are often removed if the numbers to the right of the decimal are zeros. Line up numbers at the decimal place.

Example: Add $345.89 + 23.54$

Line the numbers up at the decimal place and add.

```
    3 4 5 . 8 9
  +   2 3 . 5 4
  ─────────────
    3 6 9 . 4 3
```

Decimal Subtraction

Subtraction with decimals is done the same way as regular subtraction.

Example: Subtract $345.89 - 23.54$

Line the numbers up at the decimal place and subtract.

```
    3 4 5 . 8 9
  -   2 3 . 5 4
  ─────────────
    3 2 2 . 3 5
```

Decimal Multiplication

The simplest way to handle multiplication with decimals is to calculate the multiplication problem pretending the decimals are not there, then count how many decimal places there are in the original problem. Use that total to place the decimal the same number of places over, counting from right to left.

Example: Multiply 42.33×3.3

Line the numbers up and multiply, pretending there are no decimals.

$$
\begin{array}{r}
4\ 2\ 3\ 3 \\
\times\quad\ 3\ 3 \\
\hline
1\ 2\ 6\ 9\ 9 \\
1\ 2\ 6\ 9\ 0 \\
\hline
1\ 3\ 9\ 6\ 8\ 9
\end{array}
$$

Now look at the original problem and count how many decimal places were removed. Two decimal places were removed from 42.33 to get 4,233, and one decimal place from 3.3 to get 33. Removed were $2 + 1 = 3$ decimal places. Place the decimal three places from the right of the number 139,689. The answer is 139.689.

Another way to think of this is that when you move the decimal in the original numbers, it is like multiplying by 10. To put the decimals back, you need to divide the number by 10 the same amount of times you multiplied. It would still be three times for the above solution.

Example: Multiply 0.03×1.22

Line the numbers up and multiply, pretending there are no decimals. The zeroes in front of the 3 are unnecessary, so take them out for now.

$$
\begin{array}{r}
1\ 2\ 2 \\
\times\quad\ 3 \\
\hline
3\ 6\ 6
\end{array}
$$

Look at the original problem and count how many decimals places were removed, or how many times each number was multiplied by 10. The 1.22 moved two places (or multiplied by 10 twice), as did 0.03. That is $2 + 2 = 4$ decimal places removed. Count that number, from right to left of the number 366, and place the decimal. The result is 0.0366.

Decimal Division

Division with decimals is simplest when you eliminate some of the decimal places. Since you divide the bottom number of a fraction into the top, or divide the denominator into the numerator, the bottom number dictates the movement of the decimals. The goal is to remove the decimals from the denominator and mirror that movement in the numerator. You do not need the numerator to be decimal free, however. Divide as you would normally.

Example
Divide $\frac{4.21}{0.2}$ or $4.21 \div 0.2$

Move the decimal over one place to the right in the denominator, making 0.2 simply 2. Move the decimal in the numerator, 4.21, over the same amount, so it is now 42.1.

$$0.2\overline{)4.21}$$

25

Becomes:

$$2\overline{\smash{)}42.1}$$

Divide:

$$\begin{array}{r} 21.05 \\ 2\overline{\smash{)}42.10} \end{array}$$

The answer is 21.05 with the correct decimal placement. In decimal division, move the decimal the same amount for both numerator and denominator. There is no need to adjust anything after the problem is completed.

Fractions

A fraction is an equation that represents a part of a whole but can also be used to present ratios or division problems. An example of a fraction is $\frac{x}{y}$. In this example, x is called the **numerator**, while y is the **denominator**. The numerator represents the number of parts, and the denominator is the total number of parts. They are separated by a line or slash, known as a **fraction bar**. In simple fractions, the numerator and denominator can be nearly any integer. However, the denominator of a fraction can never be zero because dividing by zero is a function that is undefined.

Imagine that an apple pie has been baked for a holiday party, and the full pie has eight slices. After the party, there are five slices left. How could the amount of the pie that remains be expressed as a fraction? The numerator is 5 since there are 5 pieces left, and the denominator is 8 since there were eight total slices in the whole pie. Thus, expressed as a fraction, the leftover pie totals $\frac{5}{8}$ of the original amount.

Fractions come in three different varieties: proper fractions, improper fractions, and mixed numbers. **Proper fractions** have a numerator less than the denominator, such as $\frac{3}{8}$, but **improper fractions** have a numerator greater than the denominator, such as $\frac{15}{8}$. **Mixed numbers** combine a whole number with a proper fraction, such as $3\frac{1}{2}$. Any mixed number can be written as an improper fraction by multiplying the integer by the denominator, adding the product to the value of the numerator, and dividing the sum by the original denominator. For example:

$$3\frac{1}{2} = \frac{3 \times 2 + 1}{2} = \frac{7}{2}$$

Whole numbers can also be converted into fractions by placing the whole number as the numerator and making the denominator 1. For example, $3 = \frac{3}{1}$.

One of the most fundamental concepts of fractions is their ability to be manipulated by multiplication or division. This is possible since $\frac{n}{n} = 1$ for any non-zero integer. As a result, multiplying or dividing by $\frac{n}{n}$ will not alter the original fraction since any number multiplied or divided by 1 doesn't change the value of that number. Fractions of the same value are known as equivalent fractions. For example, $\frac{2}{4}, \frac{4}{8}, \frac{50}{100}$, and $\frac{75}{150}$ are equivalent, as they all equal $\frac{1}{2}$.

Although many equivalent fractions exist, they are easier to compare and interpret when reduced or simplified. The numerator and denominator of a simple fraction will have no factors in common other than 1. When reducing or simplifying fractions, divide the numerator and denominator by the **greatest common factor**. A simple strategy is to divide the numerator and denominator by low numbers, like 2, 3, or 5 until arriving at a simple fraction, but the same thing could be achieved by determining the greatest common factor for both the numerator and denominator and dividing each by it. Using the first method is preferable when both the numerator and denominator are even, end in 5, or are obviously a multiple of another number. However, if no numbers seem to work, it will be necessary to factor the numerator and denominator to find the GCF. Let's look at examples:

1) Simplify the fraction $\frac{6}{8}$:

Dividing the numerator and denominator by 2 results in $\frac{3}{4}$, which is a simple fraction.

2) Simplify the fraction $\frac{12}{36}$:

Dividing the numerator and denominator by 2 leaves $\frac{6}{18}$. This isn't a simple fraction, as both the numerator and denominator have factors in common. Dividing each by 3 results in $\frac{2}{6}$, but this can be further simplified by dividing by 2 to get $\frac{1}{3}$. This is the simplest fraction, as the numerator is 1. In cases like this, multiple division operations can be avoided by determining the greatest common factor between the numerator and denominator.

3) Simplify the fraction $\frac{18}{54}$ by dividing by the greatest common factor:

First, determine the factors for the numerator and denominator. The factors of 18 are 1, 2, 3, 6, 9, and 18. The factors of 54 are 1, 2, 3, 6, 9, 18, 27, and 54. Thus, the greatest common factor is 18. Dividing both the numerator and denominator by 18 leaves $\frac{1}{3}$, which is the simplest fraction. This method takes slightly more work, but it definitively arrives at the simplest fraction.

Operations with Fractions

Multiplication of Fractions

Of the four basic operations that can be performed on fractions, the one that involves the least amount of work is multiplication. To multiply two fractions, simply multiply the numerators together, multiply the denominators together, and place the products of each as a fraction. Whole numbers and mixed numbers can also be expressed as a fraction, as described above, to multiply with a fraction. Let's work through a couple of examples.

$$1) \frac{2}{5} \times \frac{3}{4} = \frac{6}{20} = \frac{3}{10}$$

$$2) \frac{4}{9} \times \frac{7}{11} = \frac{28}{99}$$

Division of Fractions

Dividing fractions is similar to multiplication with one key difference. To divide fractions, flip the numerator and denominator of the second fraction, and then proceed as if it were a multiplication problem:

$$1) \ \frac{7}{8} \div \frac{4}{5} = \frac{7}{8} \times \frac{5}{4} = \frac{35}{32}$$

$$2) \ \frac{5}{9} \div \frac{1}{3} = \frac{5}{9} \times \frac{3}{1} = \frac{15}{9} = \frac{5}{3}$$

Addition and Subtraction of Fractions

Addition and subtraction require more steps than multiplication and division, as these operations require the fractions to have the same denominator, also called a **common denominator**. It is always possible to find a common denominator by multiplying the denominators. However, when the denominators are large numbers, this method is unwieldy, especially if the answer must be provided in its simplest form. Thus, it's beneficial to find the **least common denominator** of the fractions—the least common denominator is incidentally also the least common multiple.

Once equivalent fractions have been found with common denominators, simply add or subtract the numerators to arrive at the answer:

$$1) \ \frac{1}{2} + \frac{3}{4} = \frac{2}{4} + \frac{3}{4} = \frac{5}{4}$$

$$2) \ \frac{3}{12} + \frac{11}{20} = \frac{15}{60} + \frac{33}{60} = \frac{48}{60} = \frac{4}{5}$$

$$3) \ \frac{7}{9} - \frac{4}{15} = \frac{35}{45} - \frac{12}{45} = \frac{23}{45}$$

$$4) \ \frac{5}{6} - \frac{7}{18} = \frac{15}{18} - \frac{7}{18} = \frac{8}{18} = \frac{4}{9}$$

Changing Fractions to Decimals

To change a fraction into a decimal, divide the denominator into the numerator until there are no remainders. There may be repeating decimals, so rounding is often acceptable. A straight line above the repeating portion denotes that the decimal repeats.

Example

Express $\frac{4}{5}$ as a decimal.

Set up the division problem.

$$5 \overline{) 4}$$

5 does not go into 4, so place the decimal and add a zero.

$$5 \overline{) 4.0}$$

28

5 goes into 40 eight times. There is no remainder.

$$
\begin{array}{r}
0\,.\,8 \\
5\overline{)4\,.\,0} \\
-\,4\,.\,0 \\
\hline
0
\end{array}
$$

The solution is 0.8.

<u>Example</u>

Express $33\frac{1}{3}$ as a decimal.

Since the whole portion of the number is known, set it aside to calculate the decimal from the fraction portion.

Set up the division problem.

$$
3\overline{)1}
$$

3 does not go into 1, so place the decimal and add zeros. 3 goes into 10 three times.

$$
\begin{array}{r}
0\,.\,3 \\
3\overline{)1\,.\,0}
\end{array}
$$

This will repeat with a remainder of 1.

$$
\begin{array}{r}
0\,.\,3\,3\,3 \\
3\overline{)1\,.\,0\,0\,0} \\
-\,9 \\
\hline
1\,0 \\
-\,9 \\
\hline
1\,0
\end{array}
$$

So, we will place a line over the 3 to denote the repetition. The solution is written $33.\overline{3}$.

Changing Decimals to Fractions

To change decimals to fractions, place the decimal portion of the number, the numerator, over the respective place value, the denominator, then reduce, if possible.

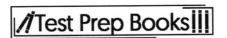

Example
Express 0.25 as a fraction.

This is read as twenty-five hundredths, so put 25 over 100. Then reduce to find the solution.

$$\frac{25}{100} = \frac{1}{4}$$

Example
Express 0.455 as a fraction

This is read as four hundred fifty-five thousandths, so put 455 over 1,000. Then reduce to find the solution.

$$\frac{455}{1000} = \frac{91}{200}$$

There are two types of problems that commonly involve percentages. The first is to calculate some percentage of a given quantity, where you convert the percentage to a decimal, and multiply the quantity by that decimal. Secondly, you are given a quantity and told it is a fixed percent of an unknown quantity. In this case, convert to a decimal, then divide the given quantity by that decimal.

Example
What is 30% of 760?

Convert the percent into a useable number. "Of" means to multiply.

$$30\% = 0.30$$

Set up the problem based on the givens, and solve.

$$0.30 \times 760 = 228$$

Example
8.4 is 20% of what number?

Convert the percent into a useable number.

$$20\% = 0.20$$

The given number is a percent of the answer needed, so divide the given number by this decimal rather than multiplying it.

$$\frac{8.4}{0.20} = 42$$

Ratios and Proportions

Ratios
Ratios are used to show the relationship between two quantities. The ratio of oranges to apples in the grocery store may be 3 to 2. That means that for every 3 oranges, there are 2 apples. This comparison

30

can be expanded to represent the actual number of oranges and apples, such as 36 oranges to 24 apples. Another example may be the number of boys to girls in a math class. If the ratio of boys to girls is given as 2 to 5, that means there are 2 boys to every 5 girls in the class. Ratios can also be compared if the units in each ratio are the same. The ratio of boys to girls in the math class can be compared to the ratio of boys to girls in a science class by stating which ratio is higher and which is lower.

Rates are used to compare two quantities with different units. *Unit rates* are the simplest form of rate. With **unit rates**, the denominator in the comparison of two units is one. For example, if someone can type at a rate of 1,000 words in 5 minutes, then their unit rate for typing is $\frac{1,000}{5} = 200$ words in one minute or 200 words per minute. Any rate can be converted into a unit rate by dividing to make the denominator one. 1,000 words in 5 minutes has been converted into the unit rate of 200 words per minute.

Ratios and rates can be used together to convert rates into different units. For example, if someone is driving 50 kilometers per hour, that rate can be converted into miles per hour by using a ratio known as the **conversion factor.** Since the given value contains kilometers and the final answer needs to be in miles, the ratio relating miles to kilometers needs to be used. There are 0.62 miles in 1 kilometer. This, written as a ratio and in fraction form, is $\frac{0.62 \text{ miles}}{1 \text{ km}}$. To convert 50 km/hour into miles per hour, the following conversion needs to be set up:

$$\frac{50 \text{ km}}{\text{hour}} \times \frac{0.62 \text{ miles}}{1 \text{ km}} = 31 \text{ miles per hour}$$

The ratio between two similar geometric figures is called the **scale factor.** For example, a problem may depict two similar triangles, A and B. The scale factor from the smaller triangle A to the larger triangle B is given as 2 because the length of the corresponding side of the larger triangle, 16, is twice the corresponding side on the smaller triangle, 8. This scale factor can also be used to find the value of a missing side, x, in triangle A. Since the scale factor from the smaller triangle (A) to larger one (B) is 2, the larger corresponding side in triangle B (given as 25) can be divided by 2 to find the missing side in A ($x = 12.5$). The scale factor can also be represented in the equation $2A = B$ because two times the lengths of A gives the corresponding lengths of B. This is the idea behind similar triangles.

Proportions

Much like a scale factor can be written using an equation like $2A = B$, a **relationship** is represented by the equation $Y = kX$. X and Y are proportional because as values of X increase, the values of Y also increase. A relationship that is inversely proportional can be represented by the equation $Y = \frac{k}{X}$, where the value of Y decreases as the value of X increases and vice versa.

Proportional reasoning can be used to solve problems involving ratios, percentages, and averages. Ratios can be used in setting up proportions and solving them to find unknowns. For example, if a student completes an average of 10 pages of math homework in 3 nights, how long would it take the student to complete 22 pages? Both ratios can be written as fractions. The second ratio would contain the unknown.

The following proportion represents this problem, where x is the unknown number of nights:

$$\frac{10 \text{ pages}}{3 \text{ nights}} = \frac{22 \text{ pages}}{x \text{ nights}}$$

Solving this proportion entails cross-multiplying (multiplying both sets of numbers that are diagonally across and setting them equal to each other) and results in the following equation: $10x = 22 \times 3$. Simplifying and solving for x results in the exact solution: $x = 6.6$ nights. The result would be rounded up to 7 because the homework would actually be completed on the 7th night.

The following problem uses ratios involving percentages:

If 20% of the class is girls and 30 students are in the class, how many girls are in the class?

To set up this problem, it is helpful to use the common proportion: $\frac{\%}{100} = \frac{is}{of}$. Within the proportion, % is the percentage of girls, 100 is the total percentage of the class, *is* is the number of girls, and *of* is the total number of students in the class. Most percentage problems can be written using this language. To solve this problem, the proportion should be set up as $\frac{20}{100} = \frac{x}{30}$ and then solved for x. Cross-multiplying results in the equation $20 \times 30 = 100x$, which results in the solution $x = 6$. There are 6 girls in the class.

Problems involving volume, length, and other units can also be solved using ratios. For example, A problem may ask for the volume of a cone that has a radius, $r = 7$ m and a height, $h = 16$ m. Referring to the formulas provided on the test, the volume of a cone is given as: $V = \pi r^2 \frac{h}{3}$, where r is the radius, and h is the height. Plugging $r = 7$ and $h = 16$ into the formula, the following is obtained:

$$V = \pi(7^2)\frac{16}{3}$$

Therefore, the volume of the cone is found to be approximately 821 m^3. Sometimes, answers in different units are sought. If this problem wanted the answer in liters, 821 m^3 would need to be converted.

Using the equivalence statement 1 m^3 = 1,000 L, the following ratio would be used to solve for liters:

$$821 \text{ m}^3 \times \frac{1,000 \text{ L}}{1 \text{ m}^3}$$

Cubic meters in the numerator and denominator cancel each other out, and the answer is converted to 821,000 liters, or 8.21×10^5 L.

Other conversions can also be made between different given and final units. If the temperature in a pool is 30°C, what is the temperature of the pool in degrees Fahrenheit? To convert these units, an equation is used relating Celsius to Fahrenheit. The following equation is used:

$$T_{°F} = 1.8T_{°C} + 32$$

Plugging in the given temperature and solving the equation for T yields the result:

$$T_{°F} = 1.8(30) + 32 = 86°F$$

Both units in the metric system and U.S. customary system are widely used.

Here are some more examples of how to solve for proportions:

1) $\frac{75\%}{90\%} = \frac{25\%}{x}$

To solve for x, the fractions must be cross multiplied: ($75\%x = 90\% \times 25\%$). To make things easier, let's convert the percentages to decimals: ($0.9 \times 0.25 = 0.225 = 0.75x$). To get rid of x's coefficient, each side must be divided by that same coefficient to get the answer $x = 0.3$. The question could ask for the answer as a percentage or fraction in lowest terms, which are 30% and $\frac{3}{10}$, respectively.

2) $\frac{x}{12} = \frac{30}{96}$

Cross-multiply: $96x = 30 \times 12$

Multiply: $96x = 360$

Divide: $x = 360 \div 96$

Answer: $x = 3.75$

3) $\frac{0.5}{3} = \frac{x}{6}$

Cross-multiply: $3x = 0.5 \times 6$

Multiply: $3x = 3$

Divide: $x = 3 \div 3$

Answer: $x = 1$

You may have noticed there's a faster way to arrive at the answer. If there is an obvious operation being performed on the proportion, the same operation can be used on the other side of the proportion to solve for x. For example, in the first practice problem, 75% became 25% when divided by 3, and upon doing the same to 90%, the correct answer of 30% would have been found with much less legwork. However, these questions aren't always so intuitive, so it's a good idea to work through the steps, even if the answer seems apparent from the outset.

Percentages

Think of percentages as fractions with a denominator of 100. In fact, **percentage** means "per hundred." Problems often require converting numbers from percentages, fractions, and decimals. The following explains how to work through those conversions.

Conversions

Decimals and Percentages: Since a percentage is based on "per hundred," decimals and percentages can be converted by multiplying or dividing by 100. Practically speaking, this always amounts to moving the decimal point two places to the right or left, depending on the conversion. To convert a percentage to a decimal, move the decimal point two places to the left and remove the % sign. To convert a decimal to a percentage, move the decimal point two places to the right and add a "%" sign. Here are some examples:

$$65\% = 0.65$$
$$0.33 = 33\%$$
$$0.215 = 21.5\%$$
$$99.99\% = 0.9999$$
$$500\% = 5.00$$
$$7.55 = 755\%$$

Fractions and Percentages: Remember that a percentage is a number per one hundred. So, a percentage can be converted to a fraction by making the number in the percentage the numerator and putting 100 as the denominator:

$$43\% = \frac{43}{100}$$

$$97\% = \frac{97}{100}$$

$$4.7\% = \frac{47}{1000}$$

Note in the last example, that the decimal can be removed by going from 100 to 1,000, because it's accomplished by multiplying the numerator and denominator by 10.

Note that the percent symbol (%) kind of looks like a 0, a 1, and another 0. So, think of a percentage like 54% as 54 over 100. Note that it's often good to simplify a fraction into the smallest possible numbers. So, $\frac{54}{100}$ would then become $\frac{27}{50}$:

$$\frac{54}{100} \div \frac{2}{2} = \frac{27}{50}$$

To convert a fraction to a percent, follow the same logic. If the fraction happens to have 100 in the denominator, you're in luck. Just take the numerator and add a percent symbol:

$$\frac{28}{100} = 28\%$$

34

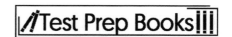
Another option is to make the denominator equal to 100. Be sure to multiply the numerator and the denominator by the same number. For example:

$$\frac{3}{20} \times \frac{5}{5} = \frac{15}{100}$$

$$\frac{15}{100} = 15\%$$

If neither of those strategies work, divide the numerator by the denominator to get a decimal:

$$\frac{9}{12} = 0.75$$

Then convert the decimal to a percentage:

$$0.75 = 75\%$$

Percent Formula

The percent formula looks like this:

$$\frac{part}{whole} = \frac{\%}{100}$$

After numbers are plugged in, multiply the diagonal numbers and then divide by the remaining one. It works every time.

So, when a question asks what percent 5 is of 10. You plug the numbers in:

$$\frac{5}{10} = \frac{\%}{100}$$

Multiply the diagonal numbers:

$$5 \times 100 = 500$$

Divide by the remaining number:

$$\frac{500}{10} = 50\%$$

The percent formula can be applied in a number of different circumstances by plugging in the numbers appropriately.

Regular Time vs. Military Time

When telling time with a regular or 12-hour clock, start counting at 12 a.m., or midnight, increasing each hour by whole numbers: 1 a.m., 2 a.m., 3 a.m., and so on. Once the count reaches 12 again, it becomes 12 p.m., or noon, and the count goes from 1 p.m., 2 p.m., 3 p.m., and so on. This switching of a.m. to p.m. and back continues in a cycle. A colon is used to separate the hours from the minutes and the minutes from the seconds.

35

Military time uses a 24-hour clock. Military time also begins at midnight and continues on to 1, 2, 3, and so on. It does not use a.m. or p.m. Midnight is the 24th hour in the count. What regular time considers 1 a.m. is called 0100, pronounced "zero one hundred hours" or "oh one hundred hours," in military time. This continues for the entire count – 0200, 0300, 0400, etc. – until you reach what regular time calls 12 p.m. or 1200, pronounced "twelve hundred hours," and then continues the count to 1300, 1400, 1500, and so on. See the following page for a comparison chart.

Regular	Military
12 a.m. Midnight	2400 Midnight/Twenty-four hundred hours
1 a.m. One o'clock	0100 Zero one hundred hours
2 a.m. Two o'clock	0200 Zero two hundred hours
3 a.m. Three o'clock	0300 Zero three hundred hours
4 a.m. Four o'clock	0400 Zero four hundred hours
5 a.m. Five o'clock	0500 Zero five hundred hours
6 a.m. Six o'clock	0600 Zero six hundred hours
7 a.m. Seven o'clock	0700 Zero seven hundred hours
8 a.m. Eight o'clock	0800 Zero eight hundred hours
9 a.m. Nine o'clock	0900 Zero nine hundred hours
10 a.m. Ten o'clock	1000 Ten hundred hours
11 a.m. Eleven o'clock	1100 Eleven hundred hours
12 p.m. Noon	1200 Noon/Twelve hundred hours
1 p.m. One o'clock	1300 Thirteen hundred hours
2 p.m. Two o'clock	1400 Fourteen hundred hours
3 p.m. Three o'clock	1500 Fifteen hundred hours
4 p.m. Four o'clock	1600 Sixteen hundred hours
5 p.m. Five o'clock	1700 Seventeen hundred hours
6 p.m. Six o'clock	1800 Eighteen hundred hours
7 p.m. Seven o'clock	1900 Nineteen hundred hours

Regular	Military
8 p.m.	2000
Eight o'clock	Twenty hundred hours
9 p.m.	2100
Nine o'clock	Twenty-one hundred hours
10 p.m.	2200
Ten o'clock	Twenty-two hundred hours
11 p.m.	2300
Eleven o'clock	Twenty-three hundred hours

A trick for converting from military to regular time is if the time is twelve hundred hours or less, it is equivalent to the a.m. version in regular time. If the time is thirteen hundred hours or more, subtract twelve and add p.m. to convert it to regular time.

Example
You are to meet someone at fourteen hundred hours. Note that the military time is more than thirteen hundred, so subtract twelve from the time.

$$14 - 12 = 2 \, \text{p.m.}$$

Example
A person needs his medicine at twenty-three hundred hours. Note the military time is more than thirteen hundred, so subtract twelve from the time.

$$23 - 12 = 11 \, \text{p.m.}$$

Properties of Exponents

Exponents are used in mathematics to express a number or variable multiplied by itself a certain number of times. For example, x^3 means x is multiplied by itself three times. In this expression, x is called the **base**, and 3 is the exponent. Exponents can be used in more complex problems when they contain fractions and negative numbers.

Order of Operations

When solving equations with multiple operations, special rules apply. These rules are known as the **Order of Operations**. The order is as follows: Parentheses, Exponents, Multiplication and Division from left to right, and Addition and Subtraction from left to right. A popular mnemonic device to help remember the order is Please Excuse My Dear Aunt Sally (PEMDAS).

Evaluate the following two problems to understand the Order of Operations:

1) $4 + (3 \times 2)^2 \div 4$

> First, solve the operation within the parentheses: $4 + 6^2 \div 4$.
> Second, solve the exponent: $4 + 36 \div 4$.
> Third, solve the division operation: $4 + 9$.
> Fourth, finish the operation with addition for the answer, 13.

2) $2 \times (6 + 3) \div (2 + 1)^2$

> $2 \times 9 \div (3)^2$
> $2 \times 9 \div 9$
> $18 \div 9$
> 2

Algebra

Algebra is used to describe things in mathematics that have differing or changeable variables. It is easily applied to real-world situations, due to its versatility. Algebra often uses **variables**, which represent unknown quantities or values. Variables are usually represented by a letter, such as X or Y. These are helpful when attempting to solve story problems. In algebra, letters are sometimes used to symbolize fixed values. In this case, the letters are called constants.

Below are some basic tips for navigating algebra.

To ensure multiplication signs (x) and unknown variables (X) are not confused, parentheses are placed around an object in an equation to signify multiplication.

Example
6×5 is the same as writing $6 (5)$.

Eliminate the multiplication sign between numbers and variables. It is understood they are multiplied.

Example
$3 (X)$ and $3 \times X$ and $3X$ all signify the same thing.

The multiplication symbol is sometimes replaced by a dot.

Example
6×5 can be written as $6 \cdot 5$.

Solving Equations in One Variable
Solving equations in one variable is the process of isolating a variable on one side of the equation. For example, in $3x - 7 = 20$, the variable is $3x$, and it needs to be isolated. The numbers (also called **constants**) are -7 and 20. That means $3x$ needs to be on one side of the equals sign (either side is fine), and all the numbers need to be on the other side of the equals sign.

To accomplish this, the equation must be manipulated by performing opposite operations of what already exists. Remember that addition and subtraction are opposites and that multiplication and

38

division are opposites. Any action taken to one side of the equation must be taken on the other side to maintain equality.

So, since the 7 is being subtracted, it can be moved to the right side of the equation by adding seven to both sides:

$$3x - 7 = 20$$

$$3x - 7 + 7 = 20 + 7$$

$$3x = 27$$

Now that the variable $3x$ is on one side and the constants (now combined into one constant) are on the other side, the 3 needs to be moved to the right side. 3 and x are being multiplied together, so 3 then needs to be divided from each side.

$$\frac{3x}{3} = \frac{27}{3}$$

$$x = 9$$

Now that x has been completely isolated, we know its value.

The solution is found to be $x = 9$. This solution can be checked for accuracy by plugging $x = 9$ in the original equation. After simplifying the equation, $20 = 20$ is found, which is a true statement:

$$3 \times 9 - 7 = 20$$

$$27 - 7 = 20$$

$$20 = 20$$

Equations that require solving for a variable (**algebraic equations**) come in many forms. Here are some more examples:

No coefficient attached to the variable:

$$x + 8 = 20$$

$$x + 8 - 8 = 20 - 8$$

$$x = 12$$

A fractional coefficient:

$$\frac{1}{2}z + 24 = 36$$

$$\frac{1}{2}z + 24 - 24 = 36 - 24$$

$$\frac{1}{2}z = 12$$

39

Now we multiply the fraction by its inverse:

$$\frac{2}{1} \times \frac{1}{2}z = 12 \times \frac{2}{1}$$

$$z = 24$$

Multiple instances of x:

$$14x + x - 4 = 3x + 2$$

All instances of x can be combined.

$$15x - 4 = 3x + 2$$

$$15x - 4 + 4 = 3x + 2 + 4$$

$$15x = 3x + 6$$

$$15x - 3x = 3x + 6 - 3x$$

$$12x = 6$$

$$\frac{12x}{12} = \frac{6}{12}$$

$$x = \frac{1}{2}$$

Evaluating Expressions

Sometimes expressions have multiple variables. For example:

$$5x + y - z$$

If you know what the variable equals, you can plug those numbers in for the variables and then solve the problem.

$$x = 3$$
$$y = 2$$
$$z = -3$$

$5(3) + 2 - (-3)$	Plug in the numbers for the variables
$15 + 2 - (-3)$	Follow the order of operations and perform multiplication first.
$15 + 2 + 3$	Subtraction of a negative can be changed to addition of a positive.
20	Add the terms

40

Algebraic **expressions** are built out of monomials. A monomial is a variable raised to some power multiplied by a constant: ax^n, where a is any constant and n is a whole number. A constant is also a monomial.

A polynomial is a sum of monomials. An example of a polynomial includes $3x^4 + 2x^2 - x - 3$.

Roman Numerals

Another form of denoting number value is through **Roman numerals**, which utilizes a finite set of letters from the alphabet to represent numbers. This numbering system doesn't account for 0, decimal, or negative numbers.

See the table below:

Arabic Numeral	Roman Numeral
1	I
5	V
10	X
50	L
100	C
500	D
1,000	M

Arabic Numeral	Roman Numeral	Arabic Numeral	Roman Numeral
1	I	6	VI
2	II	7	VII
3	III	8	VIII
4	IV	9	IX
5	V	10	X

There are two important steps to accurately reading and writing in Roman numerals. First, any smaller number immediately preceding a larger number is deducted from the larger number. For example, XC equals 90, as 10 is less than 100, so it's subtracted, as in $100 - 10 = 90$. Second, any smaller numbers after the largest one are added.

Here's an example: XLIII equals 43. In the first step, X is smaller than L, so its value is deducted from that of L, leaving 40. But the III to the right of the L is now added to the remaining 40, giving a result of 43.

Here are some more examples:

Example
XXX is what number?

Since it is the same number next to itself, add the values together.

$$10 + 10 + 10 = 30$$

Example
XL is what number?

Since X is smaller than L, and X is in front of L, it means $L - X$.

$$50 - 10 = 40$$

Example
ML is what number?

Since L is smaller than M, and L is after M, it means M + L.

$$1,000 + 50 = 1,050$$

Example
XXIX is what number?

There are two identical numbers next to each other (XX), so add them: $10 + 10 = 20$. Next, there is a smaller number (I) in front of a larger number (X), so subtract those: $10 - 1 = 9$. Finally, combine all portions to get the total $20 + 9 = 29$.

Example
What is 1988 in Roman numerals?

Break down the number into columns; $1000 + 900 + 80 + 8 = 1988$

$1000 = M, 900 = CM, 80 = LXXX, 8 = VIII$

Combine them from left to right to get the final solution: MCMLXXXVIII

Identifying Relative Sizes of Measurement Units

The United States customary system and the metric system each consist of distinct units to measure lengths and volume of liquids. The U.S. customary units for length, from smallest to largest, are: inch (in), foot (ft), yard (yd), and mile (mi). The metric units for length, from smallest to largest, are: millimeter (mm), centimeter (cm), decimeter (dm), meter (m), and kilometer (km). The relative size of each unit of length is shown below.

U.S. Customary	Metric	Conversion
12 in = 1 ft	10 mm = 1 cm	1 in = 2.54 cm
36 in = 3 ft = 1 yd	10 cm = 1 dm(decimeter)	1 m ≈ 3.28 ft ≈ 1.09 yd
5,280 ft = 1,760 yd = 1 mi	100 cm = 10 dm = 1 m	1 mi ≈ 1.6 km
	1,000 m = 1 km	

The U.S. customary units for volume of liquids, from smallest to largest, are: fluid ounces (fl oz), cup (c), pint (pt), quart (qt), and gallon (gal). The metric units for volume of liquids, from smallest to largest, are: milliliter (mL), centiliter (cL), deciliter (dL), liter (L), and kiloliter (kL). The relative size of each unit of liquid volume is shown below.

U.S. Customary	Metric	Conversion
8 fl oz = 1 c	10 mL = 1 cL	1 pt ≈ 0.473 L
2 c = 1 pt	10 cL = 1 dL	1 L ≈ 1.057 qt
4 c = 2 pt = 1 qt	1,000 mL = 100 cL = 10 dL = 1L	1 gal ≈ 3.785 L
4 qt = 1 gal	1,000 L = 1 kL	

The U.S. customary system measures weight (how strongly Earth is pulling on an object) in the following units, from least to greatest: ounce (oz), pound (lb), and ton. The metric system measures mass (the quantity of matter within an object) in the following units, from least to greatest: milligram (mg), centigram (cg), gram (g), kilogram (kg), and metric ton (MT).

The relative sizes of each unit of weight and mass are shown below.

U.S. Measures of Weight	Metric Measures of Mass
16 oz = 1 lb	10 mg = 1 cg
2,000 lb = 1 ton	100 cg = 1 g
	1,000 g = 1 kg
	1,000 kg = 1 MT

Please keep in mind that all word problems on the actual test may be hospital-related.

If you want to test your knowledge further on the math section of the HESI exam, take our online practice quiz and the practice quiz on the next page.

testprepbooks.com/hesi-quiz

43

Practice Quiz

1. After a 20% sale discount, Frank purchased a new refrigerator for $850. How much did he save from the original price?
    a. $170
    b. $212.50
    c. $105.75
    d. $200

2. A construction company is building a new housing development with the property of each house measuring 30 feet wide. If the length of the street is zoned off at 345 feet, how many houses can be built on the street?
    a. 11
    b. 115
    c. 11.5
    d. 12

3. Mo needs to buy enough material to cover the walls around the stage for a theater performance. If he needs 79 feet of wall covering, what is the minimum number of yards of material he should purchase if the material is sold only by whole yards?
    a. 23 yards
    b. 25 yards
    c. 26 yards
    d. 27 yards

4. You measure the width of your door to be 36 inches. The true width of the door is 35.75 inches. What is the relative error in your measurement?
    a. 0.7%
    b. 0.007%
    c. 0.99%
    d. 0.1%

5. A couple buys a house for $150,000. They sell it for $165,000. By what percentage did the house's value increase?
    a. 10%
    b. 13%
    c. 15%
    d. 17%

See answers on next page.

Answer Explanations

1. B: Since $850 is the price *after* a 20% discount, $850 represents 80% of the original price. To determine the original price, set up a proportion with the ratio of the sale price (850) to original price (unknown) equal to the ratio of sale percentage (where x represents the unknown original price):

$$\frac{850}{x} = \frac{80}{100}$$

To solve a proportion, cross multiply and set the products equal to each other:

$$(850)(100) = (80)(x)$$

Multiplying each side results in the equation:

$$85,000 = 80x$$

To solve for x, divide both sides by 80:

$$\frac{85,000}{80} = \frac{80x}{80}$$

$$x = 1,062.5$$

Remember that x represents the original price. Subtracting the sale price from the original price ($1,062.50 - $850) indicates that Frank saved $212.50.

2. A: 11. To determine the number of houses that can fit on the street, the length of the street is divided by the width of each house: $345 \div 30 = 11.5$. Although the mathematical calculation of 11.5 is correct, this answer is not reasonable. Half of a house cannot be built, so the company will need to either build 11 or 12 houses. Since the width of 12 houses (360 feet) will extend past the length of the street, only 11 houses can be built.

3. D: In order to solve this problem, the number of feet in a yard must be established. There are 3 feet in every yard. The equation to calculate the minimum number of yards is $79 \div 3 = 26\frac{1}{3}$.

If the material is sold only by whole yards, then Mo would need to round up to the next whole yard in order to cover the extra $\frac{1}{3}$ yard. Therefore, the answer is 27 yards. None of the other choices meets the minimum whole yard requirement.

4. A: The relative error can be found by finding the absolute error and making it a percent of the true value. The absolute error is $36 - 35.75 = 0.25$. This error is then divided by 35.75 — the true value — to find 0.7%.

5. A: The value went up by $165,000 - $150,000 = $15,000. Out of $150,000, this is $\frac{15,000}{150,000} = \frac{1}{10}$. Convert this to having a denominator of 100, the result is $\frac{10}{100}$ or 10%.

Reading Comprehension

Identifying the Main Idea

Topics and main ideas are critical parts of any writing. The **topic** is the subject matter of the piece, and it is a broader, more general term. The **main idea** is what the writer wants to say about that topic. The topic can be expressed in a word or two, but the main idea should be a complete thought.

The topic and main idea are usually easy to recognize in nonfiction writing. An author will likely identify the topic immediately in the first sentence of a passage or essay. The main idea is also typically presented in the introductory paragraph of an essay. In a single passage, the main idea may be identified in the first or the last sentence, but will likely be directly stated and easily recognized by the reader. Because it is not always stated immediately in a passage, it's important to carefully read the entire passage to identify the main idea.

Also remember that when most authors write, they want to make a point or send a message. This point or message of a text is known as the theme. Authors may state themes explicitly, like in *Aesop's Fables*. More often, especially in modern literature, readers must infer the theme based on text details. Usually after carefully reading and analyzing an entire text, the reader can identify the theme. Typically, the longer the piece, the more themes you will encounter, though often one theme dominates the rest, as evidenced by the author's purposeful revisiting of it throughout the passage.

The main idea should not be confused with the thesis statement. A thesis statement is a clear statement of the writer's specific stance, and can often be found in the introduction of a nonfiction piece. The main idea is more of an overview of the entire piece, while the thesis is a specific sentence found in that piece.

In order to illustrate the main idea, a writer will use **supporting details** in a passage. These details can provide evidence or examples to help make a point. Supporting details are most commonly found in nonfiction pieces that seek to inform or persuade the reader.

46

As a reader, you will want to carefully examine the author's supporting details to be sure they are credible. Consider whether they provide evidence of the author's point and whether they directly support the main idea. You might find that an author has used a shocking statistic to grab your attention, but that the statistic doesn't really support the main idea, so it isn't being effectively used in the piece.

Identifying Supporting Details

Supporting details help readers better develop and understand the main idea. Supporting details answer questions like *who, what, where, when, why,* and *how.* Different types of supporting details include examples, facts and statistics, anecdotes, and sensory details.

Persuasive and informative texts often use supporting details. In persuasive texts, authors attempt to make readers agree with their points of view, and supporting details are often used as "selling points." If authors make a statement, they need to support the statement with evidence in order to adequately persuade readers. Informative texts use supporting details such as examples and facts to inform readers. Review the previous "Cheetahs" passage to find examples of supporting details.

Cheetahs

Cheetahs are one of the fastest mammals on the land, reaching up to 70 miles an hour over short distances. Even though cheetahs can run as fast as 70 miles an hour, they usually only have to run half that speed to catch up with their choice of prey. Cheetahs cannot maintain a fast pace over long periods of time because their bodies will overheat. After a chase, cheetahs need to rest for approximately 30 minutes prior to eating or returning to any other activity.

In the example, supporting details include:

- Cheetahs reach up to 70 miles per hour over short distances.
- They usually only have to run half that speed to catch up with their prey.
- Cheetahs will overheat if they exert a high speed over longer distances.
- Cheetahs need to rest for 30 minutes after a chase.

Look at the diagram below (applying the cheetah example) to help determine the hierarchy of topic, main idea, and supporting details.

Finding the Meaning of Words and Phrases in Context

There will be many occasions in one's reading career in which an unknown word or a word with multiple meanings will pop up. There are ways of determining what these words or phrases mean that do not require the use of the dictionary, which is especially helpful during a test where one may not be available. Even outside of the exam, knowing how to derive an understanding of a word via **context clues** will be a critical skill in the real world. The context is the circumstances in which a story or a passage is happening, and can usually be found in the series of words directly before or directly after the word or phrase in question. The clues are the words that hint towards the meaning of the unknown word or phrase. The author may use synonyms or antonyms that you can use. **Synonyms** refer to words that have the same meaning as another word (e.g., instructor/teacher/educator, canine/dog, feline/cat, herbivore/vegetarian). **Antonyms** refer to words that have the opposite meaning as another word (e.g., true/false, up/down, in/out, right/wrong).

There may be questions that ask about the meaning of a particular word or phrase within a passage. There are a couple ways to approach these kinds of questions:

- Define the word or phrase in a way that is easy to comprehend (using context clues).
- Try out each answer choice in place of the word.

To demonstrate, here's an example from *Alice in Wonderland*:

> Alice was beginning to get very tired of sitting by her sister on the bank, and of having nothing to do: once or twice she <u>peeped</u> into the book her sister was reading, but it had no pictures or conversations in it, "and what is the use of a book," thought Alice, "without pictures or conversations?"

Q: As it is used in the selection, the word <u>peeped</u> means:

Using the first technique, before looking at the answers, define the word "peeped" using context clues and then find the matching answer. Then, analyze the entire passage in order to determine the meaning, not just the surrounding words.

To begin, imagine a blank where the word should be and put a synonym or definition there: "once or twice she ___ into the book her sister was reading." The context clue here is the book. It may be tempting to put "read" where the blank is, but notice the preposition word, "into." One does not read *into* a book, one simply reads a book, and since reading a book requires that it is seen with a pair of eyes, then "look" would make the most sense to put into the blank: "once or twice she <u>looked </u>into the book her sister was reading."

Once an easy-to-understand word or synonym has been supplanted, check to make sure it makes sense with the rest of the passage. What happened after she looked into the book? She thought to herself how a book without pictures or conversations is useless. This situation in its entirety makes sense.

Now check the answer choices for a match:
   a. To make a high-pitched cry
   b. To smack
   c. To look curiously
   d. To pout

Since the word was already defined, answer choice (c) is the best option.

Using the second technique, replace the figurative blank with each of the answer choices and determine which one is the most appropriate. Remember to look further into the passage to clarify that they work, because they could still make sense out of context.

Once or twice she <u>made a high pitched cry</u> into the book her sister was reading.

Once or twice she <u>smacked </u>the book her sister was reading.

Once or twice she <u>looked curiously</u> into the book her sister was reading.

Once or twice she <u>pouted</u> into the book her sister was reading.

For Choice *A,* it does not make much sense in any context for a person to yell into a book, unless maybe something terrible has happened in the story. Given that afterward Alice thinks to herself how useless a book without pictures is, this option does not make sense within context.

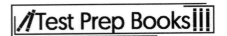

For Choice *B*, smacking a book someone is reading may make sense if the rest of the passage indicates there a reason for doing so. If Alice was angry or her sister had shoved it in her face, then maybe smacking the book would make sense within context. However, since whatever she does with the book causes her to think, "what is the use of a book without pictures or conversations?" then answer Choice *B* is not an appropriate answer.

Answer Choice *C* fits well within context, given her subsequent thoughts on the matter.

Answer Choice *D* does not make sense in context or grammatically, as people do not "pout into" things.

This is a simple example to illustrate the techniques outlined above. There may, however, be a question in which all of the definitions are correct and also make sense out of context, in which the appropriate context clues will really need to be honed in on in order to determine the correct answer. For example, here is another passage from *Alice in Wonderland*:

> ... but when the Rabbit actually took a watch out of its waistcoat pocket, and looked at it, and then hurried on, Alice <u>started</u> to her feet, for it flashed across her mind that she had never before seen a rabbit with either a waistcoat-pocket or a watch to take out of it, and burning with curiosity, she ran across the field after it, and was just in time to see it pop down a large rabbit-hole under the hedge.

Q: As it is used in the passage, the word <u>started</u> means:
   a. To turn on
   b. To begin
   c. To move quickly
   d. To be surprised

All of these words qualify as a definition of start, but using context clues, the correct answer can be identified using one of the two techniques above. It's easy to see that one does not turn on, begin, or be surprised to one's feet. The selection also states that she "ran across the field after it," indicating that she was in a hurry. Therefore, to move quickly would make the most sense in this context.

The same strategies can be applied to vocabulary that may be completely unfamiliar. In this case, focus on the words before or after the unknown word in order to determine its definition. Take this sentence, for example:

"Sam was such a <u>miser</u> that he forced Andrew to pay him twelve cents for the candy, even though he had a large inheritance and he knew his friend was poor."

Unlike with assertion questions, for vocabulary questions, it may be necessary to apply some critical thinking skills that may not be explicitly stated within the passage. Think about the implications of the passage, or what the text is trying to say. With this example, it is important to realize that it is considered unusually stingy for a person to demand so little money from someone instead of just letting their friend have the candy, especially if this person is already wealthy. Hence, a <u>miser</u> is a greedy or stingy individual.

Questions about complex vocabulary may not be explicitly asked, but this is a useful skill to know. If there is an unfamiliar word while reading a passage and its definition goes unknown, it is possible to miss out on a critical message that could inhibit the ability to appropriately answer the questions.

Practicing this technique in daily life will sharpen this ability to derive meanings from context clues with ease.

Identifying a Writer's Purpose and Tone

Purpose

Writing can be classified under four passage types: narrative, expository, descriptive (sometimes called technical), and persuasive. Though these types are not mutually exclusive, one form tends to dominate the rest. By recognizing the *type* of passage you're reading, you gain insight into *how* you should read. If you're reading a narrative, you can assume the author intends to entertain, which means you may skim the text without losing meaning. A technical document might require a close read because skimming the passage might cause the reader to miss salient details.

1. **Narrative writing**, at its core, is the art of storytelling. For a narrative to exist, certain elements must be present. First, it must have characters, While many characters are human, characters could be defined as anything that thinks, acts, and talks like a human. For example, many recent movies, such as *Lord of the Rings* and *The Chronicles of Narnia*, include animals, fantastical creatures, and even trees that behave like humans. Second, it must have a plot or sequence of events. Typically, those events follow a standard plot diagram, but recent trends start *in medias res* or in the middle (near the climax). In this instance, foreshadowing and flashbacks often fill in plot details. Finally, along with characters and a plot, there must also be conflict. Conflict is usually divided into two types: internal and external. Internal conflict indicates the character is in turmoil and is presented through the character's thoughts. External conflicts are visible. Types of external conflict include a person versus nature, another person, or society.

2. **Expository writing** is detached and to the point. Since expository writing is designed to instruct or inform, it usually involves directions and steps written in second person ("you" voice) and lacks any persuasive or narrative elements. Sequence words such as *first*, *second*, and *third*, or *in the first place*, *secondly*, and *lastly* are often given to add fluency and cohesion. Common examples of expository writing include instructor's lessons, cookbook recipes, and repair manuals.

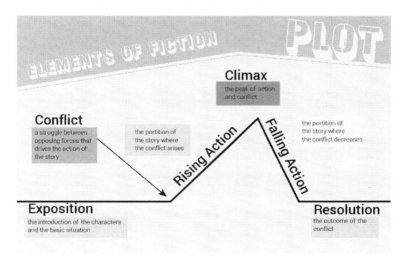

3. Due to its empirical nature, **technical writing** is filled with steps, charts, graphs, data, and statistics. The goal of technical writing is to advance understanding in a field through the scientific method.

51

Experts such as teachers, doctors, or mechanics use words unique to the profession in which they operate. These words, which often incorporate acronyms, are called *jargon*. Technical writing is a type of expository writing but is not meant to be understood by the general public. Instead, technical writers assume readers have received a formal education in a particular field of study and need no explanation as to what the jargon means. Imagine a doctor trying to understand a diagnostic reading for a car or a mechanic trying to interpret lab results. Only professionals with proper training will fully comprehend the text.

4. **Persuasive writing** is designed to change opinions and attitudes. The topic, stance, and arguments are found in the thesis, positioned near the end of the introduction. Later supporting paragraphs offer relevant quotations, paraphrases, and summaries from primary or secondary sources, which are then interpreted, analyzed, and evaluated. The goal of persuasive writers is not to stack quotes but to develop original ideas by using sources as a starting point. Good persuasive writing makes powerful arguments with valid sources and thoughtful analysis. Poor persuasive writing is riddled with bias and logical fallacies. Sometimes logical and illogical arguments are sandwiched together in the same piece. Therefore, readers should display skepticism when reading persuasive arguments.

Tone

Tone refers to the writer's attitude toward the subject matter. Tone is usually explained in terms of a work of fiction. For example, the tone conveys how the writer feels about the characters and the situations in which they're involved. Nonfiction writing is sometimes thought to have no tone at all; however, this is incorrect.

A lot of nonfiction writing has a neutral tone, which is an important one for the writer to use. A **neutral tone** demonstrates that the writer is presenting a topic impartially and letting the information speak for itself. On the other hand, nonfiction writing can be just as effective and appropriate if the tone isn't neutral. The following short passage provides an example of tone in nonfiction writing:

> Seat belts save more lives than any other automobile safety feature. Many studies show that airbags save lives as well; however, not all cars have airbags. For instance, some older cars don't. Furthermore, air bags aren't entirely reliable. For example, studies show that in 15% of accidents airbags don't deploy as designed, but, on the other hand, seat belt malfunctions are extremely rare. The number of highway fatalities has plummeted since laws requiring seat belt usage were enacted.

In this passage, the writer mostly chooses to retain a neutral tone when presenting information. If instead, the author chose to include their own personal experience of losing a friend or family member in a car accident, the tone would change dramatically. The tone would no longer be neutral and would show that the writer has a personal stake in the content, allowing him or her to interpret the information in a different way. When analyzing tone, the reader should consider what the writer is trying to achieve in the text and how they *create* the tone using style.

The following two poems and the essay concern the theme of death and are presented to demonstrate how to evaluate tone:

"Queen Mab," Percy Bysshe Shelley

How wonderful is Death,

Death, and his brother Sleep!

One, pale as yonder waning moon

With lips of lurid blue;

The other, rosy as the morn

When throned on ocean's wave

It blushes o'er the world;

Yet both so passing wonderful!

"After Great Pain, A Formal Feeling Comes," Emily Dickinson

After great pain, a formal feeling comes –

The Nerves sit ceremonious, like Tombs –

The stiff Heart questions 'was it He, that bore,'

And 'Yesterday, or Centuries before'?

The Feet, mechanical, go round –

A Wooden way

Of Ground, or Air, or Ought –

Regardless grown,

A Quartz contentment, like a stone –

This is the Hour of Lead –

Remembered, if outlived,

As Freezing persons, recollect the Snow –

First – Chill – then Stupor – then the letting go –

The Process of Dying

Death occurs in several stages. The first stage is the pre-active stage, which occurs a few days to weeks before death, in which the desire to eat and drink decreases, and the person may feel restless, irritable, and anxious. The second stage is the active stage, where the skin begins to cool, breathing becomes difficult as the lungs become congested (known as the "death rattle"), and the person loses control of their bodily fluids.

Once death occurs, there are also two stages. The first is clinical death, when the heart stops pumping blood and breathing ceases. This stage lasts approximately 4-6 minutes, and during this time, it is possible for a victim to be resuscitated via CPR or a defibrillator. After 6 minutes however, the oxygen stores within the brain begin to deplete, and the victim enters biological death. This is the point of no return, as the cells of the brain and vital organs begin to die, a process that is irreversible.

Readers should notice the differences in the word choices between the two poems. Percy Shelley's word choices—"wonderful," "rosy," "blushes," "ocean"—surrounding death indicates that he views death in a welcoming manner as his words carry positive charges. However, Dickinson's word choices—"pain," "wooden," "stone," "lead," "chill," "tombs"—carry negative connotations, which indicates an aversion to death. **Connotation** refers to the implied meaning of a word or phrase. Connotations are the ideas or feelings that words or phrases invoke other than their literal meaning. In contrast, the expository passage has no emotionally-charged words of any kind, and seems to view death simply as a process that happens, neither welcoming nor fearing it. The tone in this passage, therefore, is neutral.

Distinguishing between Fact and Opinion

It is important to distinguish between fact and opinion when reading a piece of writing. Readers should check the validity and accuracy of the facts that an author presents. When authors use opinion, they are sharing their own thoughts and feelings about the subject. You can recognize a piece that relies on opinion when the author uses words like *think, feel, believe,* or *in my opinion,* though these words won't always appear in an opinion piece, especially if it is formally written. An author's opinion may be backed up by facts, which gives it more credibility, but it should not be taken as fact. A critical reader should be wary of an author's opinion, especially if it is only supported by other opinions. Here are some examples of facts versus opinions:

Facts	Opinions
There are 9 innings in a game of baseball.	Baseball games run too long.
Eisenhower expanded Social Security.	This action was helpful for the country.
McDonalds has stores in 118 countries.	McDonalds has the best hamburgers.

As a critical reader, you must examine the facts that are used to support the author's argument. You can check the facts against other sources to be sure they are correct. You can also check the validity of the sources used to be sure they are credible, academic, and peer reviewed sources. Consider that when an author uses another person's opinion to support the argument, even if it is an expert's opinion, it is still only an opinion, and should not be taken as fact. A strong argument uses valid, measurable facts to support ideas. Even then, the reader may disagree with the argument, as it is rooted in the author's **assumptions**, which are the author's personal beliefs.

Making Logical Inferences

Critical readers should be able to make inferences. Making an **inference** requires the reader to read between the lines and look for what is implied rather than what is explicitly stated. That is, using information that *is* known from the text, the reader is able to make a logical assumption about information that is not explicitly stated but is probably true. Read the following passage:

"Hey, do you wanna meet my new puppy?" Jonathan asked.

"Oh, I'm sorry but please don't—" Jacinta began to protest, but before she could finish Jonathan had already opened the passenger side door of his car and a perfect white ball of fur came bouncing towards Jacinta.

"Isn't he the cutest?" beamed Jonathan.

"Yes—achoo!—he's pretty—aaaachooo!!—adora—aaa—aaaachoo!" Jacinta managed to say in between sneezes. "But if you don't mind, I—I—achoo!—need to go inside."

Which of the following can be inferred from Jacinta's reaction to the puppy?
a. she hates animals
b. she is allergic to dogs
c. she prefers cats to dogs
d. she is angry at Jonathan

An inference requires the reader to consider the information presented and then form their own idea about what is probably true. Based on the details in the passage, what is the best answer to the question? Important details to pay attention to include the tone of Jacinta's dialogue, which is overall polite and apologetic, as well as her reaction itself, which is a long string of sneezes. Answer Choices *A* and *D* both express strong emotions ("hates" and "angry") that are not evident in Jacinta's speech or actions. Answer Choice *C* mentions cats, but there is nothing in the passage to indicate Jacinta's feelings about cats. Answer Choice *B*, "she is allergic to dogs," is the most logical choice—based on the fact that she began sneezing as soon as a fluffy dog approached her, it makes sense to guess that Jacinta might be allergic to dogs. So even though Jacinta never directly states, "Sorry, I'm allergic to dogs!" using the clues in the passage, it is still reasonable to guess that this is true.

Making inferences is crucial for readers of literature because literary texts often avoid presenting complete and direct information to readers about characters' thoughts or feelings, or they present this information in an unclear way, leaving it up to the reader to interpret clues given in the text. In order to make inferences while reading, readers should ask themselves:

- What details are being presented in the text?
- Is there any important information that seems to be missing?
- Based on the information that the author *does* include, what else is probably true?
- Is this inference reasonable based on what is already known?

Summarizing

A **summary** is a shortened version of the original text. It focuses on the main points of the original text and includes only the relevant details. Since summaries are generally significantly shorter than the text they are about, summaries need to get straight to the point. It's important that a summary retain the original meaning of the text. Generally, a summary should follow the flow of the passage by explaining the points in the same order as the original passage; however, this is not a necessity.

Please keep in mind that passages found in the actual exam may be hospital-related.

Practice Quiz

Questions 1–5 are based on the following passage:

As long ago as 1860 it was the proper thing to be born at home. At present, so I am told, the high gods of medicine have decreed that the first cries of the young shall be uttered upon the anesthetic air of a hospital, preferably a fashionable one. So young Mr. and Mrs. Roger Button were fifty years ahead of style when they decided, one day in the summer of 1860, that their first baby should be born in a hospital. Whether this anachronism had any bearing upon the astonishing history I am about to set down will never be known.

I shall tell you what occurred, and let you judge for yourself.

The Roger Buttons held an enviable position, both social and financial, in ante-bellum Baltimore. They were related to the This Family and the That Family, which, as every Southerner knew, entitled them to membership in that enormous peerage which largely populated the Confederacy. This was their first experience with the charming old custom of having babies— Mr. Button was naturally nervous. He hoped it would be a boy so that he could be sent to Yale College in Connecticut, at which institution Mr. Button himself had been known for four years by the somewhat obvious nickname of "Cuff."

On the September morning <u>consecrated</u> to the enormous event he arose nervously at six o'clock, dressed himself, adjusted an impeccable stock, and hurried forth through the streets of Baltimore to the hospital, to determine whether the darkness of the night had borne in new life upon its bosom.

When he was approximately a hundred yards from the Maryland Private Hospital for Ladies and Gentlemen he saw Doctor Keene, the family physician, descending the front steps, rubbing his hands together with a washing movement—as all doctors are required to do by the unwritten ethics of their profession.

Mr. Roger Button, the president of Roger Button & Co., Wholesale Hardware, began to run toward Doctor Keene with much less dignity than was expected from a Southern gentleman of that picturesque period. "Doctor Keene!" he called. "Oh, Doctor Keene!"

The doctor heard him, faced around, and stood waiting, a curious expression settling on his harsh, medicinal face as Mr. Button drew near.

"What happened?" demanded Mr. Button, as he came up in a gasping rush. "What was it? How is she? A boy? Who is it? What—"

"Talk sense!" said Doctor Keene sharply. He appeared somewhat irritated.

"Is the child born?" begged Mr. Button.

Doctor Keene frowned. "Why, yes, I suppose so—after a fashion." Again he threw a curious glance at Mr. Button.

The Curious Case of Benjamin Button, F.S. Fitzgerald, 1922

57

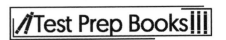
1. What major event is about to happen in this story?
   a. Mr. Button is about to go to a funeral.
   b. Mr. Button's wife is about to have a baby.
   c. Mr. Button is getting ready to go to the doctor's office.
   d. Mr. Button is about to go shopping for new clothes.

2. What kind of tone does the above passage have?
   a. Nervous and Excited
   b. Sad and Angry
   c. Shameful and Confused
   d. Grateful and Joyous

3. What is the meaning of the word "consecrated" in paragraph 4?
   a. Numbed
   b. Chained
   c. Dedicated
   d. Moved

4. What does the author mean to do by adding the following statement?

"rubbing his hands together with a washing movement—as all doctors are required to do by the unwritten ethics of their profession."

   a. Suggesting that Mr. Button is tired of the doctor.
   b. Trying to explain the detail of the doctor's profession.
   c. Hinting to readers that the doctor is an unethical man.
   d. Giving readers a visual picture of what the doctor is doing.

5. Which of the following best describes the development of this passage?
   a. It starts in the middle of a narrative in order to transition smoothly to a conclusion.
   b. It is a chronological narrative from beginning to end.
   c. The sequence of events is backwards—we go from future events to past events.
   d. To introduce the setting of the story and its characters

See answers on next page.

If you want to test your knowledge further on the reading comprehension section of the HESI exam, take our online practice quiz.

testprepbooks.com/hesi-quiz

Answer Explanations

1. B: Mr. Button's wife is about to have a baby. The passage begins by giving the reader information about traditional birthing situations. Then, we are told that Mr. and Mrs. Button decide to go against tradition to have their baby in a hospital. The next few passages are dedicated to letting the reader know how Mr. Button dresses and goes to the hospital to welcome his new baby. There is a doctor in this excerpt, as Choice *C* indicates, and Mr. Button does put on clothes, as Choice *D* indicates. However, Mr. Button is not going to the doctor's office nor is he about to go shopping for new clothes.

2. A: The tone of the above passage is nervous and excited. We are told in the fourth paragraph that Mr. Button "arose nervously." We also see him running without caution to the doctor to find out about his wife and baby—this indicates his excitement. We also see him stuttering in a nervous yet excited fashion as he asks the doctor if it's a boy or girl. Though the doctor may seem a bit abrupt at the end, indicating a bit of anger or shame, neither of these choices is the overwhelming tone of the entire passage. Despite the circumstances, joy and gratitude are not the main tone in the passage.

3. C: Dedicated. Mr. Button is dedicated to the task before him. Choice *A*, numbed, Choice *B*, chained, and Choice *D*, moved, all could grammatically fit in the sentence. However, they are not synonyms with *consecrated* like Choice *C* is.

4. D: Giving readers a visual picture of what the doctor is doing. The author describes a visual image—the doctor rubbing his hands together—first and foremost. The author may be trying to make a comment about the profession; however, the author does not "explain the detail of the doctor's profession" as Choice *B* suggests.

5. D: To introduce the setting of the story and its characters. We know we are being introduced to the setting because we are given the year in the very first paragraph along with the season: "one day in the summer of 1860." This is a classic structure of an introduction of the setting. We are also getting a long explanation of Mr. Button, what his work is, who is related to him, and what his life is like in the third paragraph.

59

Vocabulary

Identifying Roots

By analyzing and understanding Latin, Greek, and Anglo-Saxon word roots and structure, authors better convey the thoughts they want to express to the readers of their words and help them to determine their meanings within the flow and without their missing a beat. For instance, **context**—how words are used in sentences—is from the Latin for *contextus*, which means "together"+"to weave," and gives readers a graphic for the minds' eyes to see the coming together of their usage. Like every other topic discussed herein, context is needed for understanding. This element actually has a second, crucial meaning. Context is not only the *how*, but the revealed moment of the *why* a writing has been composed; it is the "Aha" moment.

The way *how* words are used in sentences is important because it also gives meaning and cohesion from sentence to sentence, paragraph to paragraph, and page after page. In other words, it gives the document continuity.

Another upside of the how side is that readers have opportunities to understand new words with which they are unfamiliar. Of course, people can always look words up if a dictionary or thesaurus, if available, but meaning might be gleaned on the spot in a piece that is well-written. **Synonyms** (words or phrases that mean about the same) and **antonyms** (words or phrases that mean the opposite of the specific word) in context give clues to meanings, and sometimes reiteration of a word might add clarification. Repetition, wisely used, can also serve as a part of how a piece flows.

The revealed moment of the *why* is important because context, up to that moment, has determined the shape of the text. This is, essentially, to bring out what it is all about.

Prefixes

A **prefix** is a word, letter, or number that is placed before another. It adjusts or qualifies the original word's meaning.

Four prefixes represent 97 percent of English words with prefixes. They are:

- *dis-* means "not" or "opposite of"; *dis*abled
- *in-, im-, il-, ir-* mean "not"; *il*literate
- *re-* means "again"; *re*turn
- *un-* means "not"; *un*predictable

Other commons prefixes include:

- *anti-* means "against"; antibacterial
- *fore-* means "before"; forefront
- *mis-* means "wrongly"; misunderstand
- *non-* means "not"; nonsense
- *over-* means "over"; overabundance

- *pre-* means "before"; preheat
- *super-* means "above"; superman

Suffixes

The official definition of a **suffix** is "a morpheme added at the end of a word to form a derivative." In English, that means a suffix is a letter or group of letters added at the end of a word to form another word. The word created with the addition is either a different tense of the same word (*help+ed=helped*) or a new word (*help+ful=helpful*).

Some common suffixes include:

- *-ed* is used to make present tense verbs into past tense verbs; wash*ed*
- *-ing* is used to make a present tense verb into a present participle verb; wash*ing*
- *-ly* is used to make characteristic of; love*ly*
- *-s* or *–es* are used to make more than one; chair*s* or box*es*
- *-able* means can be done; deplor*able*
- *-al* means having characteristics of; comic*al*
- *-est* means comparative; great*est*
- *-ful* means full of; wonder*ful*
- *-ism* means belief in; commun*ism*
- *-less* means without; faith*less*
- *-ment* means action or process; accomplish*ment*
- *-ness* means state of; happi*ness*
- *-ize* means to render, to make; terror*ize,* steril*ize*
- *-ise* is primarily the British variant of *–ize;* surpr*ise,* advert*ise*
- *-ced* means go; spelling variations include -cede (concede, recede); -ceed (only three: proceed, exceed, succeed); -sede (the only one: supersede)

(Note: In some of the examples above, the *e* has been deleted.)

Word Origins

The study of the origin of a particular word, as well as how its meaning has changed over time, is called **etymology.** As an example, one might research the word *cool* and learn when *cool* became *cool* as in meanings other than in relation to *cold.*

Here are some common terms both in general usage as well as some common in medical usage:

Abstain (v.): Decline or refuse to do something; to refrain or hold back. *Example:* The doctor abstained from giving the patient another prescription of medication, because he had concerns that the patient was exaggerating their symptoms.

Accountable (adj.): Required to justify one's decisions to another individual, organization, or institution. *Example:* Nurses need to be held accountable for their actions when mistakes are made.

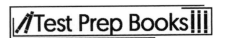

Acute (adj.): Severe or intense degree. *Example:* The doctor gave specific instructions to the patient after prescribing them a medication for their acute pain.

Adhere (v.): Listen or comply. *Example:* In order to adhere to the patient's request, the nurses and doctors only allowed family members in the room.

Adverse (adj.): Preventing success; a negative outcome. *Example:* Because of the patients' adverse reaction to the anesthesia, the surgeon had to reevaluate her treatment plan.

Ambivalent (adj.): Having contradictory ideas or a doubtful disposition. *Example:* After doing extensive research on a patient's case, the surgeon was ambivalent to performing surgery, knowing there was a lot of risk involved.

Ambulate (v.): To move around by walking. *Example:* The woman began to ambulate approximately one week after her surgery.

Apply (v.): To put on; to spread. *Example:* The doctor applied padding all the way around the patient's broken arm before applying the casting.

Assent (n.): The expression to approve or agree. *Example:* The doctor wanted the patient's assent before giving them the anesthesia.

Audible (adj.): The ability to be heard. *Example:* The patient's voice could be heard audibly throughout the hall when their shoulder was put back into its place.

Bacteria (n.): Single-celled living organisms; some can cause disease while others are essential to life. *Example:* Studies show that bacteria can live on surfaces for days; that's why it's so important for hospitals to sterilize equipment between patients.

Bilateral (adj.): Relating or affecting both sides of something. *Example:* After completing the MRI, it was discovered that the patient had bilateral tumors on both lungs.

Cardiac (adj.): Relating or referring to the heart. *Example:* Cardiac stimulants may be essential to prevent heart failure in some patients.

Cavity (n.): A hole or empty space within a solid object, specifically the human body. *Example:* The thoracic cavity, also known as the chest cavity, contains the lungs and the heart.

Cease (v.): To bring to an end, or cause to stop. *Example:* They had to cease drawing the patient's blood due to verbal discomfort and nausea expressed by the patient.

Chronic (adj.): A specification that indicates a disease is long-lasting. *Example:* The patient was diagnosed with a chronic illness; the specialist suggested the importance of learning about the illness and how to mitigate its harsher symptoms.

Chronology (n.): The arranging of events according to the ascending or descending order of dates. *Example:* the nurses referred to the patients' chart regularly in order to know the chronology of the daily medication.

Compensatory (adj.): Adjusting in order to make up for something. *Example:* A compensatory payment was put in place to make up for psychological damages.

Concave (adj.): Having a surface that curves inward. *Example:* The top of a new born baby's head is slightly concaved after birth, due to the pressure in the vaginal canal.

Concise (adj.): Giving information clearly in a comprehensive, but brief way. *Example:* The doctor needed a concise run through of all the patient's symptoms so they could treat them immediately.

Congenital (adj.): The presentation of a disease that is inherited or persistent from birth. *Example:* The symptoms in the new infant were consistent with those of congenital heart disease.

Consistency (n.): The thickness in a liquid; how a liquid holds together. *Example:* The consistency of certain foods caused the patient to present an intense gag reflex.

Constrict (v.): To become narrow, specifically by the encircling of pressure. *Example:* Smoking can cause blood vessels to constrict, which can cause circulation in extremities to be cut off.

Contingent (adj.): Occurring only under specific circumstances; dependent on. *Example:* After testing, the doctor concluded that the patient's allergic reaction was contingent on gluten consumption.

Contraindication (n.): When a medical procedure is discouraged because of a certain condition. *Example:* The surgery was contraindicated with the current medication the patient was taking.

Convulsive (adj.): Producing uncontrolled movements or spasms. *Example:* The patient explained they were experiencing multiple convulsive episodes, so the doctor prescribed them a new medication.

Cursory (adj.): Hasty; not thorough. *Example:* Because of the cursory assessment, they missed doing a full body x-ray and failed to diagnose the rib break the patient had.

Defecate (v.): To discharge feces from the body. *Example:* The patient had an abnormally difficult time defecating daily, even with medication to help, so the doctor had them stay for observation.

Deficit (n.): A lack in something. *Example:* The doctor told the teen patient that if they kept listening to their music at extreme volumes, they would risk having a hearing deficit.

Depress (v.): The motion of going downward. *Example:* The doctor used a tongue depressor to move the tongue and look down the patient's throat.

Depth (n.): The distance from the surface downward. *Example:* The depth of the glass in the patient's foot was farther than the doctors thought.

Deteriorating (adj.): Falling apart or declining in health. *Example:* After blunt trauma to the head, the patient's lucidness was deteriorating quickly.

Diagnosis (n.): An identification of the nature of an illness by the examination of a problem or of the symptoms. *Example:* After having the patient undergo multiple blood tests, the doctor diagnosed the patient with anemia.

Diffuse (v.): To spread throughout the body; not localized in a specific area. *Example:* The pain diffused from his shoulder to fingers.

Dilate (v.): To become wider, larger, or more open. *Example:* The patient's cervix was dilated 8 cm; only 2 cm more until the doctor will instruct the patient to push.

Dilute (v.): To be made thinner or weaker. *Example:* The liquid medicine was diluted in order to make the bitter taste easier to consume.

Discrete (adj.): Distinct; separate. Not joined with another. *Example:* The doctor would describe the patient's tumor as discrete from the tissues around it.

Distal (adj.): Situated away from something; specifically, the body. *Example:* The thumb is distal from the hand.

Distended (adj.): Swollen due to pressure. *Example:* The doctors were concerned because of the patients distended stomach, which didn't seem to be caused by anything obvious.

Dysfunction (n.): Impairment or abnormality in functioning. *Example:* After various tests, the doctor concluded that the patient had a bowel dysfunction.

Empathy (n.): The ability to understand the feelings of another individual. *Example:* The nurse had empathy for this patient, because, due to inconclusive results, some very uncomfortable tests had to be repeated.

Equilibrium (n.): A chemical balance in the body. *Example:* When they took the pain meds, the patient felt a difference in their equilibrium.

Etiology (n.): The set of causes in a disease. *Example:* Even though the diagnosis was accurate and confirmed, the doctor could not find the etiology of this sickness.

Exacerbate (v.): To make a problem or bad situation worse. *Example:* In students, it's common that the stress of worrying about school exacerbates any health conditions.

Expand(v.): To enlarge or stretch. *Example:* Throughout pregnancy, the skin in the torso continues to expand.

Exposure (n.): The state of being subjected to something which may have a harmful effect. *Example:* During flu season, nurses are often exposed to the flu.

Extension (n.): Returning a limb to its original position by straightening or stretching. *Example:* The doctor asked the patient for a leg extension in order to analyze the severity of the injury before an x-ray.

Fatal (adj.): Emphasizes inevitability; unable to prevent death. *Example:* The blunt force trauma to the patient was fatal, causing the heart to immediately stop.

Fatigue (n.): The vague feeling of being weak, exhausted, or tired. *Example:* The patient disclosed that her constant fatigue had been present ever since the death of her husband.

Febrile (adj.): A state of high fever. *Example:* Since the child had a febrile response to the medication, the doctor switched to something else and marked the reaction in the patient's chart.

Flexion (n.): The capacity of a limb to flex or bend. *Example:* The flexion of fingers results in a fist.

Flushed (adj.): A redness typically over the cheeks and neck. *Example:* Some people get flushed when embarrassed or nervous.

Gastrointestinal (adj.): Referring to the stomach and intestines. *Example:* The investigation of choice is endoscopy of the upper gastrointestinal tract.

Hematologic (adj.): Relating or referring to blood. *Example:* They were studying hematologic cancers in class that week.

Hydration (n.): The process of introducing additional fluid into the body. *Example:* Hydration is extremely important, especially for athletes who lose a lot of body fluid due to sweat.

Hygiene (n.): The preventative measures taken to maintain health and prevent disease. *Example:* Studies show that students who keep up proper handwashing and nail hygiene prevent the spread of sickness by approximately 20%.

Impaired (adj.): Weakened or damaged; a specific disability. *Example:* The patient explained to the doctor that they were experiencing episodes of impaired vision along with slight nausea and dizziness.

Impending (adj.): Something that is about to happen; forthcoming. *Example:* The doctor was worried about the impending necessity for insulin if the patient didn't change their diet and exercise habits.

Impervious (adj.): Not allowing the passage of any liquids or fluids through. *Example:* This blanket will keep you dry, as it's impervious to water.

Imply (v.): To insinuate or suggest something. *Example:* The patient had a distended area around the stomach and expressed discomfort; it was implied that they had an inguinal hernia.

Incidence (n.): The occurrence of something. *Example:* Incidents of nausea are common after going under general anesthesia.

Infection (n.): When pathogenic organisms such as viruses and bacteria invade the body that normally are not present. *Example:* The patient's infection was prominent because a surface wound wasn't properly treated.

Infer (v.): To make a conclusion based upon facts or events that have previously occurred. *Example:* After the patient disclosed some eating habits, and discomfort in her chest, the doctor was able to infer that the patient was experiencing mild heartburn.

Inflamed (adj.): When a part of the body is swollen or red. *Example:* Due to an allergic reaction, the patient's eyes and face were severely inflamed.

Ingest (v.): To consume, or to put in the body through absorbing or swallowing. *Example:* What you consume affects your body and how you feel throughout the day.

Initiate (v.): The action or processing of beginning something. *Example:* The nurse had to initiate CPR.

Insidious (adj.): Harmful effects, but on a gradual timeline. *Example:* According to studies, most STD's are insidious and often come with little to no symptoms.

Intact (adj.): Undamaged; completely whole. *Example:* Although there was bruising in the ribs, all of them were intact.

Intubate (v.): The act of inserting a tube into a person, usually to help with breathing. *Example:* They decided to intubate the patient after learning that their airway was not working properly.

Invasive (adj.): Something that infiltrates areas of the body. *Example:* Surgery is invasive.

Kinetic (adj.): Referring to motion or movement. *Example:* Some practices use kinetic therapy, which utilizes movement to provide a more holistic form of healing.

Labile (adj.): Changed or altered. *Example:* The man came into the ER with labile behavior and seemed very confused as to who he was.

Laceration (n.): A cut. *Example:* The young patient has a deep laceration because he played with one of the kitchen knives.

Latent (adj.): To be hidden, or lying dormant; concealed. *Example:* Oftentimes, after the initial attack of the virus that causes chicken pox, it will remain latent. Many years later, if it becomes reactivated, it will cause shingles.

Lateral (adj.): From or toward the side. *Example:* The arms are lateral to the torso.

Lethargic (adj.): Characterized by fatigue or sluggishness. *Example:* The patient explained they were feeling lethargic due to the intense lack of sleep and poor diet.

Manifestation (n.): The symptom or appearance of an ailment. *Example:* With the symptoms showing headache, a stiff neck, and a fever, the doctor concluded this was a manifestation of meningitis.

Musculoskeletal (adj.): Involving both the muscular and skeletal parts of the body. *Example:* A treatment for musculoskeletal back pain is a low intensity laser irradiation that is controlled and randomized throughout the needed areas.

Neurologic (adj.): Involving the functions of the nervous system. *Example:* A common neurologic disorder is Alzheimer's Disease.

Neurovascular (adj.): Involving or relating to blood vessels and nerves. *Example:* Migraines are described as a neurovascular condition by headache specialists.

Nutrient (adj.): Essential for the maintenance of life and provides nourishment. *Example:* Having a nutrient-rich diet is important to maintain a healthy body and lifestyle.

Occluded (v.): To obstruct or clog up. *Example:* Nurses must look out for blood clots in patients, since they can occlude the flow of oxygen through the veins.

Ongoing (adj.): Being in progress, continuing. *Example:* Some diseases, like Type I diabetes, are continuous and require ongoing treatment throughout the patient's life.

Oral (adj.): Relating to the mouth. *Example:* Oral hygiene is essential to keeping your gums and teeth healthy.

Otic (adj.): Relating to the ear. *Example:* Oftentimes, otic solutions are prescribed to treat ear infections.

Parameter (n.): A set of factors that are used to measure or express something. *Example:* Certain parameters have been set in place to decrease the spread of sickness in hospitals.

Patent (adj.): Referring to being open. *Example:* Patent surgeries typically have a higher risk because they are more invasive.

Pathogenic (adj.): An organism capable of producing disease. *Example:* Most organisms are harmless and not pathogenic.

Pathology (n.): The study of behaviors and manifestation of a disease. *Example:* She was interested in studying pathology at university.

Posterior (adj.): Situated behind in the body. *Example:* The hamstrings are located on the posterior side of the body.

Potent (adj.): Having a great influence or effect. *Example:* The doctor explained to take the directed amount of dosage since the medication was extremely potent.

Potential (adj.): The capacity or ability to develop something in the future. *Example:* The patient had a high potential to get Type II diabetes due to a poor diet and lack of exercise.

Precaution (n.): A measure taken to prevent a future occurrence. *Example:* Many precautions are taken in an operating room to prevent infection as much as possible.

Precipitous (adj.): Done suddenly or to happen without control. *Example:* The doctor explained that the condition was precipitous and would've been almost impossible to catch early.

Predispose (v.): To be inclined or prone to a specific condition. *Example:* Certain individuals can be predisposed to having heart attacks if it's common in family medical history.

Preexisting (adj.): A condition existing prior to a specific time. *Example:* The condition was preexisting, even though symptoms didn't show for several months after birth.

Primary (adj.): Referring to the first or earliest of something. *Example:* Primary care is the first point of contact between an individual and the healthcare system.

Priority (n.): Being regarded or placed as more important. *Example:* The paramedic's first priority was to make sure the patient didn't have an obstructed airway.

Prognosis (n.): The forecast or course of a disease. *Example:* The family received a good prognosis from the doctor regarding their son's illness.

Rationale (n.): The logical reason for a course of action. *Example:* The rationale for the treatment was based on years of scientific studies.

Recur (v.): Occur again repeatedly. *Example:* After the patient left the hospital, the nurse told him to call back should the rash recur.

Renal (adj.): Involving the kidneys. *Example:* Fatigue, blood in urine, swollen feet, and cramping muscles are symptoms consistent with renal disease.

Residual (n.): A substance or thing that continues or is left over from an event. *Example:* The residual cancer would need to be monitored yearly to avoid a relapse.

Respiration (n.): The act of breathing. *Example:* The patient was given artificial respiration along with cardiopulmonary resuscitation.

Retain (v.): To hold or keep in one place. *Example:* Her team noticed that she began to retain the fluids and her feet began to swell, so they immediately checked her for congestive heart failure.

Status (adj.): The description of an individual's state of being. *Example:* Before transporting the patient to a separate unit, they needed to first check his status.

Subcutaneous (adj.): Applied or lying underneath the skin. *Example:* A subcutaneous injection of insulin was given to the diabetic patient.

Sublingual (adj.): Applied underneath the tongue. *Example:* This is a sublingual medication, so place it in the mouth and let it dissolve underneath the tongue.

Supplement (n.): A substance or thing that adds to something else to make it whole. *Example:* The nurse said a vitamin supplement of B12 is necessary for individuals partaking in a plant-based diet.

Suppress (v.): To lower or inhibit the activity of something. *Example:* Since that medication suppresses the immune system, we suggest the flu vaccination as well as caution among crowded places.

Symmetric (symmetrical) (adj.): Equally distributed parts in relation to a center. *Example:* The attendant looked to see if the limbs were symmetric in order to rule out a fractured hip.

Symptom (n.): A manifestation in the body caused by an underlying illness or disease. *Example:* Her symptoms of headache, fever, and body aches were consistent with symptoms of the flu.

Syndrome (n.): Collective symptoms within a person that indicate a certain condition. *Example:* She was thought to have dry eye syndrome due to her various symptoms of dryness, irritation, and discharge in the eye.

Therapeutic (adj.): Healing, curing, or restorative. *Example:* Our therapeutic interventions include medication along with holistic treatment such as exercise and meditation.

Toxic (adj.): A substance that is poisonous or harmful to the human body. *Example:* A high dose of this medication may be toxic.

Transdermal (adj.): Absorbed through the skin. *Example:* A transdermal patch may be more comfortable for patients who are afraid of an injection.

Transmission (n.): The act of passing a thing from one place to another. *Example:* We'd like to lessen transmission of the virus through resources such as vaccination, hygiene, and public knowledge.

Trauma (n.): An experience that is distressing or damaging to an individual in a physical or emotional way. *Example:* The individual who was brought in from the car accident sustained multiple traumas, especially to the head and chest.

Triage (n.): The assignment of order of treatment determined by severity of trauma or illness. *Example:* I told the pregnant patient to call triage if she had any more concerns with the contractions.

Ubiquitous (adj.): Present or existing everywhere at once. *Example:* Bacteria is considered ubiquitous, as it can thrive anywhere in the human body.

Urinate (v.): Discharge water through the body. *Example:* After the epidural, the patient needed a catheter in order to urinate, since she could not move from the bed.

Vascular (adj.): Relating to blood vessels. *Example:* The vascular system delivers oxygen and nutrients to tissues in the human body.

Virulent (adj.): Extremely harmful or noxious. *Example:* A virulent strain of the virus has been circulating throughout the U.S., wreaking havoc on unprepared communities.

Virus (n.): An infectious microorganism that inhabits and reproduces within a human body, plant, or animal. *Example:* Cases of the flu virus have dwindled this year due to the population wearing masks, sanitizing their hands, and social distancing.

Vital (n): Essential or necessary. *Example:* The pharmacist told her it was vital that she avoid aspirin with her prescription, as the two medications were contraindicated.

Volume (n.): The space that a liquid takes up in a container. *Example:* Her low blood volume indicated that she may have hypovolemia.

If you want to test your knowledge further on the vocabulary section of the HESI exam, take our online practice quiz and the practice quiz on the next page.

testprepbooks.com/hesi-quiz

SCAN ME

Practice Quiz

1. Select the correct meaning of the italicized word in the following sentence:

   The nurse measured her *sublingual* temperature against her axillary temperature.

   a. In the ear
   b. In the rectum
   c. Under the armpit
   d. Under the tongue

2. What is the best definition of the word *dysfunction*?
   a. Exacerbate
   b. Abnormality
   c. Dilate
   d. Lethargic

3. What does *abstain* mean?
   a. To regurgitate
   b. To imbibe
   c. To refrain from something
   d. To prolong

4. Select the correct meaning of the underlined word in the following sentence:

   The surgeon was concerned about the patient's <u>prognosis</u>.

   a. Outlook
   b. Etiology
   c. Mechanism of transmission
   d. Incidence in the population

5. What word meaning "to widen or expand" best fits in the following sentence:

   The nitrous oxide was administered to _____ his blood vessels.

   a. Dilute
   b. Dilate
   c. Occlude
   d. Distill

See answers on next page.

Answer Explanations

1. D: The correct answer Choice is *D*, under the tongue. The root word of *sublingual* is *lingual,* which means *tongue*. The prefix is *sub*, which means *under*. Therefore, if we pay attention the prefix and how it relates to the root word, we get *under the tongue*. Choice *A, in the ear*, would be the word *tympanic*. Choice *B*, in the rectum, would be the word *rectal.* Choice *C*, under the armpit, would be the word *axillary*.

2. B: In the word *dysfunction*, we have the root word *function* and the prefix *dys*. *Function* means to work or operate in a particular way. The prefix *dys* denotes *bad* or *difficult*. Therefore, the word *dysfunction* would mean functioning with difficulty; the word closest to this is *abnormality*, which means the quality or state of being abnormal or defected, which is Choice *B*. Choice *A, exacerbate*, means something that becomes more intense in nature. Choice *C, dilate*, means to enlarge or extend. Choice *D, lethargic*, means sluggish or apathetic.

3. C: To refrain from something. For example, someone who chooses to *abstain* from alcohol does not drink alcohol.

4. A: Outlook. The *prognosis* is the expected likely course of an illness or injury.

5. B: Dilate. To *dilute* is to make a solution less concentrated, *occlude* means to block or obstruct, and *distill* means to purify a liquid or to extract the most important aspects or meaning of something.

Grammar

Why is grammar important? Why should we study, teach, and use proper grammar? The English language, a uniquely human achievement, deserves our consideration and examination. Language is arguably the most important tool we have for creating an impact on the world around us. Without proper grammar, language loses its efficacy for communicating well with others. Reading, writing, listening, and speaking all have a greater effect when grammar is used proficiently.

Let's begin with the basic conventions, or the **eight parts of speech**: nouns, adjectives, adverbs, pronouns, prepositions, interjections, verbs, and conjunctions.

Parts of Speech

Nouns

A **common noun** is a word that identifies any of a class of people, places, or things. Examples include numbers, objects, animals, feelings, concepts, qualities, and actions. *A, an,* or *the* usually precedes the common noun. These parts of speech are called *articles*. Here are some examples of sentences using nouns preceded by articles.

> *A* building is under construction.

> *The* girl would like to move to *the* city.

An **abstract noun** is an idea, state, or quality. It is something that can't be touched, such as happiness, courage, evil, or humor.

A **proper noun** (also called a **proper name**) is used for the specific name of an individual person, place, or organization. The first letter in a proper noun is capitalized. "My name is *Mary*." "I work for *Walmart*."

Nouns sometimes serve as adjectives (which themselves describe nouns), such as "hockey player" and "state government."

Pronouns

A word used in place of a noun is known as a **pronoun**. Pronouns are words like *I, mine, hers,* and *us.*

72

Pronouns can be split into different classifications (as shown below) which make them easier to learn; however, it's not important to memorize the classifications.

- **Personal pronouns:** refer to people

- **First person pronouns:** we, I, our, mine

- **Second person pronouns:** you, yours

- **Third person pronouns:** he, she, they, them, it

- **Possessive pronouns:** demonstrate ownership (mine, my, his, yours)

- **Interrogative pronouns:** ask questions (what, which, who, whom, whose)

- **Relative pronouns:** include the five interrogative pronouns and others that are relative (whoever, whomever, that, when, where)

- **Demonstrative pronouns:** replace something specific (this, that, those, these)

- **Reciprocal pronouns:** indicate something was done or given in return (each other, one another)

- **Indefinite pronouns:** have a nonspecific status (anybody, whoever, someone, everybody, somebody)

Indefinite pronouns such as *anybody, whoever, someone, everybody*, and *somebody* command a singular verb form, but others such as *all, none,* and *some* could require a singular or plural verb form.

Antecedents

An **antecedent** is the noun to which a pronoun refers; it needs to be written or spoken before the pronoun is used. For many pronouns, antecedents are imperative for clarity. In particular, a lot of the personal, possessive, and demonstrative pronouns need antecedents. Otherwise, it would be unclear who or what someone is referring to when they use a pronoun like *he* or *this*.

Pronoun reference means that the pronoun should refer clearly to one, clear, unmistakable noun (the antecedent).

Pronoun-antecedent agreement refers to the need for the antecedent and the corresponding pronoun to agree in gender, person, and number. Here are some examples:

The *kidneys* (plural antecedent) are part of the urinary system. *They* (plural pronoun) serve several roles.

The kidneys are part of the *urinary system* (singular antecedent). *It* (singular pronoun) is also known as the renal system.

Pronoun Cases

The **subjective pronouns** —*I, you, he/she/it, we, they,* and *who*—are the subjects of the sentence.

Example: *They* have a new house.

The **objective pronouns**—*me, you* (*singular*), *him/her, us, them,* and *whom*—are used when something is being done for or given to someone; they are objects of the action.

> Example: The teacher has an apple for *us*.

The **possessive pronouns**—*mine, my, your, yours, his, hers, its, their, theirs, our,* and *ours*—are used to denote that something (or someone) belongs to someone (or something).

> Example: It's *their* chocolate cake.

> Even Better Example: It's *my* chocolate cake!

One of the greatest challenges and worst abuses of pronouns concerns *who* and *whom*. Just knowing the following rule can eliminate confusion. *Who* is a subjective-case pronoun used only as a subject or subject complement. *Whom* is only objective-case and, therefore, the object of the verb or preposition.

> *Who* is going to the concert?

> You are going to the concert with *whom*?

Hint: When using *who* or *whom*, think of whether someone would say *he* or *him*. If the answer is *he*, use *who*. If the answer is *him*, use *whom*. This trick is easy to remember because *he* and *who* both end in vowels, and *him* and *whom* both end in the letter *M*.

Many possessive pronouns sound like contractions. For example, many people get *it's* and *its* confused. The word *it's* is the contraction for *it is*. The word *its* without an apostrophe is the possessive form of *it*.

> I love that wooden desk. It's beautiful. (contraction)

> I love that wooden desk. Its glossy finish is beautiful. (possessive)

If you are not sure which version to use, replace *it's/its* with *it is* and see if that sounds correct. If so, use the contraction (*it's*). That trick also works for *who's/whose, you're/your,* and *they're/their*.

Adjectives

"The *extraordinary* brain is the *main* organ of the central nervous system." The adjective *extraordinary* describes the brain in a way that causes one to realize it is more exceptional than some of the other organs while the adjective *main* defines the brain's importance in its system.

An **adjective** is a word or phrase that names an attribute that describes or clarifies a noun or pronoun. This helps the reader visualize and understand the characteristics—size, shape, age, color, origin, etc.—of a person, place, or thing that otherwise might not be known. Adjectives breathe life, color, and depth into the subjects they define. Life would be *drab* and *colorless* without adjectives!

Adjectives often precede the nouns they describe.

> *She drove her <u>new</u> car.*

However, adjectives can also come later in the sentence.

This material is provided for exam preparation purposes only and does not indicate an endorsement of any specific scientific, political, or religious point of view. © TPB Publishing. You have been licensed one copy of this document for personal use only. Any other reproduction or redistribution is strictly prohibited. All rights reserved.

Her car is <u>new</u>.

Adjectives using the prefix *a–* can only be used after a verb.

Correct: The dog was alive until the car ran up on the curb and hit him.

Incorrect: The alive dog was hit by a car that ran up on the curb.

Other examples of this rule include *awake, ablaze, ajar, alike,* and *asleep.*

Other adjectives used after verbs concern states of health.

The girl was finally *well* after a long bout of pneumonia.

The boy was *fine* after the accident.

An adjective phrase is not a bunch of adjectives strung together, but a group of words that describes a noun or pronoun and, thus, functions as an adjective. Very happy is an adjective phrase; so are way too hungry and passionate about traveling.

Possessives

In grammar, *possessive nouns* show ownership, which was seen in previous examples like *mine, yours,* and *theirs.*

Singular nouns are generally made possessive with an apostrophe and an *s* (*'s*).

My *uncle's* new car is silver.

The *dog's* bowl is empty.

James's ties are becoming outdated.

Plural nouns ending in *s* are generally made possessive by just adding an apostrophe (*'*):

The pistachio nuts' saltiness is added during roasting. (The saltiness of pistachio nuts is added during roasting.)

The students' achievement tests are difficult. (The achievement tests of the students are difficult.)

If the plural noun does not end in an *s* such as *women,* then it is made possessive by adding an *apostrophe s* (*'s*)—*women's.*

Indefinite possessive pronouns such as *nobody* or *someone* become possessive by adding an *apostrophe s*— *nobody's* or *someone's.*

Verbs

A **verb** is the part of speech that describes an action, state of being, or occurrence.

75

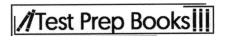

A verb forms the main part of a predicate of a sentence. This means that the verb explains what the noun (which will be discussed shortly) is doing. A simple example is *time flies*. The verb *flies* explains what the action of the noun, *time*, is doing. This example is a *main* verb.

Helping (auxiliary) verbs are words like *have, do, be, can, may, should, must,* and *will.* "I *should* go to the store." Helping verbs assist main verbs in expressing tense, ability, possibility, permission, or obligation.

Particles are minor function words like *not, in, out, up,* or *down* that become part of the verb itself. "I might *not*."

Participles are words formed from verbs that are often used to modify a noun, noun phrase, verb, or verb phrase.

> The *running* teenager collided with the cyclist.

Participles can also create compound verb forms.

> He is *speaking*.

Participial phrases are made up of the participle and modifiers, complements, or objects.

> *Crying for most of an hour*, the baby didn't seem to want to nap.

> *Having already taken this course*, the student was bored during class.

Verbs have five basic forms: the **base** form, the **-s** form, the **-ing** form, the **past** form, and the **past participle** form.

The past forms are either **regular** (*love/loved; hate/hated*) or **irregular** because they don't end by adding the common past tense suffix "-ed" (*go/went; fall/fell; set/set*).

Adverbs

Adverbs have more functions than adjectives because they modify or qualify verbs, adjectives, or other adverbs as well as word groups that express a relation of place, time, circumstance, or cause. Therefore, adverbs answer any of the following questions: *How, when, where, why, in what way, how often, how much, in what condition,* and/or *to what degree. How good looking is he? He is very handsome.*

Here are some examples of adverbs for different situations:

- how: quickly
- when: daily
- where: there
- in what way: easily
- how often: often
- how much: much
- in what condition: badly
- what degree: hardly

As one can see, for some reason, many adverbs end in *-ly*.

76

Adverbs do things like emphasize (*really, simply,* and *so*), amplify (*heartily, completely,* and *positively*), and tone down (*almost, somewhat,* and *mildly*).

Adverbs also come in phrases.

The dog ran as <u>though his life depended on it.</u>

Prepositions

Prepositions are connecting words and, while there are only about 150 of them, they are used more often than any other individual groups of words. They describe relationships between other words. They are placed before a noun or pronoun, forming a phrase that modifies another word in the sentence. **Prepositional phrases** begin with a preposition and end with a noun or pronoun, the **object of the preposition.** *A pristine lake is <u>near the store</u> and <u>behind the bank.</u>*

Some commonly used prepositions are *about, after, anti, around, as, at, behind, beside, by, for, from, in, into, of, off, on, to,* and *with.*

Complex prepositions, which also come before a noun or pronoun, consist of two or three words such as *according to, in regards to,* and *because of.*

Interjections

Interjections are words used to express emotion. Examples include *wow, ouch,* and *hooray.* Interjections are often separate from sentences; in those cases, the interjection is directly followed by an exclamation point. In other cases, the interjection is included in a sentence and followed by a comma. The punctuation plays a big role in the intensity of the emotion that the interjection is expressing. Using a comma or semicolon indicates less excitement than using an exclamation mark.

Conjunctions

Conjunctions are vital words that connect words, phrases, thoughts, and ideas. Conjunctions show relationships between components. There are two types:

Coordinating conjunctions are the primary class of conjunctions placed between words, phrases, clauses, and sentences that are of equal grammatical rank; the coordinating conjunctions are *for, and, nor, but, or, yet,* and *so.* A useful memorization trick is to remember that all the first letters of these conjunctions collectively spell the word fanboys.

I need to go shopping, *but* I must be careful to leave enough money in the bank.

She wore a black, red, *and* white shirt.

Subordinating conjunctions are the secondary class of conjunctions. They connect two unequal parts, one **main** (or **independent**) and the other **subordinate** (or **dependent**). I must go to the store *even though* I do not have enough money in the bank.

Because I read the review, I do not want to go to the movie.

Notice that the presence of subordinating conjunctions makes clauses dependent. *I read the review* is an independent clause, but *because* makes the clause dependent. Thus, it needs an independent clause to complete the sentence.

Sentences

First, let's review the basic elements of sentences.

A **sentence** is a set of words that make up a grammatical unit. The words must have certain elements and be spoken or written in a specific order to constitute a complete sentence that makes sense.

> 1. A sentence must have a **subject** (a noun or noun phrase). The subject tells whom or what the sentence is addressing (i.e., what it is about).

> 2. A sentence must have an **action** or **state of being** (*a* verb). To reiterate: A verb forms the main part of the predicate of a sentence. This means that it explains what the noun is doing.

> 3. A sentence must convey a complete thought.

When examining writing, be mindful of grammar, structure, spelling, and patterns. Sentences can come in varying sizes and shapes; so, the point of grammatical correctness is not to stamp out creativity or diversity in writing. Rather, grammatical correctness ensures that writing will be enjoyable and clear. One of the most common methods for catching errors is to mouth the words as you read them. Many typos are fixed automatically by our brain, but mouthing the words often circumvents this instinct and helps one read what's actually on the page. Often, grammar errors are caught not by memorization of grammar rules but by the training of one's mind to know whether something *sounds* right or not.

Types of Sentences

There isn't an overabundance of absolutes in grammar, but here is one: every sentence in the English language falls into one of four categories.

- Declarative: a simple statement that ends with a period

    The price of milk per gallon is the same as the price of gasoline.

- Imperative: a command, instruction, or request that ends with a period

    Buy milk when you stop to fill up your car with gas.

- Interrogative: a question that ends with a question mark

    Will you buy the milk?

- Exclamatory: a statement or command that expresses emotions like anger, urgency, or surprise and ends with an exclamation mark

    Buy the milk now!

Declarative sentences are the most common type, probably because they are comprised of the most general content, without any of the bells and whistles that the other three types contain. They are, simply, declarations or statements of any degree of seriousness, importance, or information.

Imperative sentences often seem to be missing a subject. The subject is there, though; it is just not visible or audible because it is *implied*. Look at the imperative example sentence.

> Buy the milk when you fill up your car with gas.

You is the implied subject, the one to whom the command is issued. This is sometimes called *the understood you* because it is understood that *you* is the subject of the sentence.

Interrogative sentences—those that ask questions—are defined as such from the idea of the word *interrogation*, the action of questions being asked of suspects by investigators. Although that is serious business, interrogative sentences apply to all kinds of questions.

To exclaim is at the root of **exclamatory sentences**. These are made with strong emotions behind them. The only technical difference between a declarative or imperative sentence and an exclamatory one is the exclamation mark at the end. The example declarative and imperative sentences can both become an exclamatory one simply by putting an exclamation mark at the end of the sentences.

> The price of milk per gallon is the same as the price of gasoline!
> Buy milk when you stop to fill up your car with gas!

After all, someone might be really excited by the price of gas or milk, or they could be mad at the person that will be buying the milk! However, as stated before, exclamation marks in abundance defeat their own purpose! After a while, they begin to cause fatigue! When used only for their intended purpose, they can have their expected and desired effect.

Independent and Dependent Clauses

Independent and dependent clauses are strings of words that contain both a subject and a verb. An **independent clause** *can* stand alone as complete thought, but a **dependent clause** *cannot*. A dependent clause relies on other words to be a complete sentence.

> Independent clause: The keys are on the counter.
> Dependent clause: If the keys are on the counter

Notice that both clauses have a subject (*keys*) and a verb (*are*). The independent clause expresses a complete thought, but the word *if* at the beginning of the dependent clause makes it *dependent* on other words to be a complete thought.

> Independent clause: If the keys are on the counter, please give them to me.

This example constitutes a complete sentence since it includes at least one verb and one subject and is a complete thought. In this case, the independent clause has two subjects (*keys* & an implied *you*) and two verbs (*are* & *give*).

> Independent clause: I went to the store.
> Dependent clause: Because we are out of milk,

Complete Sentence: Because we are out of milk, I went to the store.

Complete Sentence: I went to the store because we are out of milk.

Sentence Structures

A **simple sentence** has one independent clause.

I am going to win.

A **compound sentence** has two independent clauses. A comma and a conjunction—*for, and, nor, but, or, yet, so*—links them together. Note that each of the independent clauses has a subject and a verb.

I am going to win, but the odds are against me.

A **complex sentence** has one independent clause and one or more dependent clauses.

I am going to win, even though I don't deserve it.

Even though I don't deserve it is a dependent clause. It does not stand on its own. Some conjunctions that link an independent and a dependent clause are *although, because, before, after, that, when, which,* and *while.*

A **compound-complex sentence** has at least three clauses, two of which are independent and at least one that is a dependent clause.

While trying to dance, I tripped over my partner's feet, but I regained my balance quickly.

The dependent clause is *While trying to dance.*

Run-Ons and Fragments

Run-Ons

A common mistake in writing is the run-on sentence. A **run-on** is created when two or more independent clauses are joined without the use of a conjunction, a semicolon, a colon, or a dash. We don't want to use commas where periods belong. Here is an example of a run-on sentence:

Making wedding cakes can take many hours I am very impatient, I want to see them completed right away.

There are a variety of ways to correct a run-on sentence. The method you choose will depend on the context of the sentence and how it fits with neighboring sentences:

Making wedding cakes can take many hours. I am very impatient. I want to see them completed right away. (Use periods to create more than one sentence.)

Making wedding cakes can take many hours; I am very impatient—I want to see them completed right away. (Correct the sentence using a semicolon, colon, or dash.)

Making wedding cakes can take many hours, and I am very impatient and want to see them completed right away. (Correct the sentence using coordinating conjunctions.)

80

I am very impatient because I would rather see completed wedding cakes right away than wait for it to take many hours. (Correct the sentence by revising.)

Fragments

Remember that a complete sentence must have both a subject and a verb. Complete sentences consist of at least one independent clause. Incomplete sentences are called **sentence fragments**. A sentence fragment is a common error in writing. Sentence fragments can be independent clauses that start with subordinating words, such as *but, as, so that,* or *because,* or they could simply be missing a subject or verb.

You can correct a fragment error by adding the fragment to a nearby sentence or by adding or removing words to make it an independent clause. For example:

Dogs are my favorite animals. Because cats are too lazy. (Incorrect; the word because creates a sentence fragment)

Dogs are my favorite animals because cats are too lazy. (Correct; this is a dependent clause.)

Dogs are my favorite animals. Cats are too lazy. (Correct; this is a simple sentence.)

Subject and Predicate

Every complete sentence can be divided into two parts: the subject and the predicate.

Subjects: We need to have subjects in our sentences to tell us who or what the sentence describes. Subjects can be simple or complete, and they can be direct or indirect. There can also be compound subjects.

Simple subjects are the noun or nouns the sentence describes, without modifiers. The simple subject can come before or after the verb in the sentence:

The big brown <u>dog</u> is the calmest one.

Complete subjects are the subject together with all of its describing words or modifiers.

The <u>big brown dog</u> is the calmest one. (The complete subject is big brown dog.)

Direct subjects are subjects that appear in the text of the sentence, as in the example above. **Indirect subjects** are implied. The subject is "you," but the word *you* does not appear.

Indirect subjects are usually in imperative sentences that issue a command or order:

Feed the short skinny dog first. (The understood you is the subject.)

Watch out—he's really hungry! (The sentence warns you to watch out.)

Compound subjects occur when two or more nouns join together to form a plural subject.

<u>Carson</u> and <u>Emily</u> make a great couple.

Predicates: Once we have identified the subject of the sentence, the rest of the sentence becomes the predicate. Predicates are formed by the verb, the direct object, and all words related to it.

We <u>went to see the Cirque du' Soleil performance</u>.

The gigantic green character <u>was funnier than all the rest</u>.

A **predicate nominative** renames the subject:

John is a <u>carpenter</u>.

A **predicate adjective** describes the subject:

Margaret is <u>beautiful</u>.

Direct objects are the nouns in the sentence that are receiving the action. Sentences don't necessarily need objects. Sentences only need a subject and a verb.

The clown brought the acrobat the <u>hula-hoop</u>. (What is getting brought? the hula-hoop)

Then he gave the trick pony a <u>soapy bath</u>. (What is being given? (a soapy bath)

Indirect objects are words that tell us to or for whom or what the action is being done. For there to be an indirect object, there first must always be a direct object.

The clown brought <u>the acrobat</u> the hula-hoop. (Who is getting the direct object? the hula-hoop)

Then he gave <u>the trick pony</u> a soapy bath. (What is getting the bath? a trick pony)

Phrases

A **phrase** is a group of words that go together but do not include both a subject and a verb. We use them to add information, explain something, or make the sentence easier for the reader to understand. Unlike clauses, phrases can never stand alone as their own sentence. They do not form complete thoughts. There are noun phrases, prepositional phrases, verbal phrases, appositive phrases, and absolute phrases. Here are some examples of phrases:

I know <u>all the shortest routes</u>.

<u>Before the sequel</u>, we wanted to watch the first movie. (introductory phrase)

The jumpers have hot cocoa <u>to drink right away</u>.

Subject-Verb Agreement

The subject of a sentence and its verb must agree. The cornerstone rule of subject-verb agreement is that subject and verb must agree in number. Whether the subject is singular or plural, the verb must follow suit.

> Incorrect: The houses is new.
>
> Correct: The houses are new.
>
> Also Correct: The house is new.

In other words, a singular subject requires a singular verb; a plural subject requires a plural verb.

The words or phrases that come between the subject and verb do not alter this rule.

> Incorrect: The houses built of brick is new.
>
> Correct: The houses built of brick are new.
>
> Incorrect: The houses with the sturdy porches is new.
>
> Correct: The houses with the sturdy porches are new.

The subject will always follow the verb when a sentence begins with *here* or *there.* Identify these with care.

> Incorrect: Here *is* the *houses* with sturdy porches.
>
> Correct: Here *are* the *houses* with sturdy porches.

The subject in the sentences above is not *here,* it is *houses.* Remember, *here* and *there* are never subjects. Be careful that contractions such as *here's* or *there're* do not cause confusion!

Two subjects joined by *and* require a plural verb form, except when the two combine to make one thing:

> Incorrect: Garrett and Jonathan is over there.
>
> Correct: Garrett and Jonathan are over there.
>
> Incorrect: Spaghetti and meatballs are a delicious meal!
>
> Correct: Spaghetti and meatballs is a delicious meal!

In the example above, *spaghetti and meatballs* is a compound noun. However, *Garrett and Jonathan* is not a compound noun.

Two singular subjects joined by *or, either/or,* or *neither/nor* call for a singular verb form.

> Incorrect: Butter or syrup are acceptable.
>
> Correct: Butter or syrup is acceptable.

83

Plural subjects joined by *or*, *either/or*, or *neither/nor* are, indeed, plural.

The chairs or the boxes are being moved next.

If one subject is singular and the other is plural, the verb should agree with the closest noun.

Correct: The chair or the boxes are being moved next.

Correct: The chairs or the box is being moved next.

Some plurals of money, distance, and time call for a singular verb.

Incorrect: Three dollars *are* enough to buy that.

Correct: Three dollars *is* enough to buy that.

For words declaring degrees of quantity such as *many of, some of,* or *most of,* let the noun that follows *of* be the guide:

Incorrect: Many of the books is in the shelf.

Correct: Many of the books are in the shelf.

Incorrect: Most of the pie *are* on the table.

Correct: Most of the pie *is* on the table.

For indefinite pronouns like anybody or everybody, use singular verbs.

Everybody *is* going to the store.

However, the pronouns *few, many, several, all, some,* and *both* have their own rules and use plural forms.

Some *are* ready.

Some nouns like *crowd* and *congress* are called *collective nouns* and they require a singular verb form.

Congress *is* in session.

The news *is* over.

Books and movie titles, though, including plural nouns such as *Great Expectations*, also require a singular verb. Remember that only the subject affects the verb. While writing tricky subject-verb arrangements, say them aloud. Listen to them. Once the rules have been learned, one's ear will become sensitive to them, making it easier to pick out what's right and what's wrong.

Dangling and Misplaced Modifiers

A **modifier** is a word or phrase meant to describe or clarify another word in the sentence. When a sentence has a modifier but is missing the word it describes or clarifies, it's an error called a **dangling modifier**. We can fix the sentence by revising to include the word that is being modified.

84

Consider the following examples with the modifier underlined:

Incorrect: <u>Having walked five miles</u>, this bench will be the place to rest. (This implies that the bench walked the miles, not the person.)

Correct: <u>Having walked five miles</u>, Matt will rest on this bench. (*Having walked five miles* correctly modifies *Matt*, who did the walking.)

Incorrect: <u>Since midnight</u>, my dreams have been pleasant and comforting. (The adverb clause *since midnight* cannot modify the noun *dreams*.)

Correct: <u>Since midnight</u>, I have had pleasant and comforting dreams. (*Since midnight* modifies the verb have had, telling us when the dreams occurred.)

Sometimes the modifier is not located close enough to the word it modifies for the sentence to be clearly understood. In this case, we call the error a **misplaced modifier**. Here is an example with the modifier underlined.

Incorrect: We gave the hot cocoa to the children <u>that was filled with marshmallows</u>. (This sentence implies that the children are what are filled with marshmallows.)

Correct: We gave the hot cocoa <u>that was filled with marshmallows</u> to the children. (The cocoa is filled with marshmallows. The modifier is near the word it modifies.)

Parallel Structure in a Sentence

Parallel structure, also known as **parallelism**, refers to using the same grammatical form within a sentence. This is important in lists and for other components of sentences.

Incorrect: At the recital, the boys and girls were dancing, singing, and played musical instruments.
Correct: At the recital, the boys and girls were dancing, singing, and playing musical instruments.

Notice that in the second example, *played* is not in the same verb tense as the other verbs, nor is it compatible with the helping verb *were*. To test for parallel structure in lists, try reading each item as if it were the only item in the list.

The boys and girls were dancing.
The boys and girls were singing.
The boys and girls were played musical instruments.

85

Suddenly, the error in the sentence becomes very clear. Here's another example:

Incorrect: After the accident, I informed the police *that Mrs. Holmes backed* into my car, *that Mrs. Holmes got out* of her car to look at the damage, and *she was driving* off without leaving a note.

Correct: After the accident, I informed the police *that Mrs. Holmes backed* into my car, *that Mrs. Holmes got out* of her car to look at the damage, and *that Mrs. Holmes drove off* without leaving a note.

Correct: After the accident, I informed the police that Mrs. Holmes *backed* into my car, *got out* of her car to look at the damage, and *drove off* without leaving a note.

Note that there are two ways to fix the nonparallel structure of the first sentence. The key to parallelism is consistent structure.

Punctuation

Commas

A **comma** (,) is the punctuation mark that signifies a pause—breath—between parts of a sentence. It denotes a break of flow. As with so many aspects of writing structure, authors will benefit by reading their writing aloud or mouthing the words. This can be particularly helpful if one is uncertain about whether the comma is needed.

In a complex sentence—one that contains a subordinate (dependent) clause or clauses—the use of a comma is dictated by where the subordinate clause is located. If the subordinate clause is located before the main clause, a comma is needed between the two clauses.

I will not pay for the steak, *because I don't have that much money.*

Generally, if the subordinate clause is placed after the main clause, no punctuation is needed. I did well on my exam because I studied two hours the night before. Notice how the last clause is dependent because it requires the earlier independent clauses to make sense.

Use a comma on both sides of an interrupting phrase.

I will pay for the ice cream, chocolate and vanilla, and then will eat it all myself.

The words forming the phrase in italics are nonessential (extra) information. To determine if a phrase is nonessential, try reading the sentence without the phrase and see if it's still coherent.

A comma is not necessary in this next sentence because no interruption—nonessential or extra information—has occurred. Read sentences aloud when uncertain.

I will pay for his chocolate and vanilla ice cream and then will eat it all myself.

If the nonessential phrase comes at the beginning of a sentence, a comma should only go at the end of the phrase. If the phrase comes at the end of a sentence, a comma should only go at the beginning of the phrase.

Other types of interruptions include the following:

- interjections: Oh no, I am not going.
- abbreviations: Barry Potter, M.D., specializes in heart disorders.
- direct addresses: Yes, Claudia, I am tired and going to bed.
- parenthetical phrases: His wife, lovely as she was, was not helpful.
- transitional phrases: Also, it is not possible.

The second comma in the following sentence is called an Oxford comma.

> I will pay for ice cream, syrup, and pop.

It is a comma used after the second-to-last item in a series of three or more items. It comes before the word *or* or *and*. Not everyone uses the Oxford comma; it is optional, but many believe it is needed. The comma functions as a tool to reduce confusion in writing. So, if omitting the Oxford comma would cause confusion, then it's best to include it.

Commas are used in math to mark the place of thousands in numerals, breaking them up so they are easier to read. Other uses for commas are in dates (*March 19, 2016*), letter greetings (*Dear Sally,*), and in between cities and states (*Louisville, KY*).

Apostrophes

This punctuation mark, the apostrophe ('), is a versatile little mark. It has a few different functions:

- Quotes: Apostrophes are used when a second quote is needed within a quote.

- In my letter to my friend, I wrote, "The girl had to get a new purse, and guess what Mary did? She said, 'I'd like to go with you to the store.' I knew Mary would buy it for her."

- Contractions: Another use for an apostrophe in the quote above is a contraction. *I'd* is used for *I would*.

  The basic rule for making *contractions* is one area of spelling that is pretty straightforward: combine the two words by inserting an apostrophe (') in the space where a letter is omitted. For example, to combine *you* and *are*, drop the *a* and put the apostrophe in its place: *you're*.

    he+is=he's

    you+all=y'all (informal but often misspelled)

- Possession: An apostrophe followed by the letter *s* shows possession (*Mary's* purse). If the possessive word is plural, the apostrophe generally just follows the word.

- The trees' leaves are all over the ground.

Ellipses

An **ellipsis** (...) consists of three handy little dots that can speak volumes on behalf of irrelevant material. Writers use them in place of words, lines, phrases, list content, or paragraphs that might just as easily

87

have been omitted from a passage of writing. This can be done to save space or to focus only on the specifically relevant material.

> Exercise is good for some unexpected reasons. Watkins writes, "Exercise has many benefits such as...reducing cancer risk."

In the example above, the ellipsis takes the place of the other benefits of exercise that are more expected.

The ellipsis may also be used to show a pause in sentence flow.

> "I'm wondering...how this could happen," Dylan said in a soft voice.

Semicolons

The **semicolon** (;) might be described as a heavy-handed comma. Take a look at these two examples:

> I will pay for the ice cream, but I will not pay for the steak.
> I will pay for the ice cream; I will not pay for the steak.

What's the difference? The first example has a comma and a conjunction separating the two independent clauses. The second example does not have a conjunction, but there are two independent clauses in the sentence, so something more than a comma is required. In this case, a semicolon is used.

Two independent clauses can only be joined in a sentence by either a comma and conjunction or a semicolon. If one of those tools is not used, the sentence will be a run-on. Remember that while the clauses are independent, they need to be closely related in order to be contained in one sentence.

Another use for the semicolon is to separate items in a list when the items themselves require commas.

> The family lived in Phoenix, Arizona; Oklahoma City, Oklahoma; and Raleigh, North Carolina.

Colons

Colons (:) have many miscellaneous functions. Colons can be used to proceed further information or a list. In these cases, a colon should only follow an independent clause.

> Humans take in sensory information through five basic senses: sight, hearing, smell, touch, and taste.

The meal includes the following components:

- Caesar salad
- spaghetti
- garlic bread
- cake

The family got what they needed: a reliable vehicle.

While a comma is more common, a colon can also proceed a formal quotation.

He said to the crowd: "Let's begin!"

The colon is used after the greeting in a formal letter.

> Dear Sir:
> To Whom It May Concern:

In the writing of time, the colon separates the minutes from the hour (*4:45 p.m.*). The colon can also be used to indicate a ratio between two numbers (*50:1*).

Hyphens

The **hyphen** (-) is a little hash mark that can be used to join words to show that they are linked.

Hyphenate two words that work together as a single adjective (a compound adjective).

> honey-covered biscuits

Some words always require hyphens, even if not serving as an adjective.

> merry-go-round

Hyphens always go after certain prefixes like *anti-* & *all-*.

Hyphens should also be used when the absence of the hyphen would cause a strange vowel combination (*semi-engineer*) or confusion. For example, *re-collect* should be used to describe something being gathered twice rather than being written as *recollect*, which means to remember.

Parentheses and Dashes

Parentheses are half-round brackets that look like this: ( ). They set off a word, phrase, or sentence that is an afterthought, explanation, or side note relevant to the surrounding text but not essential. A pair of commas is often used to set off this sort of information, but parentheses are generally used for information that would not fit well within a sentence or that the writer deems not important enough to be structurally part of the sentence.

> The picture of the heart (see above) shows the major parts you should memorize.
> Mount Everest is one of three mountains in the world that are over 28,000 feet high (K2 and Kanchenjunga are the other two).

See how the sentences above are complete without the parenthetical statements? In the first example, *see above* would not have fit well within the flow of the sentence. The second parenthetical statement could have been a separate sentence, but the writer deemed the information not pertinent to the topic.

The **em-dash** (—) is a mark longer than a hyphen used as a punctuation mark in sentences and to set apart a relevant thought. Even after plucking out the line separated by the dash marks, the sentence will be intact and make sense.

> Looking out the airplane window at the landmarks—Lake Clarke, Thompson Community College, and the bridge—she couldn't help but feel excited to be home.

The dashes use is similar to that of parentheses or a pair of commas. So, what's the difference? Many believe that using dashes makes the clause within them stand out while using parentheses is subtler. It's advised to not use dashes when commas could be used instead.

Quotation Marks

Here are some instances where *quotation marks* should be used:

- Dialogue for characters in narratives. When characters speak, the first word should always be capitalized and the punctuation goes inside the quotes. For example:

    Janie said, "The tree fell on my car during the hurricane."

- Around titles of songs, short stories, essays, and chapters in books
- To emphasize a certain word
- To refer to a word as the word itself

Capitalization

Here's a non-exhaustive list of things that should be capitalized.

- The first word of every sentence
- The first word of every line of poetry
- The first letter of proper nouns (World War II)
- Holidays (Valentine's Day)
- The days of the week and months of the year (Tuesday, March)
- The first word, last word, and all major words in the titles of books, movies, songs, and other creative works (In the novel, *To Kill a Mockingbird*, note that *a* is lowercase since it's not a major word, but *to* is capitalized since it's the first word of the title.)
- Titles when preceding a proper noun (President Roberto Gonzales, Aunt Judy)

When simply using a word such as president or secretary, though, the word is not capitalized.

    Officers of the new business must include a *president* and *treasurer*.

Seasons—spring, fall, etc.—are not capitalized.

North, *south*, *east*, and *west* are capitalized when referring to regions but are not when being used for directions. In general, if it's preceded by *the* it should be capitalized.

    I'm from the South.
    I drove south.

Writing Tips

Conciseness

Unfortunately, writers often include extra words and phrases that seem necessary at the time but add nothing to the main idea. This confuses the reader and creates unnecessary repetition. Writing that lacks conciseness is usually guilty of excessive wordiness and redundant phrases.

Here's an example containing both of these issues:

> When legislators decided to begin creating legislation making it mandatory for automobile drivers and passengers to make use of seat belts while in cars, a large number of them made those laws for reasons that were political reasons.

There are several empty or "luff words here that take up too much space. These can be eliminated while still maintaining the writer's meaning. For example:

- "Decided to begin" could be shortened to "began"
- "Making it mandatory for" could be shortened to "requiring"
- "Make use of" could be shortened to "use"
- "A large number" could be shortened to "many"

In addition, there are several examples of redundancy that can be eliminated:

- "Legislators decided to begin creating legislation" and "made those laws"
- "Automobile drivers and passengers" and "while in cars"
- "Reasons that were political reasons"

These changes are incorporated as follows:

> When legislators began requiring drivers and passengers to use seat belts, many of them did so for political reasons.

Euphemisms
Eliminating **euphemisms** can be helpful in writing more concisely. Euphemisms are terms or phrases used to say something indirectly. Often times it's to soften an expression, be polite, or in some cases to be impolite.

Normal expression: He is very short.

Euphemism: He is vertically challenged.

Clichés
A **cliché** is an old, often-used phrase that has lost all originality or humor due to it's overuse. These idioms are all *clichés*:

A penny for your thoughts

Head over heels in love

91

Give your two cents

It's best to avoid clichés since they are overused and because their elimination can help you be more concise.

Distinguishing Between Formal and Informal Language

It can be helpful to distinguish whether a writer or speaker is using formal or informal language because it can give the reader or listener clues to whether the text is informative, nonfiction, argumentative, or the intended tone or audience. Formal and informal language in written or verbal communication serve different purposes and are often intended for different audiences. Consequently, their tone, word choices, and grammatical structures vary. These differences can be used to identify which form of language is used in a given piece and to determine which type of language should be used for a certain context. Understanding the differences between formal and informal language will also allow a writer or speaker to implement the most appropriate and effective style for a given situation.

Formal language is less personal and more informative and pragmatic than informal language. It is more "buttoned-up" and business-like, adhering to proper grammatical rules. It is used in professional or academic contexts, to convey respect or authority. For example, one would use formal language to write an informative or argumentative essay for school and to address a superior or esteemed professional like a potential employer, a professor, or a manager. Formal language avoids contractions, slang, colloquialisms, and first-person pronouns.

Informal language is often used when communicating with family members, friends, peers, and those known more personally. It is more casual, spontaneous, and forgiving in its conformity to grammatical rules and conventions. Informal language is used for personal emails, some light fiction stories, and some correspondence between coworkers or other familial relationships.

Slang refers to non-standard expressions that are not used in elevated speech and writing. Slang creates linguistic in-groups and out-groups of people, those who can understand the slang terms and those who can't. Slang is often tied to a specific time period. For example, "groovy" and "far out" are connected to the 1970s, and "as if!" and "4-1-1-" are connected to the 1990s. **Colloquial language** is language that is used conversationally or familiarly—e.g., "What's up?"—in contrast to formal, professional, or academic language—"How are you this evening?" Formal language uses sentences that are usually more complex and often in passive voice. Punctuation can differ as well. For example, exclamation points are used to show strong emotion or can be used as an interjection but should be used sparingly in formal writing situations.

Textspeak is a term used to refer to the informal language used in text messages and similar messaging mediums. While often appropriate for use in those contexts, it should be avoided in more formal settings.

Outside of casual conversations, it's important to use formal language both in speaking and writing.

Sensitivity

In speech and writing, it's important to be cognizant as to how your words are perceived by others. Racist, sexist, and other derogatory language should be avoided because it is rude, demeaning, and can severely hurt career opportunities. It may be helpful to adopt a position of being "above reproach", meaning that your words and actions are so pure they cannot be criticized for being insensitive.

Word Confusion

That/Which

The pronouns *that* and *which* are both used to refer to animals, objects, ideas, and events—but they are not interchangeable. The rule is to use the word *that* in essential clauses and phrases that help convey the meaning of the sentence. Use the word *which* in nonessential (less important) clauses. Typically, *which* clauses are enclosed in commas.

The morning <u>that I fell asleep in class</u> caused me a lot of trouble.

This morning's coffee, <u>which had too much creamer</u>, woke me up.

Who/Whom

We use the pronouns *who* and *whom* to refer to people. We always use *who* when it is the subject of the sentence or clause. We never use *whom* as the subject; it is always the object of a verb or preposition.

<u>Who</u> hit the baseball for the home run? (subject)

The baseball fell into the glove of <u>whom</u>? (object of the preposition of)

The umpire called <u>whom</u> "out"? (object of the verb called)

To/Too/Two

to: a preposition or infinitive (*to walk, to run, walk to the store, run to the tree*)
too: means also, as well, or very (*She likes cookies, too.; I ate too much.*)
two: a number (*I have two cookies. She walked to the store two times.*)

There/Their/They're

there: an adjective, adverb, or pronoun used to start a sentence or indicate place (*There are four vintage cars over there.*)
their: a possessive pronoun used to indicate belonging (*Their car is the blue and white one.*)
they're: a contraction of the words "they are" (*They're going to enter the vintage car show.*)

Your/You're

your: a possessive pronoun (*Your artwork is terrific.*)
you're: a contraction of the words "you are" (*You're a terrific artist.*)

Its/It's

its: a possessive pronoun (*The elephant had its trunk in the water.*)
it's: a contraction of the words "it is" (*It's an impressive animal.*)

Affect/Effect

affect: as a verb means "to influence" (*How will the earthquake affect your home?*); as a noun means "emotion or mood" (*Her affect was somber.*)

effect: as a verb means "to bring about" (*She will effect a change through philanthropy.*); as a noun means "a result of" (*The effect of the earthquake was devastating.*)

Other pairs of words cause mix-ups but are not necessarily homonyms. Here are a few of those:

Bring/Take

bring: when the action is coming toward (*Bring me the money.*)
take: when the action is going away from (*Take her the money.*)

Can/May

can: means "able to" (*The child can ride a bike.*)
may: asks permission (*The child asked if he may ride his bike.*)

Than/Then

than: a conjunction used for comparison (*I like tacos better than pizza.*)
then: an adverb telling when something happened (*I ate and then slept.*)

Disinterested/Uninterested

disinterested: used to mean "neutral" (*The jury remains disinterested during the trial.*)
uninterested: used to mean "bored" (*I was uninterested during the lecture.*)

Percent/Percentage

percent: used when there is a number involved (*Five percent of us like tacos.*)
percentage: used when there is no number (*That is a low percentage.*)

Fewer/Less

fewer: used for things you can count (*He has fewer playing cards.*)
less: used for things you cannot count, as well as time (*He has less talent. You have less than a minute.*)

Farther/Further

farther: used when discussing distance (*His paper airplane flew farther than mine.*)
further: used to mean "more" (*He needed further information.*)

Lend/Loan

lend: a verb used for borrowing (*Lend me your lawn mower. He will lend it to me.*)
loan: a noun used for something borrowed (*She applied for a student loan.*)

Among/Between

among: used when referring to more than two things (*Surfing is among my favorite hobbies.*)
between: usually used when referring to just two things, or when naming specific distinct items, even if more than two (*She sat between Bill and Ronald.*)

Good/Well

good: an adjective, which modifies a noun or pronoun (*She is a good pianist.*)
well: an adverb that answers the question "how?" (*She plays piano well.*)

94

Bad/Badly

bad: an adjective, which modifies a noun or pronoun (*That was a bad storm.*)

badly: an adverb that answers the question "how?" (*Donna was hurt badly in the car accident.*)

Hear/Here

hear: a verb that means to perceive sound by using one's ears (*I can hear the birds chirping.*)

here: an adverb meaning at, on, or in this place (*The book was found here.*)

i.e./e.g.

i.e.: short for the Latin phrase *id est,* which means "in other words." (*Our new house is a money pit – i.e., things are constantly breaking and we have spent tens of thousands of dollars on repairs.*)

e.g.: short for the Latin phrase *exempli gratia*, which means "for example." (*The textbook also comes with online features (e.g., interactive quizzes, instructional videos)*).

Lie/Lay

lie: a verb meaning to recline in a flat position, and using it does not require a direct object (*I'm going to lie down after I call Terry.*)

lay: a verb that means to place something in its resting position, and using it requires a direct object (*I usually lay my sweater on the back of the chair.*)

Who's/Whose

who's: a contraction of "who is" (*Who's coming to dinner?*)

whose: indicates possession (*Whose sweater is this?*)

Look at the following sentence:

Who's job is it to protect America's drivers?

The easiest way to check for correct usage is to replace the word *who's* with "who is" and see if the sentence makes sense:

Who is job is it to protect America's drivers?

By changing the contraction to "Who is" the sentence no longer makes sense. Therefore, the correct word must be *whose*.

Your/You're

your: indicates possession (*Your desk is very organized.*)

you're: a contraction for "you are" (*You are our pick for next VP.*)_

Look at the following example:

Your going to have to write your congressman if you want to see action.

Again, the easiest way to check correct usage is to replace the word *Your* with "You are" and see if the sentence still makes sense.

You are going to have to write your congressman if you want to see action.

95

By replacing Your with "You are," the sentence still makes sense. Thus, in this case, the writer should have used "You're."

Note
Some people have problems with these:

- regardless/irregardless
- a lot/alot

Irregardless and *alot* are always incorrect. Don't use them.

Please keep in mind that grammar questions on the actual exam may be hospital related.

Practice Quiz

1. Which sentence that contains an error in punctuation or capitalization?
    a. "The show is on," Jackson said.
    b. The Grand Canyon is a national park.
    c. Lets celebrate tomorrow.
    d. Oliver, a social worker, got a new job this month.

2. Which of the following sentences contains an error in usage?
    a. Their words was followed by a signing document.
    b. No one came to the theater that evening.
    c. Several cats were living in the abandoned house down the road.
    d. It rained that morning; they had to cancel the kayaking trip.

3. What type of grammatical error does the following sentence contain?

    It was true, Lyla ate the last cupcake.

    a. Subject-verb agreement error
    b. Punctuation error
    c. Shift in verb tense
    d. Split infinitive

4. Which sentence below contains an error in punctuation or capitalization?
    a. Afterwards, we got ice cream down the road.
    b. The word "slacken" means to decrease.
    c. They started building the Hoover dam in 1931.
    d. Matthew got married to his best friend, Maria.

5. Choose the sentence that contains an error in usage. If there are no errors, select Choice *D*.
    a. After her swim, Jeanine saw a blue kid's shovel.
    b. Pistachios are my favorite kind of nut, although they're expensive.
    c. One apple is better than two lemons.
    d. We found three five-dollar bills on the way home.

See answers on next page.

If you want to test your knowledge further on the
grammar section of the HESI exam,
take our online practice quiz.

testprepbooks.com/hesi-quiz

SCAN ME

Answer Explanations

1. C: The correct answer choice is "Lets celebrate tomorrow." "Lets" is supposed to be short for "let us," and therefore needs an apostrophe between the "t" and the "s": "Let's."

2. A: This error is marked by a subject/verb agreement. "Words" is plural, so the verb must be plural as well. The correct usage would be: "Their words were followed by a signing document."

3. B: There is a punctuation error. The comma creates a comma splice where a period or a semicolon should be since we have two independent clauses on either side of the comma.

4. C: Choice *C* is the problematic answer; the whole phrase "Hoover Dam" should be capitalized, not just "Hoover."

5. A: Choice *A* has the error in usage because we have a dangling modifier with the phrase "blue kid's shovel." The sentence indicates the kid is blue. We want the sentence to say that the shovel is blue. Therefore, it should be: "After her swim, Jeanine saw a kid's blue shovel."

Biology

Biology is the study of living organisms and the processes that are vital for life.

Biology Basics

Taxonomy is the science behind the biological names of organisms. Biologists often refer to organisms by their Latin scientific names to avoid confusion with common names, such as with fish. Jellyfish, crayfish, and silverfish all have the word "fish" in their name, but belong to three different species. In the eighteenth century, Carl Linnaeus invented a naming system for species that included using the Latin scientific name of a species, called the *binomial*, which has two parts: the *genus*, which comes first, and the *specific epithet*, which comes second. Similar species are grouped into the same genus. The Linnaean system is the commonly used taxonomic system today and, moving from comprehensive similarities to more general similarities, classifies organisms into their species, genus, family, order, class, phylum, and kingdom. *Homo sapiens* is the Latin scientific name for humans.

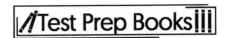
Scientific Method

Human beings are, by nature, very curious. Long before the scientific method was established, people have been making observations and predicting outcomes, manipulating the physical world to create extraordinary things—from the first man-made fire in 6000 B.C.E. to the satellite that orbited Pluto in 2016. Although the history of the scientific method is sporadic and attributed to many different people, it remains the most reliable way to obtain and utilize knowledge about the observable universe. The scientific method consists of the following steps:

- **Make an observation:** An **observation** is the analysis of information using basic human senses: sight, sound, touch, taste, and smell. Observations can be two different types—qualitative or quantitative. A *qualitative observation* describes what is being observed, such as the color of a house or the smell of a flower. *Quantitative observations* measure what is being observed, such as the number of windows on a house or the intensity of a flower's smell on a scale of 1-5.

- **Create a question:** Observations lead to the identification of a problem, also called an **inference**. Inferences are logical predictions based on experience or education that lead to the formation of a hypothesis.

- **Form a hypothesis:** A **hypothesis** is a testable explanation of an observed scenario and is presented in the form of a statement. It's an attempt to answer a question based on an observation, and it allows a scientist to predict an outcome. A hypothesis makes assumptions on the relationship between two different variables, and answers the question: "If I do this, what happens to that?"

- **Conduct an experiment:** Once a hypothesis has been formed, it must be tested to determine whether it's true or false. To test a hypothesis, one must conduct a carefully designed experiment.

- **Collect and analyze data:** Once the experiment begins, a disciplined scientist must always record the observations in meticulous detail, usually in a journal. Upon reading this journal, a different scientist should be able to clearly understand the experiment and recreate it exactly. The journal includes all **collected data**, or any observed changes.

- **Form a conclusion:** The final step of the scientific method is to make inferences from observed data, which is also known as forming a **conclusion**.

Water

Most cells are primarily composed of water and live in water-rich environments. Since water is such a familiar substance, it is easy to overlook its unique properties. Chemically, water is made up of two hydrogen atoms bonded to one oxygen atom by covalent bonds. The three atoms join to make a V-shaped molecule. Water is a polar molecule, meaning it has an unevenly distributed overall charge due to an unequal sharing of electrons. Due to oxygen's electronegativity and its more substantial positively charged nucleus, hydrogen's electrons are pulled closer to the oxygen. This causes the hydrogen atoms to have a slight positive charge and the oxygen atom to have a slight negative charge. In a glass of water, the molecules constantly interact and link for a fraction of a second due to intermolecular bonding between the slightly positive hydrogen atoms of one molecule and the slightly negative oxygen of a different molecule. These weak intermolecular bonds are called **hydrogen bonds**.

Water has several important qualities, including: cohesive and adhesive behaviors, temperature moderation ability, expansion upon freezing, and diverse use as a solvent.

Cohesion is the interaction of many of the same molecules. In water, cohesion occurs when there is hydrogen bonding between water molecules. Water molecules use this bonding ability to attach to each other and can work against gravity to transport dissolved nutrients to the top of a plant. A network of water-conducting cells can push water from the roots of a plant up to the leaves. Adhesion is the linking of two different substances. Water molecules can form a weak hydrogen bond with, or adhere to, plant cell walls to help fight gravity. The cohesive behavior of water also causes surface tension. If a glass of water is slightly overfull, water can still stand above the rim. This is because of the unique bonding of water molecules at the surface—they bond to each other and to the molecules below them, making it seem like it is covered with an impenetrable film. A raft spider could actually walk across a small body of water due to this surface tension.

Another important property of water is its ability to moderate temperature. Water can moderate the temperature of air by absorbing or releasing stored heat into the air. Water has the distinctive capability of being able to absorb or release large quantities of stored heat while undergoing only a small change in temperature. This is because of the relatively high **specific heat** of water, where specific heat is the amount of heat it takes for one gram of a material to change its temperature by 1 degree Celsius. The specific heat of water is one calorie per gram per degree Celsius, meaning that for each gram of water, it takes one calorie of heat to raise or lower the temperature of water by 1 degree Celsius.

When the temperature of water is reduced to freezing levels, water displays another interesting property: It expands instead of contracts. Most liquids become denser as they freeze because the molecules move around slower and stay closer together. Water molecules, however, form hydrogen bonds with each other as they move together. As the temperature lowers and they begin to move slower, these bonds become harder to break apart. When water freezes into ice, molecules are frozen with hydrogen bonds between them and they take up about 10 percent more volume than in their liquid state. The fact that ice is less dense than water is what makes ice float to the top of a glass of water.

Lastly, the **polarity** of water molecules makes it a versatile solvent. **Ionic compounds**, such as salt, are made up of positively- and negatively-charged atoms, called **cations** and **anions**, respectively. Cations and anions are easily dissolved in water because of their individual attractions to the slight positive charge of the hydrogen atoms or the slight negative charge of the oxygen atoms in water molecules. Water molecules separate the individually charged atoms and shield them from each other so they don't bond to each other again, creating a homogenous solution of the cations and anions. Nonionic compounds, such as sugar, have polar regions, so are easily dissolved in water. For these compounds, the water molecules form hydrogen bonds with the polar regions (hydroxyl groups) to create a homogenous solution. Any substance that is attracted to water is termed **hydrophilic**. Substances that repel water are termed **hydrophobic**.

Biological Molecules

Basic units of organic compounds are often called **monomers**. Repeating units of linked monomers are called **polymers**. The most important large molecules, or polymers, found in all living things can be divided into four categories: carbohydrates, lipids, proteins, and nucleic acids. This may be surprising since there is so much diversity in the outward appearance and physical abilities of living things present on Earth. Carbon (C), hydrogen (H), oxygen (O), nitrogen (N), sulfur (S), and phosphorus (P) are the major elements of most biological molecules. Carbon is a common backbone of large molecules because of its ability to form four covalent bonds.

Carbohydrates

Carbohydrates consist of sugars and polymers of sugars. The simplest sugar are **monosaccharide**, which have the empirical formula of CH_2O. The formula for the monosaccharide glucose, for example, is $C_6H_{12}O_6$. Glucose is an important molecule for cellular respiration, the process of cells extracting energy by breaking bonds through a series of reactions. The individual atoms are then used to rebuild new small molecules. **Polysaccharides** are made up of a few hundred to a few thousand monosaccharides linked together. These larger molecules have two major functions. The first is that they can be stored as starches, such as **glycogen**, and then broken down later for energy. Secondly, they may be used to form strong materials, such as **cellulose**, which is the firm wall that encloses plant cells, and **chitin**, the carbohydrate insects use to build exoskeletons.

Classification of Carbs

Monosaccharides

CHO
|
H — C — OH
|
CH₂OH

Trioses

CHO
|
H — C — OH
|
H — C — OH
|
CH₂OH

Tetroses

CHO
|
HO — C — H
|
HO — C — H
|
H — C — OH
|
CH₂OH

Pentoses

CHO
|
H — C — OH
|
HO — C — H
|
HO — C — H
|
H — C — OH
|
CH₂OH

Hexoses or Heptoses

Lipids

Lipids are a class of biological molecules that are **hydrophobic**, meaning they don't mix well with water. They are mostly made up of large chains of carbon and hydrogen atoms, termed **hydrocarbon chains**. When lipids mix with water, the water molecules bond to each other and exclude the lipids because they are unable to form bonds with the long hydrocarbon chains. Because the structure of different lipids is so diverse, they have a wide range of functions, which include energy storage, signaling, structure, protection, and making up the cell membrane. The three most important types of lipids are fats, phospholipids, and steroids.

Fats are made up of two types of smaller molecules: glycerol and fatty acids. **Glycerol** is a chain of three carbon atoms, with a **hydroxyl group** attached to each carbon atom. A hydroxyl group is made up of an oxygen and hydrogen atom bonded together. **Fatty acids** are long hydrocarbon chains that have a backbone of sixteen or eighteen carbon atoms. The carbon atom on one end of the fatty acid is part of a **carboxyl group.** A carboxyl group is a carbon atom that uses two of its four bonds to bond to one oxygen atom (double bond) and uses another one of its bonds to link to a hydroxyl group.

Fats are made by joining three fatty acid molecules and one glycerol molecule.

These energy-storage molecules can exist as any of the following types.

- **Saturated fats** have no double bonds within their fatty acid tails. These are solid at room temperature and are mostly animal fats like bacon fat.

- **Unsaturated fats** have double bonds within any of their fatty acid tails. Due to the kinks caused by the double bonds, these fats are liquid at room temperature and are mostly plant fats like olive oil.

Phospholipids are made of two fatty acid molecules linked to one glycerol molecule. A **phosphate group** is attached to a third hydroxyl group of the glycerol molecule. A phosphate group consists of a phosphate atom connected to four oxygen atoms and has an overall negative charge.

103

Phospholipids have an interesting structure because their fatty acid tails are hydrophobic, but their phosphate group heads are hydrophilic. When phospholipids mix with water, they create double-layered structures, called **bilayers,** that shield their hydrophobic regions from water molecules. Cell membranes are made of phospholipid bilayers, which allow the cells to mix with aqueous solutions outside and inside, while forming a protective barrier and a semi-permeable membrane around the cell.

Steroids are lipids that consist of four fused carbon rings. The different chemical groups that attach to these rings are what make up the many types of steroids. **Cholesterol** is a common type of steroid found in animal cell membranes. Steroids are mixed in between the phospholipid bilayer and help maintain the structure of the membrane and aids in cell signaling.

Proteins

Proteins are essential for most all functions in living beings. The term *protein* is derived from the Greek word *proteios*, meaning *first* or *primary*. All proteins are made from a set of twenty **amino acids**, molecules that are linked in unbranched polymers. The combinations are numerous, which accounts for the diversity of proteins. Amino acids are linked by peptide bonds, while polymers of amino acids are called **polypeptides**. These polypeptides, either individually or in linked combination with each other, fold up to form coils of biologically-functional molecules, called proteins.

There are four levels of protein structure: primary, secondary, tertiary, and quaternary. The **primary structure** is the sequence of amino acids, similar to the letters in a long word. The **secondary structure** is beta sheets, or alpha helices, formed by hydrogen bonding between the polar regions of the polypeptide backbone. **Tertiary structure** is the overall shape of the molecule that results from the interactions between the side chains linked to the polypeptide backbone. **Quaternary structure** is the overall protein structure that occurs when a protein is made up of two or more polypeptide chains.

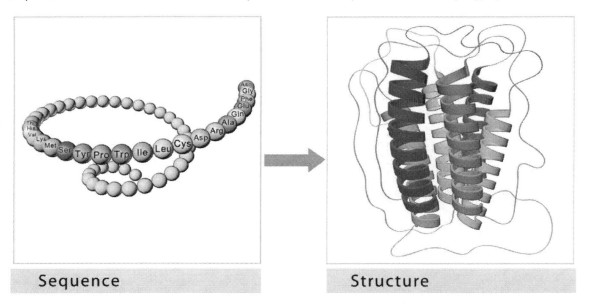

Sequence   Structure

Nucleic Acids

Nucleic acids can also be called **polynucleotides** because they are made up of chains of monomers called **nucleotides.** Nucleotides consist of a five-carbon sugar, a nitrogen-containing base, and a phosphate group. There are two types of nucleic acids: **deoxyribonucleic acid (DNA)** and **ribonucleic acid (RNA)**. Both DNA and RNA enable living organisms to pass on their genetic information and complex components to subsequent generations. While DNA is made up of two strands of nucleotides coiled together in a double-helix structure, RNA is made up of a single strand of nucleotides that folds onto itself.

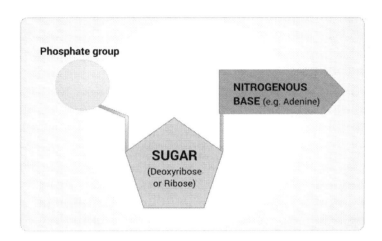

Metabolism

Metabolism is the set of chemical processes that occur within a cell for the maintenance of life. It includes both the synthesizing and breaking down of substances. A **metabolic pathway** begins with a molecule and ends with a specific product after going through a series of reactions, often involving an enzyme at each step. An **enzyme** is a protein that aids in the reaction. **Catabolic pathways** are metabolic pathways in which energy is released by complex molecules being broken down into simpler molecules. Contrast to catabolic pathways are **anabolic pathways**, which use energy to build complex molecules out of simple molecules. With cell metabolism, remember the **first law of thermodynamics**: Energy can be transformed, but it cannot be created or destroyed. Therefore, the energy released in a cell by a catabolic pathway is used up in anabolic pathways.

The reactions that occur within metabolic pathways are classified as either exergonic reactions or endergonic reactions. **Exergonic reactions** end in a release of free energy, while **endergonic reactions** absorb free energy from its surroundings. **Free energy** is the portion of energy in a system, such as a living cell, that can be used to perform work, such as a chemical reaction. It is denoted as the capital letter G and the change in free energy from a reaction or set of reactions is denoted as delta G (ΔG). When reactions do not require an input of energy, they are said to occur spontaneously. Exergonic reactions are considered spontaneous because they result in a negative delta G ($-\Delta$G), where the products of the reaction have less free energy within them than the reactants. Endergonic reactions require an input of energy and result in a positive delta G ($+\Delta$G), with the products of the reaction containing more free energy than the individual reactants. When a system no longer has free energy to do work, it has reached **equilibrium**. Since cells always work, they are no longer alive if they reach equilibrium.

Cells balance their energy resources by using the energy from exergonic reactions to drive endergonic reactions forward, a process called **energy coupling**. **Adenosine triphosphate**, or ATP, is a molecule that is an immediate source of energy for cellular work. When it is broken down, it releases energy used in endergonic reactions and anabolic pathways. ATP breaks down into adenosine diphosphate, or ADP, and a separate phosphate group, releasing energy in an exergonic reaction. As ATP is used up by reactions, it is also regenerated by having a new phosphate group added onto the ADP products within the cell in an endergonic reaction.

Enzymes are special proteins that help speed up metabolic reactions and pathways. They do not change the overall free energy release or consumption of reactions; they just make the reactions occur more quickly as it lowers the activation energy required. Enzymes are designed to act only on specific substrates. Their physical shape fits snugly onto their matched substrates, so enzymes only speed up reactions that contain the substrates to which they are matched.

The Cell

Cells are the basic structural and functional unit of all organisms. They are the smallest unit of matter that is living. While there are many single-celled organisms, most biological organisms are more complex and made up of many different types of cells. There are two distinct types of cells: prokaryotic and eukaryotic.

Prokaryotic cells include bacteria, while **eukaryotic cells** include animal and plant cells. Both types of cells are enclosed by a cell membrane, which is selectively permeable. Selective permeability means essentially that it is a a **cell membrane**, which is selectively permeable. Selective permeability means essentially that it is a gatekeeper, allowing certain molecules and ions in and out, and keeping unwanted ones at bay, at least until they are ready for use. Both contain ribosomes, which are complexes that make protein inside the cell, and DNA. One major difference is that the DNA in eukaryotic cells are enclosed in a membrane-bound **nucleus**, where in prokaryotic cells, DNA is in the **nucleoid**, a region that is not enclosed by a membrane. Another major difference is that eukaryotic cells contain **organelles,** which are membrane-enclosed structures, each with a specific function, while prokaryotic cells do not have organelles.

Organelles Found in Eukaryotic Cells

The following cell organelles are found in both animal and plant cells unless otherwise noted:

Nucleus: The nucleus consists of three parts: nuclear envelope, nucleolus, and chromatin. The **nuclear envelope** is the double membrane that surrounds the nucleus and separates its contents from the rest of the cell. It is porous so substances can pass back and forth between the nucleus and the other parts of the cell. It is also continuous, with the endoplasmic reticulum that is present within the cytosol of the cell. The **nucleolus** is in charge of producing ribosomes. **Chromosomes** are comprised of tightly coiled proteins, RNA, and DNA and are collectively called **chromatin**.

Endoplasmic Reticulum (ER): The ER is a network of membranous sacs and tubes responsible for membrane synthesis and other metabolic and synthetic activities of the cell. There are two types of ER, rough and smooth. **Rough ER** is lined with ribosomes and is the location of protein synthesis. This provides a separate compartment for site-specific protein synthesis and is important for the intracellular transport of proteins. **Smooth ER** does not contain ribosomes and is the location of lipid synthesis.

Flagellum: The flagellum is found in protists and animal cells. It is a cluster of microtubules projected out of the plasma membrane and aids in cell motility.

Centrosome: The centrosome is the area of the cell where microtubules are created and organized for mitosis. Each centrosome contains two **centrioles.**

Cytoskeleton: The cytoskeleton in animal cells is made up of microfilaments, intermediate filaments, and microtubules. In plant cells, the cytoskeleton is made up of only microfilaments and microtubules. These structures reinforce the cell's shape and aid in cell movements.

Microvilli: Microvilli are found only in animal cells. They are protrusions in the cell membrane that increase the cell's surface area. They have a variety of functions, including absorption, secretion, and cellular adhesion.

Peroxisome: A peroxisome contains enzymes that are involved in many of the cell's metabolic functions, one of the most important being the breakdown of fatty acid chains. It produces hydrogen peroxide as a by-product of these processes and then converts the hydrogen peroxide to water.

Mitochondrion: The mitochondrion, considered the cell's powerhouse, is one of the most important structures for maintaining regular cell function. It is where cellular respiration occurs and where most of the cell's ATP is generated.

Lysosome: Lysosomes are found exclusively in animal cells. They are responsible for digestion and can hydrolyze macromolecules.

Golgi Apparatus: The Golgi apparatus is responsible for synthesizing, modifying, sorting, transporting, and secreting cell products. Because of its large size, it was one of the first organelles studied in detail.

Ribosomes: Ribosomes are found either free in the cytosol, bound to the rough ER, or bound to the nuclear envelope. They are also found in prokaryotes. Ribosomes make up a complex that forms proteins within the cell.

Plasmodesmata: Found only in plant cells, plasmodesmata are cytoplasmic channels, or tunnels, that go through the cell wall and connect the cytoplasm of adjacent cells.

Chloroplast: Chloroplasts are plastids found in protists, such as algae and plant cells. It is responsible for photosynthesis, which is the process of converting sunlight to chemical energy that is stored and used later to drive cellular activities.

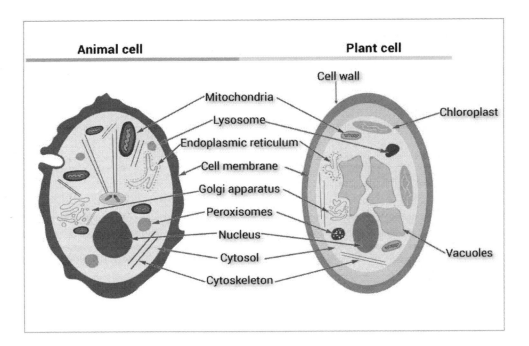

Vacuoles: Vacuoles are membrane-bound organelles found primarily in plant and fungi cells, but also in some animal cells. Vacuoles are filled with water and some enzymes and are important for intracellular digestion and waste removal. The membrane-bound nature of the vacuole allows for the storage of harmful material and poisonous substances. The pressure from the water inside the vacuole also contributes to the structure of plant cells. Animals have food vacuoles that contain the contents of phagocytosis. **Phagocytosis**, or "cellular eating," occurs when a cell engulfs large particles and internalizes them by using vacuoles.

Central Vacuole: A central vacuole is found only in plant cells, and is responsible for storage, breakdown of waste products, and hydrolysis of macromolecules.

Plasma Membrane: The plasma membrane is a phospholipid bilayer that encloses the cell. It is also found in prokaryotes.

Cell Wall: Cell walls are present in fungi, plant cells, and some protists. The cell wall is made up of strong fibrous substances, including cellulose (plants), chitin (fungi) and other polysaccharides, and protein. It is a layer outside of the plasma membrane that protects the cell from mechanical damage and helps maintain the cell's shape.

Cellular Respiration

Cellular respiration is a set of metabolic processes that converts energy from nutrients into ATP. Respiration can either occur aerobically, using oxygen, or anaerobically, without oxygen. While

108

prokaryotic cells carry out respiration in the cytosol, most of the respiration in eukaryotic cells occurs in the mitochondria.

Aerobic Respiration

There are three main steps in aerobic cellular respiration: glycolysis, the citric acid cycle (also known as the Krebs cycle), and oxidative phosphorylation. **Glycolysis** is an essential metabolic pathway that converts glucose to pyruvate and allows for cellular respiration to occur. It does not require oxygen to be present. Glucose is a common molecule used for energy production in cells. During glycolysis, two three-carbon sugars are generated from the splitting of a glucose molecule. These smaller sugars are then converted into pyruvate molecules via oxidation and atom rearrangement. Glycolysis requires two ATP molecules to drive the process forward, but the end product of the process has four ATP molecules, for a net production of two ATP molecules. Also, two reduced nicotinamide adenine dinucleotide (NADH) molecules are created from when the electron carrier oxidized nicotinamide adenine dinucleotide (NAD+) peels off two electrons and a hydrogen atom.

In aerobically-respiring eukaryotic cells, the pyruvate molecules then enter the mitochondrion. Pyruvate is oxidized and converted into a compound called acetyl-CoA. This molecule enters the **citric acid cycle** to begin the process of aerobic respiration.

The citric acid cycle has eight steps. Remember that glycolysis produces two pyruvate molecules from each glucose molecule. Each pyruvate molecule oxidizes into a single acetyl-CoA molecule, which then enters the citric acid cycle. Therefore, two citric acid cycles can be completed and twice the number of ATP molecules are generated per glucose molecule.

Eight Steps of the Citric Acid Cycle

Step 1: Acetyl-CoA adds a two-carbon acetyl group to an oxaloacetate molecule and produces one citrate molecule.

Step 2: Citrate is converted to its isomer isocitrate by removing one water molecule and adding a new water molecule in a different configuration.

Step 3: Isocitrate is oxidized and converted to α-ketoglutarate. A carbon dioxide (CO_2) molecule is released and one NAD+ molecule is converted to NADH.

Step 4: α-Ketoglutarate is converted to succinyl-CoA. Another carbon dioxide molecule is released and another NAD+ molecule is converted to NADH.

Step 5: Succinyl-CoA becomes succinate by the addition of a phosphate group to the cycle. The oxygen molecule of the phosphate group attaches to the succinyl-CoA molecule and the CoA group is released. The rest of the phosphate group transfers to a guanosine diphosphate (GDP) molecule, converting it to guanosine triphosphate (GTP). GTP acts similarly to ATP and can actually be used to generate an ATP molecule at this step.

Step 6: Succinate is converted to fumarate by losing two hydrogen atoms. The hydrogen atoms join a flavin adenine dinucleotide (FAD) molecule, converting it to $FADH_2$, which is a hydroquinone form.

Step 7: A water molecule is added to the cycle and converts fumarate to malate.

Step 8: Malate is oxidized and converted to oxaloacetate. One lost hydrogen atom is added to an NAD molecule to create NADH. The oxaloacetate generated here then enters back into step one of the cycle.

At the end of glycolysis and the citric acid cycles, four ATP molecules have been generated. The NADH and $FADH_2$ molecules are used as energy to drive the next step of oxidative phosphorylation.

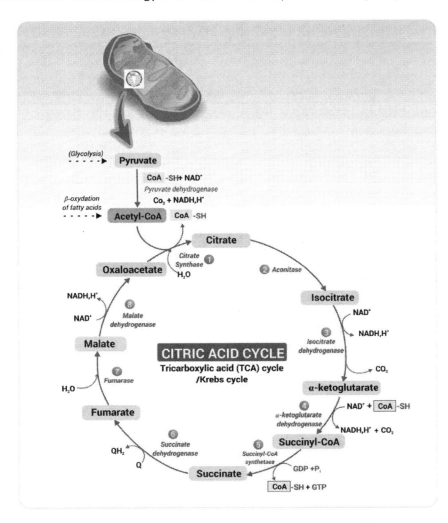

Oxidative Phosphorylation

Oxidative phosphorylation includes two steps: the electron transport chain and chemiosmosis. The inner mitochondrial membrane has four protein complexes, sequenced I to IV, used to transport protons and electrons through the inner mitochondrial matrix. Two electrons and a proton (H+) are passed from each NADH and $FADH_2$ to these channel proteins, pumping the hydrogen ions to the inner-membrane space using energy from the high-energy electrons to create a concentration gradient. NADH and $FADH_2$ also drop their high-energy electrons to the electron transport chain. NAD+ and FAD molecules in the mitochondrial matrix return to the Krebs cycle to pick up materials for the next delivery. From here, two processes happen simultaneously:

1. **Electron Transport Chain:** In addition to complexes I to IV, there are two mobile electron carriers present in the inner mitochondrial membrane, called **ubiquinone** and **cytochrome C.** At the end of this transport chain, electrons are accepted by an O_2 molecule in the matrix, and water is formed with the addition of two hydrogen atoms from chemiosmosis.

2. **Chemiosmosis:** This occurs in an ATP synthase complex that sits next to the four electron transporting complexes. ATP synthase uses **facilitated diffusion** (passive transport) to deliver protons across the concentration gradient from the inner mitochondrial membrane to the matrix. As the protons travel, the ATP synthase protein physically spins, and the kinetic energy generated is invested into phosphorylation of ADP molecules to generate ATP. Oxidative phosphorylation produces twenty-six to twenty-eight ATP molecules, bringing the total number of ATP generated through glycolysis and cellular respiration to thirty to thirty-two molecules.

Anaerobic Respiration

Some organisms do not live in oxygen-rich environments and must find alternate methods of respiration. Anaerobic respiration occurs in certain prokaryotic organisms. They utilize an electron transport chain similar to the aerobic respiration pathway; however, the terminal acceptor molecule is an electronegative substance that is not O_2. Some bacteria, for example, use the sulfate ion (SO_4^{2-}) as the final electron accepting molecule and the resulting byproduct is hydrogen sulfide (H_2S) instead of water.

Muscle cells that reach anaerobic threshold go through lactic acid respiration, while yeasts go through alcohol fermentation. Both processes only make two ATP.

Photosynthesis

Photosynthesis is the process of converting light energy into chemical energy that is then stored in sugar and other organic molecules. It can be divided into two stages: the light-dependent reactions and the Calvin cycle. In plants, the photosynthetic process takes place in the chloroplast. Inside the chloroplast are membranous sacs, called **thylakoids**. Chlorophyll is a green pigment that lives in the thylakoid membranes and absorbs the light energy, starting the process of photosynthesis. The **Calvin cycle** takes place in the **stroma,** or inner space, of the chloroplasts. The complex series of reactions that take place in photosynthesis can be simplified into the following equation:

$$6CO_2 + 12H_2O + \text{Light Energy} \rightarrow C_6H_{12}O_6 + 6O_2 + 6H_2O$$

Basically, carbon dioxide and water mix with light energy inside the chloroplast to produce organic molecules, oxygen, and water. Note that water is on both sides of the equation. Twelve water molecules are consumed during this process and six water molecules are newly formed as byproducts.

The Light Reactions

During the **light reactions**, chlorophyll molecules absorb light energy, or solar energy. In the thylakoid membrane, chlorophyll molecules, together with other small molecules and proteins, form photosystems, which are made up of a reaction-center complex surrounded by a light-harvesting complex. In the first step of photosynthesis, the light-harvesting complex from photosystem II (PSII) absorbs a photon from light, passes the photon from one pigment molecule to another within itself, and then transfers it to the reaction-center complex. Inside the reaction-center complex, the energy from

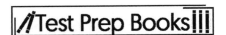

the photon enables a special pair of chlorophyll *a* molecules to release two electrons. These two electrons are then accepted by a primary electron acceptor molecule. Simultaneously, a water molecule is split into two hydrogen atoms, two electrons and one oxygen atom. The two electrons are transferred one by one to the chlorophyll *a* molecules, replacing their released electrons.

The released electrons are then transported down an electron transport chain by attaching to the electron carrier plastoquinone (Pq), a cytochrome complex, and then a protein called plastocyanin (Pc) before they reach photosystem I (PS I). As the electrons pass through the cytochrome complex, protons are pumped into the thylakoid space, providing the concentration gradient that will eventually travel through ATP synthase to make ATP (like in aerobic respiration). PS I absorbs photons from light, similar to PS II. However, the electrons that are released from the chlorophyll *a* molecules in PS I are replaced by the electrons coming down the electron transport chain (from PS II). A primary electron acceptor molecule accepts the released electrons in PS I and passes the electrons onto another electron transport chain involving the protein ferredoxin (Fd).

In the final steps of the light reactions, electrons are transferred from Fd to Nicotinamide adenine dinucleotide phosphate (NADP+) with the help of the enzyme NADP+ reductase and NADPH is produced. The ATP and nicotinamide adenine dinucleotide phosphate-oxidase (NADPH) produced from the light reactions are used as energy to form organic molecules in the Calvin cycle.

The Calvin Cycle

There are three phases in the Calvin cycle: carbon fixation, reduction, and regeneration of the CO_2 acceptor. **Carbon fixation** is when the first carbon molecule is introduced into the cycle, when CO_2 from the air is absorbed by the chloroplast. Each CO_2 molecule enters the cycle and attaches to ribulose bisphosphate (RuBP), a five-carbon sugar. The enzyme RuBP carboxylase-oxygenase, also known as rubisco, catalyzes this reaction. Next, two three-carbon 3-phosphoglycerate sugar molecules are formed immediately from the splitting of the six-carbon sugar.

Next, during the **reduction** phase, an ATP molecule is reduced to ADP and the phosphate group attaches to 3-phosphoglycerate, forming 1,3-bisphosphoglycerate. An NADPH molecule then donates two high-energy electrons to the newly formed 1,3-bisphosphate, causing it to lose the phosphate group and become glyceraldehyde 3-phosphate (G3P), which is a high-energy sugar molecule. At this point in the cycle, one G3P molecule exits the cycle and is used by the plant. However, to regenerate RuBP molecules, which are the CO_2 acceptors in the cycle, five G3P molecules continue in the cycle. It takes three turns of the cycle and three CO_2 molecules entering the cycle to form one G3P molecule.

In the final phase of the Calvin cycle, three RuBP molecules are formed from the rearrangement of the carbon skeletons of five G3P molecules. It is a complex process that involves the reduction of three ATP molecules. At the end of the process, RuBP molecules are again ready to enter the first phase and accept CO_2 molecules.

Although the Calvin cycle is not dependent on light energy, both steps of photosynthesis usually occur during daylight, as the Calvin cycle is dependent upon the ATP and NADPH produced by the light reactions, because that energy can be invested into bonds to create high-energy sugars. The Calvin cycle invests nine ATP molecules and six NADPH molecules into every one molecule of G3P that it produces. The G3P that is produced can be used as the starting material to build larger organic compounds, such as glucose.

Cellular Reproduction

Cellular reproduction is the process that cells use to divide into two new cells. The ability of a multi-cellular organism to generate new cells to replace dying and damaged cells is vital for sustaining its life. Bacteria reproduce via **binary fission,** which is a simpler process than eukaryotic division because it doesn't involve splitting a nucleus and doesn't have a web of proteins to pull chromosomes apart. Bacteria copy their DNA in a process called DNA replication, grow, and then the replicated DNA moves to either side, and two new cells are made.

There are two processes by which a eukaryotic cell can divide: mitosis and meiosis. In **mitosis,** the daughter cells produced from parental cell division are identical to each other and the parent. **Meiosis** produces genetically unique haploid cells due to two stages of cell division. Meiosis produces **haploid** cells, or **gametes** (sperm and egg cells), which only have one set of chromosomes. Humans are **diploid** because we have two sets of chromosomes – one from each parent. **Somatic** (body) cells are all diploid and are produced via mitosis.

Mitosis

Mitosis is the division of the genetic material in the nucleus of a cell, and is immediately followed by **cytokinesis,** which is the division of the cytoplasm of the cell. The two processes make up the mitotic phase of the cell cycle. Mitosis can be broken down into five stages: prophase, prometaphase, metaphase, anaphase, and telophase. Mitosis is preceded by **interphase**, where the cell spends the majority of its life while growing and replicating its DNA.

Prophase: During this phase, the mitotic spindles begin to form. They are made up of centrosomes and microtubules. As the microtubules lengthen, the centrosomes move farther away from each other. The nucleolus disappears and the chromatin fibers begin to coil up and form chromosomes. Two sister **chromatids**, which are two identical copies of one chromosome, are joined together at the centromere.

113

Prometaphase: The nuclear envelope begins to break down and the microtubules enter the nuclear area. Each pair of chromatin fibers develops a **kinetochore**, which is a specialized protein structure in the middle of the adjoined fibers. The chromosomes are further condensed.

Metaphase: The microtubules are stretched across the cell and the centrosomes are at opposite ends of the cell. The chromosomes align at the **metaphase plate**, which is a plane that is exactly between the two centrosomes. The centromere of each chromosome is attached to the kinetochore microtubules that are stretching from each centrosome to the metaphase plate.

Anaphase: The sister chromatids break apart, forming individual chromosomes. The two daughter chromosomes move to opposite ends of the cell. The microtubules shorten toward opposite ends of the cell as well. The cell elongates and, by the end of this phase, there is a complete set of chromosomes at each end of the cell.

Telophase: Two nuclei form at each end of the cell and nuclear envelopes begin to form around each nucleus. The nucleoli reappear and the chromosomes become less condensed. The microtubules are broken down by the cell and mitosis is complete.

Cytokinesis divides the cytoplasm by pinching off the cytoplasm, forming a cleavage furrow, and the two daughter cells then enter interphase, completing the cycle.

Plant cell mitosis is similar except that it lacks centromeres, and instead has a microtubule organizing center. Cytokinesis occurs with the formation of a cell plate.

Meiosis

Meiosis is a type of cell division in which the parent cell has twice as many sets of chromosomes as the daughter cells into which it divides. Although the first stage of meiosis involves the duplication of chromosomes, similar to that of mitosis, the parent cell in meiosis divides into four cells, as opposed to the two produced in mitosis.

Meiosis has the same phases as mitosis, except that they occur twice: once in meiosis I and again in meiosis II. The diploid parent has two sets of homologous chromosomes, one set from each parent. During meiosis I, each chromosome set goes through a process called **crossing over**, which jumbles up the genes on each chromatid. In anaphase one, the separated chromosomes are no longer identical and, once the chromosomes pull apart, each daughter cell is haploid (one set of chromosomes with two non-identical sister chromatids). Next, during meiosis II, the two intermediate daughter cells divide again, separating the chromatids, producing a total of four total haploid cells that each contains one set of chromosomes.

Genetics

Genetics is the study of heredity, which is the transmission of traits from one generation to the next, and hereditary variation. The chromosomes passed from parent to child contain hereditary information in the form of genes. Each gene has specific sequences of DNA that encode proteins, start pathways, and result in inherited traits. In the human life cycle, one haploid sperm cell joins one haploid egg cell to form a diploid cell. The diploid cell is the zygote, the first cell of the new organism, and from then on mitosis takes over and nine months later, there is a fully developed human that has billions of identical cells.

The monk Gregor Mendel is referred to as the father of genetics. In the 1860s, Mendel came up with one of the first models of inheritance, using peapods with different traits in the garden at his abbey to test his theory and develop his model. His model included three laws to determine which traits are inherited; his theories still apply today, after genetics has been studied more in depth.

> 1. The **Law of Dominance**: Each characteristic has two versions that can be inherited. The gene that encodes for the characteristic has two variations, or alleles, and one is dominant over the other.

> 2. The **Law of Segregation:** When two parent cells form daughter cells, the alleles segregate and each daughter cell only inherits one of the alleles from each parent.

> 3. The **Law of Independent Assortment:** Different traits are inherited independent of one another because in metaphase, the set of chromosomes line up in random fashion – mom's set of chromosomes do not line up all on the left or right, there is a random mix.

Organisms contain a **genotype** and a **phenotype**. The genotype is the DNA present in the cells that code for the genes, and the phenotype is the set of observable traits that are expressed. For example, a brown-eyed girl may have genes for both blue and brown eyes, but the actual physical trait expressed is brown eyes. So, the genotype is blue and brown eyes, but the phenotype is brown eyes.

Dominant and Recessive Traits

Each gene has two **alleles**, one inherited from each parent. **Dominant alleles** are noted in capital letters (A) and **recessive alleles** are noted in lower case letters (a). There are three possible combinations of alleles among dominant and recessive alleles: AA, Aa, and aa. If both alleles are identical, the individual is considered **homozygous**; if the two alleles have different sequences, the individual is considered **heterozygous**. In most genes, one allele is considered more dominant than the other and will mask the appearance of the less dominant, or recessive, allele when there is a heterozygous situation. Dominant alleles, when mixed with recessive alleles, will mask the recessive trait. The recessive trait would only appear as the phenotype when the allele combination is aa because a dominant allele is not present to mask it.

Although most genes follow the standard dominant/recessive rules, there are some genes that defy them. Examples include cases of co-dominance, multiple alleles, incomplete dominance, sex-linked traits, and polygenic inheritance.

In cases of **co-dominance**, both alleles are expressed equally. For example, blood type has three alleles: I^A, I^B, and i. I^A and I^B are both dominant to i, but co-dominant with each other. An $I^A I^B$ has AB blood. With incomplete dominance, the allele combination Aa actually makes a third phenotype. An example: certain flowers can be red (AA), white (aa), or pink (Aa).

Punnett Square

For simple genetic combinations, a **Punnett square** can be used to assess the phenotypes of subsequent generations. In a 2 x 2 cell square, one parent's alleles are set up in columns and the other parent's alleles are in rows. The resulting allele combinations are shown in the four internal cells.

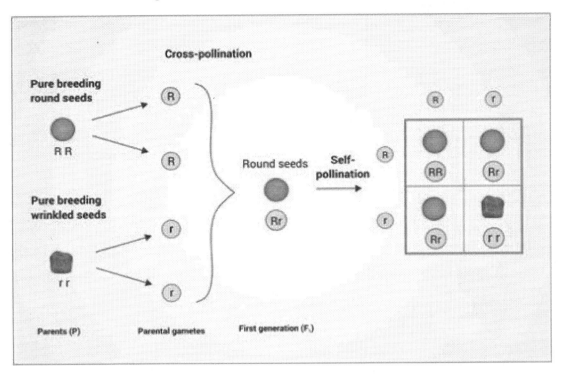

In the example above, two parents with alleles RR and rr, have a 50% chance (2 in 4) of having an offspring with alleles Rr.

Mutations

Genetic **mutations** occur when there is a permanent alteration in the DNA sequence that codes for a specific gene. They can be small, affecting only one base pair, or large, affecting many genes on a chromosome. Mutations are classified as either hereditary, which means they were also present in the parent gene, or acquired, meaning they occurred after the genes were passed down from the parents. Although mutations are not common, they are an important aspect of genetics and variation in the general population.

DNA

DNA is made of nucleotide, and contains the genetic information of a living organism. It consists of two polynucleotide strands that are twisted and linked together in a double-helix structure. The polynucleotide strands are made up of four nitrogenous bases: adenine (A), thymine (T), guanine (G), and cytosine (C). Adenine and guanine are purines while thymine and cytosine are pyrimidines. These bases have specific pairings of A with T, and G with C. The bases are ordered so that these specific pairings will occur when the two polynucleotide strands coil together to form a DNA molecule. The two strands of DNA are described as antiparallel because one strand runs 5' → 3' while the other strand of the helix runs 3' → 5'.

Before chromosome replication and cell division can occur, DNA replication must happen in interphase. There are specific base pair sequences on DNA, called origins of replication, where DNA replication begins. The proteins that begin the replication process attach to this site and begin separating the two strands and creating a replication bubble. Each end of the bubble has a replication fork, which is a Y-shaped area of the DNA that is being unwound. Several types of proteins are important to the beginning of DNA replication. **Helicases** are enzymes responsible for untwisting the two strands at the replication fork. Single-strand binding proteins bind to the separated strands so that they do not join back together during the replication process. While part of the DNA is unwound, the remainder of the molecule becomes even more twisted in response. Topoisomerase enzymes help relieve this strain by breaking, untwisting, and rejoining the DNA strands.

Once the DNA strand is unwound, an initial primer chain of RNA from the enzyme primase is made to start replication. Replication of DNA can only occur in the 5' → 3' direction. Therefore, during replication, one strand of the DNA template creates the leading strand in the 5' → 3' direction and the other strand creates the lagging strand. While the leading strand is created efficiently and in one piece, the lagging strand is generated in fragments, called **Okazaki fragments**, then are pieced together to form a complete strand by DNA ligase. Following the primer chain of RNA, DNA polymerases are the enzymes responsible for extending the DNA chains by adding on base pairs.

DNA forms the genetic code in the nucleus of eukaryotes, and RNA is the interpreter of that code. RNA exists in the following subtypes:

- **Messenger RNA (mRNA)** copies the DNA into a complementary transcript. This process is called **transcription**.

- **Ribosomal RNA (rRNA)** makes up the protein-making structure called the ribosome, which reads the transcript in a process called **translation**.

- **Transfer RNA (tRNA)** carries amino acids and delivers them to the ribosome. Each three letters of the mRNA transcript, or **codon**, recruits the anti-codon of a tRNA molecule that carries the corresponding amino acid.

Only when a **stop codon** is reached will the ribosome disassemble, thus releasing the assembled protein.

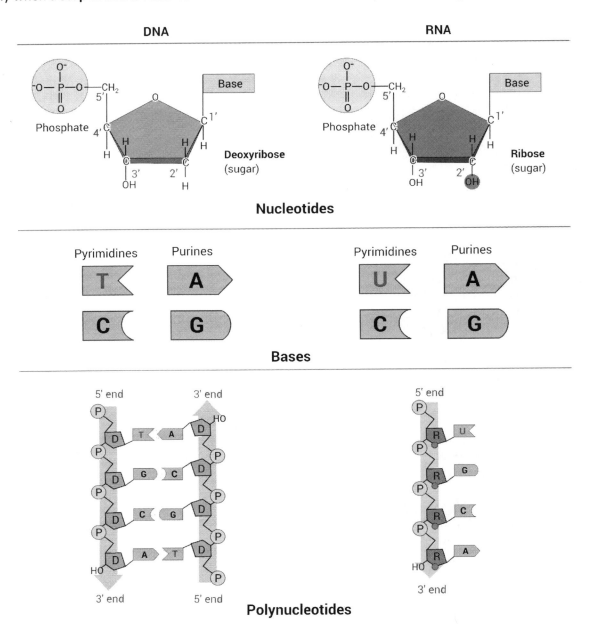

Nucleotides

Bases

Polynucleotides

Practice Quiz

1. What is an adaptation?
    a. The original traits found in a common ancestor
    b. Changes that occur in the environment
    c. When one species begins behaving like another species
    d. An inherited characteristic that enhances survival and reproduction

2. If a person with AB blood and a person with O blood have children, what is the probability that their children will have the same phenotype as either parent?
    a. 0%
    b. 25%
    c. 50%
    d. 75%

3. What organelle is the site of protein synthesis?
    a. Nucleus
    b. Smooth ER
    c. Ribosome
    d. Lysosome

4. Which of the following structures is unique to eukaryotic cells?
    a. Cell walls
    b. Nuclei
    c. Cell membranes
    d. Ribosomes

5. Which level of protein structure is defined by the folds and coils of the protein's polypeptide backbone?
    a. Primary
    b. Secondary
    c. Tertiary
    d. Quaternary

See answers on next page.

If you want to test your knowledge further on the biology section of the HESI exam, take our online practice quiz.

testprepbooks.com/hesi-quiz

119

Answer Explanations

1. D: Charles Darwin based the idea of adaptation around his original concept of natural selection. He believed that evolution occurred based on three observations: the unity of life, the diversity of life, and the suitability of organisms to their environments. There was unity in life based on the idea that all organisms descended from a common ancestor. Then, as the descendants of common ancestors faced changes in their environments or moved to new environments, they began adapting new features to help them. This concept explained the diversity of life and how organisms were matched to their environments. Natural selection helps to improve the fit between organisms and their environments by increasing the frequency of features that enhance survival and reproduction.

2. A: 0%. There is no chance that an offspring will be O blood or AB blood (see Punnett square).

	I^A	I^B
i	$I^A i$	$I^B i$
i	$I^A i$	$I^B i$

3. C: Proteins are synthesized on ribosomes. The ribosome uses messenger RNA as a template and transfer RNA brings amino acids to the ribosome where they are synthesized into peptide strands using the genetic code provided by the messenger RNA.

4. B: The structure exclusively found in eukaryotic cells is the nucleus. Animal, plant, fungi, and protist cells are all eukaryotic. DNA is contained within the nucleus of eukaryotic cells, and they also have membrane-bound organelles that perform complex intracellular metabolic activities. Prokaryotic cells (archaea and bacteria) do not have a nucleus or other membrane-bound organelles and are less complex than eukaryotic cells.

5. B: The secondary structure of a protein refers to the folds and coils that are formed by hydrogen bonding between the slightly charged atoms of the polypeptide backbone. The primary structure is the sequence of amino acids, similar to the letters in a long word. The tertiary structure is the overall shape of the molecule that results from the interactions between the side chains that are linked to the polypeptide backbone. The quaternary structure is the complete protein structure that occurs when a protein is made up of two or more polypeptide chains.

Chemistry

Scientific Notation, the Metric System, and Temperature Scales

Scientific Notation

Scientific notation is the conversion of extremely small or large numbers into a format that is easier to comprehend and manipulate. It changes the number into three separate parts: a mathematical sign (+/−), a digit term (known as a **significand**), and an exponential term.

$$Scientific\ notation = (+\ or\ -)\ significand \times exponential\ term$$

To put a number into scientific notation, one should use the following steps:

- Move the decimal point to after the first non-zero number to find the digit number.
- Count how many places the decimal point was moved in step 1.
- Determine if the exponent is positive or negative.
- Create an exponential term using the information from steps 2 and 3.
- Combine the digit term and exponential term to get scientific notation.

For example, to put 0.0000098 into scientific notation, the decimal should be moved so that it lies between the last two numbers: 000009.8. This creates the digit number:

$$9.8$$

Next, the number of places that the decimal point moved is determined; to get between the 9 and the 8, the decimal was moved six places to the right. It may be helpful to remember that a decimal moved to the right creates a negative exponent, and a decimal moved to the left creates a positive exponent. Because the decimal was moved six places to the right, the exponent is negative.

Now, the exponential term can be created by using the base 10 (this is *always* the base in scientific notation) and the number of places moved as the exponent, in this case:

$$10^{-6}$$

Finally, the digit term and the exponential term can be combined as a product. Therefore, the scientific notation for the number 0.0000098 is:

$$9.8 \times 10^{-6}$$

Standard vs. Metric Systems

The measuring system used today in the United States developed from the British units of measurement during colonial times. The most typically used units in this customary system are those used to measure weight, liquid volume, and length, whose common units are found below. In the customary system, the basic unit for measuring weight is the ounce (oz); there are 16 ounces (oz) in 1 pound (lb) and 2000 pounds in 1 ton. The basic unit for measuring liquid volume is the ounce (oz); 1 ounce is equal to 2 tablespoons (tbsp) or 6 teaspoons (tsp), and there are 8 ounces in 1 cup, 2 cups in 1 pint (pt), 2 pints in 1 quart (qt), and 4 quarts in 1 gallon (gal). For measurements of length, the inch (in) is the base unit; 12 inches make up 1 foot (ft), 3 feet make up 1 yard (yd), and 5280 feet make up 1 mile (mi). However, as there are only a set number of units in the customary system, with extremely large or extremely small amounts of material, the numbers can become awkward and difficult to compare.

Common Customary Measurements		
Length	**Weight**	**Capacity**
1 foot = 12 inches	1 pound = 16 ounces	1 cup = 8 fluid ounces
1 yard = 3 feet	1 ton = 2,000 pounds	1 pint = 2 cups
1 yard = 36 inches		1 quart = 2 pints
1 mile = 1,760 yards		1 quart = 4 cups
1 mile = 5,280 feet		1 gallon = 4 quarts
		1 gallon = 16 cups

Aside from the United States, most countries in the world have adopted the **metric system** embodied in the International System of Units (SI). The three main SI base units used in the metric system are the meter (m), the gram (g), and the liter (L); meters measure length, grams measure mass, and liters measure volume. These are known as the **basic units of measure.**

These three units can use different **prefixes**, which indicate larger or smaller versions of the unit by powers of ten. This can be thought of as making a new unit, which is sized by multiplying the original unit in size by a factor.

These prefixes and associated factors are:

Metric Prefixes			
Prefix	**Symbol**	**Multiplier**	**Exponential**
kilo	k	1,000	10^3
hecto	h	100	10^2
deca	da	10	10^1
no prefix		1	10^0
deci	d	0.1	10^{-1}
centi	c	0.01	10^{-2}
milli	m	0.001	10^{-3}

The correct prefix is then attached to the base. Some examples:

1 milliliter equals .001 liters.

1 kilogram equals 1,000 grams.

Some units of measure are represented as square or cubic units depending on the solution. For example, perimeter is measured in linear units, area is measured in square units, and volume is measured in cubic units.

Also be sure to use the most appropriate unit for the thing being measured. A building's height might be measured in feet or meters while the length of a nail might be measured in inches or centimeters. Additionally, for SI units, the prefix should be chosen to provide the most succinct available value. For

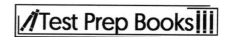

example, the mass of a bag of fruit would likely be measured in kilograms rather than grams or milligrams, and the length of a bacteria cell would likely be measured in micrometers rather than centimeters or kilometers.

Temperature Scales

There are three main temperature scales used in science. The scale most often used in the United States is the **Fahrenheit** scale. This scale is based on the measurement of water freezing at 32°F and water boiling at 212°F. The **Celsius** scale uses 0°C as the temperature for water freezing and 100°C for water boiling. The Celsius scale is the most widely used in the scientific community. The Celsius scale is the most widely used in the scientific community. The accepted measurement by the International System of Units (from the French Système international d'unités), or SI, for temperature is the Kelvin scale. This is the scale employed in thermodynamics, since its zero is the basis for absolute zero, or the unattainable temperature, when matter no longer exhibits degradation.

The conversions between the temperature scales are as follows:

°Fahrenheit to °Celsius: $°C = \frac{5}{9}(°F - 32)$

°Celsius to °Fahrenheit: $°F = \frac{9}{5}(°C) + 32$

°Celsius to Kelvin: $K = °C + 273.15$

Accuracy and Precision

For a hypothesis to be proven true or false, all experiments are subject to multiple trials in order to verify accuracy and precision. A measurement is **accurate** if the observed value is close to the "true value." For example, if someone measured the pH of water at 6.9, this measurement would be considered accurate (the pH of water is 7). On the other hand, a measurement is **precise** if the measurements are consistent—that is, if they are reproducible. If someone had a series of values for a pH of water that were 6.9, 7.0, 7.2, and 7.3, their measurements would not be precise. However, if all measured values were 6.9, or the average of these values was 6.9 with a small range, then their measurements would be precise. Measurements can fall into the following categories:

- Both accurate and precise
- Accurate but not precise
- Precise but not accurate
- Neither accurate nor precise

Atomic Structure and the Periodic Table

Atomic Structure

The structure of an atom has two major components: the atomic nucleus and the atomic shells (also known as **orbitals**). The **nucleus** is found in the center of an atom. The three major subatomic particles are protons, neutrons, and electrons and are found in the atomic nucleus and shells.

Protons are found in the atomic nucleus and are positively charged particles. The addition or removal of protons from an atom's nucleus creates an entirely different element. **Neutrons** are also found in the atomic nucleus and are neutral particles, meaning they have no net electrical charge. The addition or removal of neutrons from an atom's nucleus does not create a different element but instead creates a lighter or heavier form of that element called an isotope. **Electrons** are found orbiting in the atomic shells around the nucleus and are negatively charged particles. A proton or a neutron has nearly 2,000 times the mass of an electron.

Electrons orbit the nucleus in **atomic shells,** or **electron clouds**, each of which can accommodate a certain number of electrons. For example, the first atomic shell can accommodate two electrons, the second atomic shell can hold a maximum of eight electrons, and the third atomic shell can house a maximum of eight electrons. The negatively charged electrons orbiting the nucleus are attracted to the positively charged protons in the nucleus via electromagnetic force. The attraction of opposite electrical charges gives rise to chemical bonds, which refers to the ways atoms are attached to each other.

The **atomic number** of an atom is determined by the number of protons within the nucleus. When a substance is composed of atoms that all have the same atomic number, it is called an **element**. Elements are arranged by atomic number and grouped by properties in the **Periodic table.**

An atom's **mass number** is determined by the sum of the total number of protons and neutrons in the atom. Most nuclei have a net neutral charge, and all atoms of one type have the same atomic number. However, there are some atoms of the same type that have a different mass number, due to an imbalance of neutrons. These are called **isotopes**. In isotopes, the atomic number, which is determined

124

by the number of protons, is the same, but the mass number, which is determined by adding the protons and neutrons, is different due to the irregular number of neutrons.

An atom can gain a charge by having greater or fewer electrons than protons, and any atom with a charge is referred to as an **ion**. If an ion has more electrons than protons, it has a negative charge and is an **anion**. If an atom has fewer electrons than protons, it has a positive charge and is a **cation**.

Chemical Bonding

Chemical bonding typically results in the formation of a new substance, called a **compound**. Only the electrons in the outermost atomic shell are able to form chemical bonds. These electrons are known as **valence electrons**, and they are what determines the chemical properties of an atom.

Chemical bonding occurs between two or more atoms that are joined together. There are three types of chemical bonds: ionic, covalent, and metallic. The characteristics of the different bonds are determined by how electrons behave in a compound. **Lewis structures** were developed to help visualize the electrons in molecules; they are a method of writing a compound structure formula and including its electron composition. A Lewis symbol for an element consists of the element symbol and a dot for each valence electron. The dots are located on all four sides of the symbol, with a maximum of two dots per side, and eight dots, or electrons, total. The octet rule states that atoms tend to gain, lose, or share electrons until they have a total of eight valence electrons.

Ionic bonds are formed from the electrostatic attractions between oppositely charged atoms. They result from the transfer of electrons from a metal on the left side of the periodic table to a nonmetal on the right side. The metallic substance often has low ionization energy and will transfer an electron easily to the nonmetal, which has a high electron affinity. An example of this is the compound NaCl, which is sodium chloride or table salt, where the Na atom transfers an electron to the Cl atom. Due to strong bonding, ionic compounds have several distinct characteristics. They have high melting and boiling points and are brittle and crystalline. They are arranged in rigid, well-defined structures, which allow them to break apart along smooth, flat surfaces. The formation of ionic bonds is a reaction that is exothermic. In the opposite scenario, the energy it takes to break up a one mole quantity of an ionic compound is referred to as lattice energy, which is generally endothermic. The Lewis structure for NaCl is written as follows:

$$Na + \cdot \overset{\cdot \cdot}{\underset{\cdot \cdot}{Cl}} : \rightarrow Na^+ + : \overset{\cdot \cdot}{\underset{\cdot \cdot}{Cl}} :^-$$

Covalent bonds are formed when two atoms share electrons, instead of transferring them as in ionic compounds. The atoms in covalent compounds have a balance of attraction and repulsion between their protons and electrons, which keeps them bonded together. Two atoms can be joined by single, double, or even triple covalent bonds. As the number of electrons that are shared increases, the length of the bond decreases. Covalent substances have low melting and boiling points and are poor conductors of heat and electricity.

The Lewis structure for Cl_2 is written as follows:

Metallic bonds are formed by electrons that move freely through metal. They are the product of the force of attraction between electrons and metal ions. The electrons are shared by many metal cations and act like glue that holds the metallic substance together, similar to the attraction between oppositely-charged atoms in ionic substances, except the electrons are more fluid and float around the bonded metals and form a sea of electrons. Metallic compounds have characteristic properties that include strength, conduction of heat and electricity, and malleability. They can conduct electricity by passing energy through the freely moving electrons, creating a **current**. These compounds also have high melting and boiling points. Lewis structures are not common for metallic structures because of the free-roaming ability of the electrons.

Periodic Table

The periodic table catalogues all of the elements known to man, currently 118. It is one of the most important references in the science of chemistry. Information that can be gathered from the periodic table includes the element's atomic number, atomic mass, and chemical symbol. The first periodic table was rendered by Mendeleev in the mid-1800s and was ordered according to increasing atomic mass. The modern periodic table is arranged in order of increasing atomic number. It is also arranged in horizontal rows known as **periods,** and vertical columns known as **families,** or **groups**. The periodic table contains seven periods and eighteen families. Elements in the periodic table can also be classified into three major groups: metals, metalloids, and nonmetals. **Metals** are concentrated on the left side of the periodic table, while **nonmetals** are found on the right side. **Metalloids** occupy the area between the metals and nonmetals.

Due to the fact the periodic table is ordered by increasing atomic number, the electron configurations of the elements show periodicity. As the atomic number increases, electrons gradually fill the shells of an atom. In general, the start of a new period corresponds to the first time an electron inhabits a new shell.

Periodic Table of the Elements

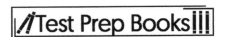

Other trends in the properties of elements in the periodic table are:

Atomic radius: One-half the distance between the nuclei of atoms of the same element.

Electronegativity: A measurement of the tendency of an atom to form a chemical bond.

Ionization energy: The amount of energy needed to remove an electron from a gas or ion.

Electron affinity: The ability of an atom to accept an electron.

Trends in the Periodic Table

Chemical Equations

Chemical reactions are represented by **chemical equations**. The equations help to explain how the molecules change during the reaction. For example, when hydrogen gas (H_2) combines with oxygen gas (O_2), two molecules of water are formed. The equation is written as follows, where the "+" sign means *reacts with* and the "→" means *produces*:

$$2H_2 + O_2 \rightarrow 2H_2O$$

128

Two hydrogen molecules react with an oxygen molecule to produce two water molecules. In all chemical equations, the quantity of each element on the reactant side of the equation should equal the quantity of the same element on the product side of the equation due to the law of conservation of matter. If this is true, the equation is described as balanced. To figure out how many of each element there is on each side of the equation, the coefficient of the element should be multiplied by the subscript next to the element. Coefficients and subscripts are noted for quantities larger than one. The **coefficient** is the number located directly to the left of the element. The **subscript** is the small-sized number directly to the right of the element.

In the previous equation, on the left side, the coefficient of the hydrogen is two and the subscript is also two, which makes a total of four hydrogen atoms. Using the same method, there are two oxygen atoms. On the right side, the coefficient two is multiplied by the subscript in each element of the water molecule, making four hydrogen atoms and two oxygen atoms. This equation is balanced because there are four hydrogen atoms and two oxygen atoms on each side. The states of the reactants and products can also be written in the equation: gas (g), liquid (l), solid (s), and dissolved in water (aq). If they are included, they are noted in parentheses on the right side of each molecule in the equation.

Reaction Rates, Equilibrium, and Reversibility

Chemical reactions are conveyed using chemical equations. Chemical equations must be balanced with equivalent numbers of atoms for each type of element on each side of the equation. Antoine Lavoisier, a French chemist, was the first to propose the **Law of Conservation of Mass** for the purpose of balancing a chemical equation. The law states, "Matter is neither created nor destroyed during a chemical reaction."

The **reactants** are located on the left side of the arrow, while the **products** are located on the right side of the arrow. Coefficients are the numbers in front of the chemical formulas. Subscripts are the numbers to the lower right of chemical symbols in a formula. To tally atoms, one should multiply the formula's coefficient by the subscript of each chemical symbol. For example, the chemical equation $2\ H_2 + O_2 \rightarrow 2H_2O$ is balanced. For H, the coefficient of 2 multiplied by the subscript 2=4 hydrogen atoms. For O, the coefficient of 1 multiplied by the subscript 2=2 oxygen atoms. Coefficients and subscripts of 1 are understood and never written.

States of Matter and Factors that Affect Phase Changes

Matter is most commonly found in three distinct states or phases: solid, liquid, and gas. A solid has a distinct shape and a defined volume. A liquid has a more loosely defined shape and a definite volume, while a gas has no definite shape or volume. The *Kinetic Theory of Matter* states that matter is composed of a large number of small particles (specifically, atoms and molecules) that are in constant motion. The distance between the separations in these particles determines the state of the matter: solid, liquid, or gas. In gases, the particles have a large separation and no attractive forces. In liquids, there is moderate separation between particles and some attractive forces to form a loose shape. Solids have almost no separation between their particles, causing a defined and set shape. The constant movement of particles causes them to bump into each other, thus allowing the particles to transfer energy between each other. This bumping and transferring of energy helps explain the transfer of heat and the relationship between pressure, volume, and temperature.

The *Ideal Gas Law* states that pressure, volume, and temperature are all related through the equation: $PV=nRT$, where P is pressure, V is volume, n is the amount of the substance in moles, R is the gas constant, and T is temperature.

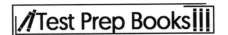

Through this relationship, volume and pressure are both proportional to temperature, but pressure is inversely proportional to volume. Therefore, if the equation is balanced, and the volume decreases in the system, pressure needs to proportionately increase to keep both sides of the equation balanced. In contrast, if the equation is unbalanced and the pressure increases, then the temperature would also increase, since pressure and temperature are directly proportional.

When pressure, temperature, or volume change in matter, a change in state can occur. Changes in state include solid to liquid (melting), liquid to gas (evaporation), solid to gas (sublimation), gas to solid (deposition), gas to liquid (condensation), and liquid to solid (freezing). There is one other state of matter called *plasma*, which is seen in lightning, television screens, and neon lights. Plasma is most commonly converted from the gas state at extremely high temperatures.

The amount of energy needed to change matter from one state to another is labeled by the terms for phase changes. For example, the temperature needed to supply enough energy for matter to change from a liquid to a gas is called the *heat of vaporization*. When heat is added to matter in order to cause a change in state, there will be an increase in temperature until the matter is about to change its state. During its transition, all of the added heat is used by the matter to change its state, so there is no increase in temperature. Once the transition is complete, then the added heat will again yield an increase in temperature.

Reaction Rates

The rate of a reaction is the measure of the change in concentration of the reactants or products over a certain period of time. Many factors affect how fast or slow a reaction occurs, such as concentration, pressure, or temperature. As the concentration of a reactant increases, the rate of the reaction also increases, because the frequency of collisions between elements increases. High-pressure situations for reactants that are gases cause the gas to compress and increase the frequency of gas molecule collisions, similar to solutions with higher concentrations. Reactions rates are then increased with the higher frequency of gas molecule collisions. Higher temperatures usually increase the rate of the reaction, adding more energy to the system with heat and increasing the frequency of molecular collisions.

Equilibrium

Equilibrium is described as the state of a system when no net changes occur. Chemical equilibrium occurs when opposing reactions occur at equal rates. In other words, the rate of reactants forming products is equal to the rate of the products breaking down into the reactants — the concentration of reactants and products in the system doesn't change. This happens in **reversible chemical reactions** as opposed to irreversible chemical reactions. In **irreversible chemical reactions**, the products cannot be changed back to reactants. Although the concentrations are not changing in equilibrium, the forward and reverse reactions are likely still occurring. This type of equilibrium is called a **dynamic equilibrium**. In situations where all reactions have ceased, a **static equilibrium** is reached. Chemical equilibriums are also described as homogeneous or heterogeneous. **Homogeneous equilibrium** involves substances that are all in the same phase, while **heterogeneous equilibrium** means the substances are in different phases when equilibrium is reached.

When a reaction reaches equilibrium, the conditions of the equilibrium are described by the following equation, based on the chemical equation $aA + bB \leftrightarrow cC + dD$:

Catalysts are substances that accelerate the speed of a chemical reaction. A catalyst remains unchanged throughout the course of a chemical reaction. In most cases, only small amounts of a catalyst are needed. Catalysts increase the rate of a chemical reaction by providing an alternate path requiring less activation energy. Activation energy refers to the amount of energy required for the initiation of a chemical reaction.

Catalysts can be homogeneous or heterogeneous. Catalysts in the same phase of matter as its reactants are homogeneous, while catalysts in a different phase than reactants are heterogeneous. It is important to remember catalysts are selective. They don't accelerate the speed of all chemical reactions, but catalysts do accelerate specific chemical reactions.

Solutions and Solution Concentrations

A homogeneous mixture, also called a **solution,** has uniform properties throughout a given sample. An example of a homogeneous solution is salt (the **solute,** or what is being dissolved) fully dissolved in warm water (the **solvent,** the material dissolving the solute). In this example, salt is the **solute,** or the material being dissolved, and water is the **solvent,** or the material dissolving the solute. In this case, any number of samples taken from the parent solution would be identical.

One **mole** is the amount of matter contained in 6.02×10^{23} of any object, such as atoms, ions, or molecules. It is a useful unit of measure for items in large quantities. This number is also known as **Avogadro's number.** One mole of ^{12}C atoms is equivalent to 6.02×10^{23} ^{12}C atoms. Avogadro's number is often written as an inverse mole, or as $6.02 \times 10^{23}/mol$.

Molarity is the concentration of a solution. It is based on the number of moles of solute in one liter of solution and is written as the capital letter M. A 1.0 molar solution, or 1.0 M solution, has one mole of solute per liter of solution. The molarity of a solution can be determined by calculating the number of moles of the solute and dividing it by the volume of the solution in liters. The resulting number is the mol/L or M for molarity of the solution. Alternatively, **percent concentration** can be written as parts of solute per 100 parts of solvent.

Chemical Reactions

Chemical reactions are characterized by a chemical change in which the starting substances, or reactants, differ from the substances formed, or products. Chemical reactions may involve a change in color, the production of gas, the formation of a precipitate, or changes in heat content. The following are the basic types of chemical reactions:

- **Decomposition Reactions:** A compound is broken down into smaller elements. For example, $2H_2O \rightarrow 2H_2 + O_2$. This is read as, "2 molecules of water decompose into 2 molecules of hydrogen and 1 molecule of oxygen."

- **Synthesis Reactions:** Two or more elements or compounds are joined together. For example, $2H_2 + O_2 \rightarrow 2H_2O$. This is read as, "2 molecules of hydrogen react with 1 molecule of oxygen to produce 2 molecules of water."

- **Single Displacement Reactions:** A single element or ion takes the place of another element in a compound. It is also known as a substitution reaction. For example, $Zn + 2HCl \rightarrow ZnCl_2 + H_2$. This is read as, "zinc reacts with 2 molecules of hydrochloric acid to produce one molecule of zinc chloride and one molecule of hydrogen." In other words, zinc replaces the hydrogen in hydrochloric acid.

- **Double Displacement Reactions:** Two elements or ions exchange a single element to form two different compounds, resulting in different combinations of cations and anions in the final compounds. It is also known as a metathesis reaction. For example, $H_2SO_4 + 2NaOH \rightarrow Na_2SO_4 + 2H_2O$

  - Special types of double displacement reactions include:

    - **Oxidation-Reduction (or Redox) Reactions:** Elements undergo a change in oxidation number. For example, $2S_2O_3{}^{2-}$ (aq) $+ I_2$ (aq) $\rightarrow S_4O_6{}^{2-}$ (aq) $+ 2I^-$ (aq).

    - **Acid-Base Reactions:** Involves a reaction between an acid and a base, which produces a salt and water. For example, $HBr + NaOH \rightarrow NaBr + H_2O$.

    - **Combustion Reactions:** A hydrocarbon (a compound composed of only hydrogen and carbon) reacts with oxygen (O_2) to form carbon dioxide (CO_2) and water (H_2O). For example, $CH_4 + 2O_2 \rightarrow CO_2 + 2H_2O$.

Stoichiometry

Stoichiometry investigates the quantities of chemicals that are consumed and produced in chemical reactions. Chemical equations are made up of reactants and products; stoichiometry helps elucidate how the changes from reactants to products occur, as well as how to ensure the equation is balanced.

Chemical reactions are limited by the amount of starting material, or reactants, available to drive the process forward. The reactant that has the smallest amount of substance is called the limiting reactant. The **limiting reactant** is completely consumed by the end of the reaction. The other reactants are called **excess reactants**. For example, gasoline is used in a combustion reaction to make a car move and is the limiting reactant of the reaction. If the gasoline runs out, the combustion reaction can no longer take place, and the car stops.

The quantity of product that should be produced after using up all of the limiting reactant can be calculated and is called the **theoretical yield of the reaction**. Since the reactants do not always act as they should, the actual amount of resulting product is called the **actual yield**. The actual yield is divided by the theoretical yield and then multiplied by 100 to find the **percent yield** for the reaction.

Solution stoichiometry deals with quantities of solutes in chemical reactions that occur in solutions. The quantity of a solute in a solution can be calculated by multiplying the molarity of the solution by the volume. Similar to chemical equations involving simple elements, the number of moles of the elements that make up the solute should be equivalent on both sides of the equation.

When the concentration of a particular solute in a solution is unknown, a **titration** is used to determine that concentration. In a titration, the solution with the unknown solute is combined with a standard solution, which is a solution with a known solute concentration. The point at which the unknown solute has completely reacted with the known solute is called the **equivalence point**. Using the known information about the standard solution, including the concentration and volume, and the volume of the unknown solution, the concentration of the unknown solute is determined in a balanced equation. For example, in the case of combining acids and bases, the equivalence point is reached when the resulting solution is neutral. HCl, an acid, combines with NaOH, a base, to form water, which is neutral, and a solution of Cl^- ions and Na^+ ions. Before the equivalence point, there are an unequal number of cations and anions and the solution is not neutral.

Oxidation and Reduction

Oxidation and reduction reactions, also known as **redox reactions**, are those in which electrons are transferred from one element to another. Batteries and fuel cells are two energy-related technologies that utilize these reactions. When an atom, ion, or molecule loses its electrons and becomes more positively charged, it is described as being oxidized. When a substance gains electrons and becomes more negatively charged, it is reduced. In chemical reactions, if one element or molecule is oxidized, another must be reduced for the equation to be balanced. Although the transfer of electrons is obvious in some reactions where ions are formed, redox reactions also include those in which electrons are transferred but the products remain neutral.

Keep track of oxidation states or oxidation numbers to ensure the chemical equation is balanced. **Oxidation numbers** are assigned to each atom in a neutral substance or ion. For ions made up of a single atom, the oxidation number is equal to the charge of the ion. For atoms in their original elemental form, the oxidation number is always zero. Each hydrogen atom in an H_2 molecule, for example, has an oxidation number of zero. The sum of the oxidation numbers in a molecule should be equal to the overall charge of the molecule. If the molecule is a positively charged ion, the sum of the oxidation number should be equal to overall positive charge of the molecule. In ionic compounds that have a cation and anion joined, the sum of the oxidation numbers should equal zero.

All chemical equations must have the same number of elements on each side of the equation to be balanced. Redox reactions have an extra step of counting the electrons on both sides of the equation to be balanced. Separating redox reactions into oxidation reactions and reduction reactions is a simple way to account for all of the electrons involved. The individual equations are known as **half-reactions**. The number of electrons lost in the oxidation reaction must be equal to the number of electrons gained in the reduction reaction for the redox reaction to be balanced.

The oxidation of tin (Sn) by iron (Fe) can be balanced by the following half-reactions:

Oxidation: $Sn^{2+} \rightarrow Sn^{4+} + 2e^-$

Reduction: $2Fe^{3+} + 2e^- \rightarrow 2Fe^{2+}$

Complete redox reaction: $Sn^{2+} + 2Fe^{3+} \rightarrow Sn^{4+} + 2Fe^{2+}$

Acids and Bases

Acids and bases are defined in many different ways. An **acid** can be described as a substance that increases the concentration of H^+ ions when it is dissolved in water, as a proton donor in a chemical equation, or as an electron-pair acceptor. A **base** can be a substance that increases the concentration of

133

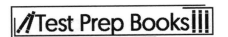
OH^- ions when it is dissolved in water, accepts a proton in a chemical reaction, or is an electron-pair donor.

pH refers to the power or potential of hydrogen atoms and is used as a scale for a substance's acidity. In chemistry, pH represents the hydrogen ion concentration (written as $[H^+]$) in an aqueous, or watery, solution. The hydrogen ion concentration, $[H^+]$, is measured in moles of H^+ per liter of solution.

The pH scale is a logarithmic scale used to quantify how acidic or basic a substance is. pH is the negative logarithm of the hydrogen ion concentration: $pH=-\log[H^+]$. A one-unit change in pH correlates with a ten-fold change in hydrogen ion concentration. The pH scale typically ranges from zero to 14, although it is possible to have pHs outside of this range. Pure water has a pH of 7, which is considered **neutral**. pH values less than 7 are considered **acidic**, while pH values greater than 7 are considered **basic**, or **alkaline**.

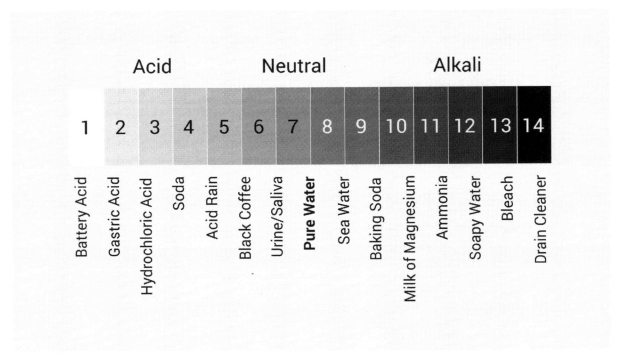

Generally speaking, an acid is a substance capable of donating hydrogen ions, while a base is a substance capable of accepting hydrogen ions. A **buffer** is a molecule that can act as either a hydrogen ion donor or acceptor. Buffers are crucial in the blood and body fluids, and prevent the body's pH from fluctuating into dangerous territory. pH can be measured using a pH meter, test paper, or indicator sticks.

Water can act as either an acid or a base. When mixed with an acid, water can accept a proton and become an H_3O^+ ion. When mixed with a base, water can donate a proton and become an OH^- ion. Sometimes water molecules donate and accept protons from each other; this process is called **autoionization**. The chemical equation is written as follows: $H_2O + H_2O \rightarrow OH^- + H_3O^+$.

Acids and bases are characterized as strong, weak, or somewhere in between. Strong acids and bases completely or almost completely ionize in aqueous solution. The chemical reaction is driven completely forward, to the right side of the equation, where the acidic or basic ions are formed. Weak acids and bases do not completely disassociate in aqueous solution. They only partially ionize and the solution becomes a mixture of the acid or base, water, and the acidic or basic ions. Strong acids are complemented by weak bases, and vice versa. A **conjugate acid** is an ion that forms when its base pair gains a proton. For example, the conjugate acid NH_4^+ is formed from the base NH_3. The **conjugate base** that pairs with an acid is the ion that is formed when an acid loses a proton. NO_2^- is the conjugate base of the acid HNO_2.

Nuclear Chemistry

Nuclear chemistry is the study of reactions in which the nuclei of atoms are transformed and their identities are changed. These reactions can involve large changes in energy—much larger than the energy changes that occur when chemical bonds between atoms are made or broken. Nuclear chemistry is also used to create electricity.

Nuclear reactions are described by nuclear equations, which have different notations than regular chemical equations. Nuclear equations are written as follows, with the top number being the **atomic mass** and the bottom number being the atomic number for each element:

$$^{238}_{92}U \longrightarrow {}^{234}_{90}Th + {}^{4}_{2}He$$

The equation describes the spontaneous decomposition of uranium into thorium and helium via alpha decay. When this happens, the process is referred to as nuclear decay. Similar to chemical equations, nuclear equations must be balanced on each side; the sum of the mass numbers and the sum of the atomic numbers should be equal on both sides of the equation.

In some cases, the nucleus of an atom is unstable and constantly emits particles due to this instability. These atoms are described as radioactive and the isotopes are referred to as **radioisotopes.** There are three types of radioactive decay that occur most frequently: alpha (α), beta (β), and gamma (γ). **Alpha radiation** is emitted when a nucleus releases a stream of alpha particles, which are helium-4 nuclei. **Beta radiation** occurs when a stream of high-speed electrons is emitted by an unstable nucleus. The beta particles are often noted as β^-. **Gamma radiation** occurs when the nucleus emits high-energy photons. In gamma radiation, the atomic number and the mass remain the same for the unstable nucleus. This type of radiation represents a rearrangement of an unstable nucleus into a more stable one and often accompanies other types of radioactive emission. **Radioactive decay** is often described in terms of its half-life, which is the time that it takes for half of the radioactive substance to react. For example, the radioisotope strontium-90 has a half-life of 28.8 years. If there are 10 grams of strontium-90 to start with, after 28.8 years, there would be 5 grams left.

There are two distinct types of nuclear reactions: fission and fusion reactions. Both involve a large energy release. In **fission** reactions, a large atom is split into two or more smaller atoms. The nucleus absorbs slow-moving neutrons, resulting in a larger nucleus that is unstable. The unstable nucleus then undergoes fission. Nuclear power plants depend on nuclear fission reactions for energy. **Fusion** reactions involve the combination of two or more lighter atoms into a larger atom. Fusion reactions do not occur in Earth's nature due to the extreme temperature and pressure conditions required to make

135

them happen. Fusion products are generally not radioactive. Fusion reactions are responsible for the energy that is created by the Sun.

Biochemistry

Biochemistry deals with the chemistry of organisms. There are four classes of macromolecules that allow organisms to exist: carbohydrates, lipids, proteins, and nucleic acids. Carbon is the backbone of these organic molecules because of its ability to form up to four covalent bonds.

Carbon (C), hydrogen (H), oxygen (O), nitrogen (N), sulfur (S), and phosphorus (P) are the most prevalent elements in these biological molecules. The following chart gives an overview of each organic molecule.

Organic Molecule	Example	Monomer (smallest repeating unit)	Structure	Function
Carbohydrate	• Sugar • Cellulose	Monosaccharide	Glucose Fructose Galactose	• Energy • Structure
Protein	• Actin • Insulin	Amino Acid		• Structure • Support • Some hormones
Lipid	• Fat • Oil	Technically none because the glycerol and fatty acids are not repeating.	Glycerol Triglyceride-Saturated	• Long-term energy • Steroid Hormones • Cell membranes

136

Organic Molecule	Example	Monomer (smallest repeating unit)	Structure	Function
Nucleic Acid	• DNA • RNA	Nucleotide	Phosphate group NITROGENOUS BASE (e.g. Adenine) SUGAR (Deoxyribose or Ribose)	• Genetic code • Makes Protein

Carbohydrates

Carbohydrates are usually sweet, ring-like sugar molecules that are built from carbon (carbo-), oxygen, and hydrogen (-hydrates, meaning water). They can exist as one-ring **monosaccharides,** like glucose, fructose, and galactose, or as two-ring **disaccharides**, like lactose, maltose, and sucrose. These simple sugars can be easily broken down and used via glycolysis to provide a source of quick energy. **Polysaccharides** are repeating chains of monosaccharide rings. They are more complex carbohydrates, and there are several types. For example:

- Plants store energy in the form of **starch**.
- Animals store energy in the form of **glycogen**. Vertebrates store glycogen in the liver and muscles.
- **Cellulose** is the chief structural component of plant cell walls.
- **Chitin** is the chief structural component of fungi cell walls and the exoskeletons of arthropods.

Glycolysis is an essential metabolic pathway that converts glucose to pyruvate and allows for cellular respiration to occur. It does not require oxygen to be present. Glucose is a common molecule used for energy production in cells. During glycolysis, two three-carbon sugars are generated from the splitting of a glucose molecule. These smaller sugars are then converted into pyruvate molecules via oxidation and atom rearrangement. Glycolysis requires two ATP molecules to drive the process forward, but the end product of the process has four ATP molecules, for a net production of two ATP molecules. Also, two reduced nicotinamide adenine dinucleotide (NADH) molecules are created from when the electron carrier oxidized nicotinamide adenine dinucleotide (NAD +) peels off two electrons and a hydrogen atom.

Proteins

Proteins are composed of chains of amino acids. There are several different kinds.

Enzymes catalyze chemical reactions in the body.

Storage proteins like albumin in eggs are important for development.

Hormonal proteins are responsible for initiating signal transduction cascades that regulate gene expression.

Motor proteins like actin and myosin are responsible for movement.

Immune proteins like antibodies and antigens are important for fighting disease.

Transport proteins like channel proteins and protein pumps move molecules.

Receptor proteins receive chemical messages like neurotransmitters.

Marker proteins serve as a cell's identification or fingerprint that distinguishes between cells of different types and sources.

Structural proteins like keratin are important for things like spider webs, hair, and feathers.

All proteins are made from a combination of some of all of the same 20 amino acids. The varying amino acids are linked by **peptide bonds** and form the primary structure of the polypeptide, or chain of amino acids. The primary structure is just the string of amino acids. It is the secondary, tertiary, and quaternary structure that determines protein shape and function. The secondary structure can be beta sheets or alpha helices formed by hydrogen bonding between the polar regions of the polypeptide backbone. Tertiary structure results from the interactions between the side chains. Quaternary structure is the overall protein structure that occurs when subunits merge, take the correct shape, and become functional.

The process of breaking down proteins to produce glucose is **gluconeogenesis.**

Lipids

Lipids are mostly nonpolar, hydrophobic molecules that are not soluble in water. **Triglycerides** are a type of lipid with a glycerol backbone attached to three long fatty acid chains.

Phospholipids are also composed of glycerol except they have two fatty acid tails. The third tail is replaced with a hydrophilic phosphate group. The amphipathic nature of this molecule results in a lipid bilayer where the "water-loving" hydrophilic heads face the extracellular matrix and cytoplasm and the "water-hating" hydrophobic tails face each other on the inside.

138

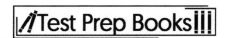

Steroids are another type of lipid. Cholesterol is a steroid that is embedded in animal cell membranes and acts as a fluidity buffer. Steroid hormones such as testosterone and estrogen are responsible for transcriptional regulation in certain cells.

Nucleic acids

Nucleic acids are made of **nucleotides**. Nucleotides consist of a five-carbon sugar, a nitrogen-containing base, and a phosphate group. Deoxyribonucleic acid (DNA) exists as two nucleotide chains arranged in a double helix. Each **deoxyribose** sugar is connected to a nitrogenous base and an electrically-negative phosphate group. The nitrogenous bases are adenine and guanine, the two-ringed purines, and cytosine and thymine, the one-ringed pyrimidines. The double helix is held together by weak hydrogen bonds that connect adenine to thymine and cytosine to guanine. Ribonucleic acid (RNA) has a slightly different structure. It is usually single-stranded, has a **ribose** sugar as opposed to deoxyribose, and contains uracil instead of thymine.

Practice Quiz

1. Which of the following shows the correct order of strength of intermolecular bonds?
    a. London dispersion > hydrogen > dipole-dipole
    b. Hydrogen > London dispersion > dipole-dipole
    c. London dispersion > dipole-dipole > hydrogen
    d. Hydrogen > dipole-dipole > London dispersion

2. Which property of liquids describes how water defies gravity to move upward from the root of a plant through the stem and into the leaves?
    a. Capillary action
    b. Surface tension
    c. High vapor pressure
    d. Solubility

3. Which element's atoms have the greatest number of electrons?
    a. Hydrogen
    b. Iron
    c. Copper
    d. Iodine

4. Which coefficient would fill in the blank in the following equation to correctly balance the chemical reaction between iron oxide and carbon monoxide: $FeO_3 + 3CO \rightarrow Fe + \_\_CO_2$?
    a. 1
    b. 3
    c. 2
    d. 6

5. Which characteristic is NOT a property of water?
    a. If it acts as a base, it donates a proton.
    b. It is amphoteric and can act as an acid or a base.
    c. If it donates a proton, it becomes a conjugate base in the form of hydroxide ions.
    d. If it accepts a proton, it becomes a conjugate acid in the form of hydronium ions.

See answers on next page.

If you want to test your knowledge further on the chemistry section of the HESI exam, take our online practice quiz.

testprepbooks.com/hesi-quiz

SCAN ME

Answer Explanations

1. D: London dispersion forces are the weakest type of intermolecular attraction. They form between induced dipoles that are temporary and break apart easily. Hydrogen bonds are the strongest type of weak intermolecular attraction. When hydrogen bonds to a highly electronegative atom, the interaction becomes exaggerated and creates a stronger bond than expected. Dipole-dipole interactions are stronger than London dispersion forces because the dipoles are permanently present in the molecular configuration, but are weaker than hydrogen bonds.

2. A: Capillary action is a combination of adhesion and cohesion and allows water to move up the stem of a plant, so Choice *A* is correct. Adhesion is the attraction of liquid to the container that it is in and cohesion is the attraction of liquid molecules to each other. These intermolecular forces combine to move water upward throughout the plant from the roots. Surface tension, Choice *B*, occurs when the molecules at the surface of a liquid are pulled down into the body of the liquid and a strong interface is created at the surface. Vapor pressure, Choice *C*, involves the ability of a liquid to become a gas. Water does not dissolve the plant stem, so solubility is not involved in the travel of water up the stem, making Choice *D* incorrect.

3. D: Iodine has the greatest number of electrons at 53 electrons. The number of electrons increases in elements going from left to right across the periodic table. Hydrogen, Choice *A*, is at the top left corner of the periodic table, so it has the fewest electrons (one electron). Iron has 26 electrons, copper has 29 electrons, Choices *B*, and *C*, respectively.

4. B: For a chemical equation to be balanced, the same quantity of each element must be present on each side of the equation. On the left side of the equation, there is one Fe atom, and there are six oxygen atoms and three carbon atoms. On the right side of the equation, there is one iron atom and the rest of the oxygen and carbon atoms must be accounted for by the carbon dioxide molecules. Having three carbon dioxide molecules would give three carbon atoms and six oxygen atoms, which is equivalent to the reactants' side of the equation.

5. A: Choice *A* is the correct answer because it is the only one that contains an incorrect statement about the properties of water. Water is amphoteric and can act as an acid or a base, as stated in Choice *B*. When it acts as an acid, it donates a proton to the molecule it is reacting with, and then becomes hydroxide ions and acts as a conjugate base, Choice *C*. When it acts like a base, it accepts a proton, Choice *D*, and becomes hydronium ions, which act as a conjugate acid. When water acts as a base, it does not donate a proton, making Choice *A* the correct answer.

Anatomy and Physiology

General Terminology

Anatomy may be defined as the structural makeup of an organism. The study of anatomy may be divided into microscopic/fine anatomy and macroscopic/gross anatomy. **Fine anatomy** concerns itself with viewing the features of the body with the aid of a microscope, while **gross anatomy** concerns itself with viewing the features of the body with the naked eye. **Physiology** refers to the functions of an organism, and it examines the chemical or physical functions that help the body function appropriately.

Levels of Organization of the Human Body

All the parts of the human body are built of individual units called **cells.** Groups of similar cells are arranged into **tissues,** different tissues are arranged into **organs,** and organs working together form entire **organ systems.** The human body has twelve organ systems that govern circulation, digestion, immunity, hormones, movement, support, coordination, urination & excretion, reproduction (male and female), respiration, and general protection.

Body Cavities

The body is partitioned into different hollow spaces that house organs. The human body contains the following cavities:

- **Cranial cavity:** The cranial cavity is surrounded by the skull and contains organs such as the brain and pituitary gland.

- **Thoracic cavity:** The thoracic cavity is encircled by the sternum (breastbone) and ribs. It contains organs such as the lungs, heart, trachea (windpipe), esophagus, and bronchial tubes.

- **Abdominal cavity:** The abdominal cavity is separated from the thoracic cavity by the diaphragm. It contains organs such as the stomach, gallbladder, liver, small intestines, and large intestines. The abdominal organs are held in place by a membrane called the peritoneum.

- **Pelvic cavity:** The pelvic cavity is enclosed by the pelvis, or bones of the hip. It contains organs such as the urinary bladder, urethra, ureters, anus, and rectum. It contains the reproductive organs as well. In females, the pelvic cavity also contains the uterus.

- **Spinal cavity:** The spinal cavity is surrounded by the vertebral column. The vertebral column has five regions: cervical, thoracic, lumbar, sacral, and coccygeal. The spinal cord runs through the middle of the spinal cavity.

Three Primary Body Planes

A **plane** is an imaginary flat surface. The three primary planes of the human body are frontal, sagittal, and transverse. The **frontal,** or **coronal,** plane is a vertical plane that divides the body or organ into front (anterior) and back (posterior) portions. The **sagittal,** or **lateral,** plane is a vertical plane divides the body or organ into right and left sides. The **transverse** plane is a horizontal plane that divides the body or organ into upper and lower portions. In medical imaging, computed tomography (CT) scans are oriented only in the transverse plane; while magnetic resonance imaging (MRI) scans may be oriented in any of the three planes.

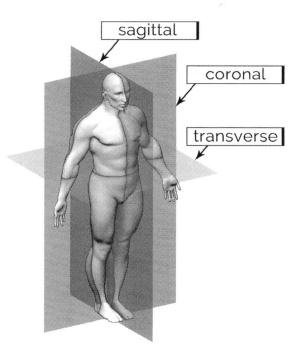

Note the body above is in the **anatomic position**. In anatomic position, the body and head are straight up and down, the feet are close but not touching, and the hands are pointed forward.

Terms of Direction

Medial refers to a structure being closer to the midline of the body. For example, the nose is medial to the eyes.

Lateral refers to a structure being farther from the midline of the body, and it is the opposite of medial. For example, the eyes are lateral to the nose.

Proximal refers to a structure or body part located near an attachment point. For example, the elbow is proximal to the wrist.

Distal refers to a structure or body part located far from an attachment point, and it is the opposite of proximal. For example, the wrist is distal to the elbow.

Anterior means toward the front in humans. For example, the lips are anterior to the teeth. The term **ventral** can be used in place of anterior.

Posterior means toward the back in humans, and it is the opposite of anterior. For example, the teeth are posterior to the lips. The term **dorsal** can be used in place of posterior.

Superior means above and refers to a structure closer to the head. For example, the head is superior to the neck. The terms **cephalic** or **cranial** may be used in place of superior.

Inferior means below and refers to a structure farther from the head, and it is the opposite of superior. For example, the neck is inferior to the head. The term **caudal** may be used in place of inferior.

Superficial refers to a structure closer to the surface. For example, the muscles are superficial because they are just beneath the surface of the skin.

Deep refers to a structure farther from the surface, and it is the opposite of superficial. For example, the femur is a deep structure lying beneath the muscles.

Body Regions

Terms for general locations on the body include:

- Cervical: relating to the neck
- Clavicular: relating to the clavicle, or collarbone
- Ocular: relating to the eyes
- Acromial: relating to the shoulder
- Cubital: relating to the elbow
- Brachial: relating to the arm
- Carpal: relating to the wrist
- Thoracic: relating to the chest
- Abdominal: relating to the abdomen
- Pubic: relating to the groin
- Pelvic: relating to the pelvis, or bones of the hip
- Femoral: relating to the femur, or thigh bone
- Geniculate: relating to the knee
- Pedal: relating to the foot
- Palmar: relating to the palm of the hand
- Plantar: relating to the sole of the foot

Abdominopelvic Regions and Quadrants

The **abdominopelvic region** may be defined as the combination of the abdominal and the pelvic cavities. The region's upper border is the breasts and its lower border is the groin region. The region is divided into the following nine sections:

- Right hypochondriac: region below the cartilage of the ribs
- Epigastric: region above the stomach between the hypochondriac regions
- Left hypochondriac: region below the cartilage of the ribs
- Right lumbar: region of the waist
- Umbilical: region between the lumbar regions where the umbilicus, or belly button (navel), is located
- Left lumbar: region of the waist
- Right inguinal: region of the groin
- Hypogastric: region below the stomach between the inguinal regions
- Left inguinal: region of the groin

A simpler way to describe the abdominopelvic area is to divide it into the following quadrants:

- Right upper quadrant (RUQ): Encompasses the right hypochondriac, right lumbar, epigastric, and umbilical regions.

- Right lower quadrant (RLQ): Encompasses the right lumbar, right inguinal, hypogastric, and umbilical regions.

- Left upper quadrant (LUQ): Encompasses the left hypochondriac, left lumbar, epigastric, and umbilical regions.

- Left lower quadrant (LLQ): Encompasses the left lumbar, left inguinal, hypogastric, and umbilical regions.

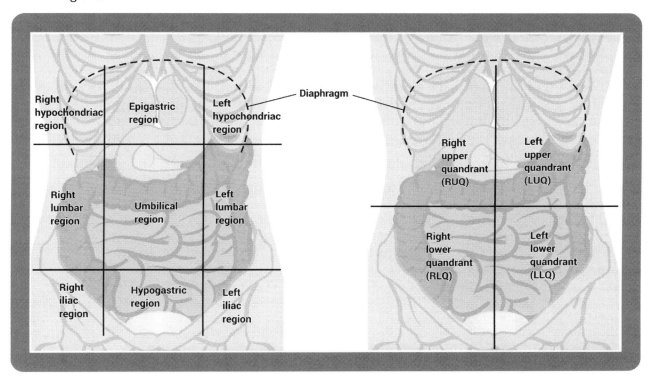

Cytology

Every living organism consists of cells, and cells are the basic unit of life. **Cytology** is the study of cells (usually eukaryotic cells), and is somewhat similar to **histology** (the study of cells and tissues in living organisms). Cells must contain a cell membrane, cytoplasm, and genetic information (usually in a nucleus). The cell membrane forms a barrier between the inside and outside of the cell, envelops the cellular contents, and interfaces with the extracellular fluid through proteins and other structures found in and on the cell membrane.

Eukaryotic cells—those found in plants, animals, and fungi—possess functional units called **organelles**. Each organelle performs one or more specific tasks in the cell. The nucleus contains the cell's genetic material, deoxyribonucleic acid, or DNA, which contains the necessary information for assembling all of the cell's proteins. The rough ER has embedded ribosomes, and it assembles enzymes and proteins. The

145

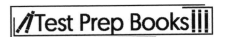

smooth ER lacks ribosomes, and creates and stores lipids. The Golgi apparatus contains many enzymes; these enzymes allow it to process incoming proteins and package them into small membranous sacs called **vesicles** for transport into and out of the cell. Mitochondria are involved in aerobic cellular respiration, which generates ATP.

There are several other important cellular components that aren't usually classified as organelles, because they lack membranes. Ribosomes serve a vital role by assembling proteins based on the sequence in RNA in a process known as **translation**. The cytoskeleton is a collection of protein filaments; it provides a lattice for intracellular transport and helps maintain the cell's shape. The cytosol is the fluid inside the cell and membrane-bound organelles. Vesicles transport material in or out of the cell. Vacuoles are large, amorphous cell compartments, mostly found in plants and fungi, that store fluid, proteins, and other materials, and maintain the cell's rigidity. Cilia and flagella move fluids past the cell's surface or help with mobility.

Mitosis and Meiosis

The **cell cycle** is the process by which a cell divides and duplicates itself. There are two processes by which a cell can divide itself: mitosis and meiosis. In **mitosis,** the daughter cells that are produced from parental cell division are identical to each other and the parent. **Meiosis** is a unique process that involves two stages of cell division and produces haploid cells, which are cells containing only one set of chromosomes, from diploid parent cells, which are cells containing two sets of chromosomes.

Histology

Histology is the examination of specialized cells and cell groups that perform a specific function by working together. Although there are trillions of cells in the human body, there are only 200 different types of cells. Groups of cells form biological tissues, and tissues combine to form organs, such as the heart and kidney. Organs are structures that have many different functions that are vital to living creatures. There are four primary types of tissue: epithelial, connective, muscle, and neural. Each tissue type has specific characteristics that enable organs and organ systems to function properly.

Muscle: Muscle tissue supports the body and allows it to move, and muscles are special because their cells have the ability to contract. There are three distinct types of muscle tissue: skeletal, smooth, and cardiac. **Skeletal muscle** is voluntary, or under conscious control, and is usually attached to bones. Most body movement is directly caused by the contraction of skeletal muscle. **Smooth muscle** is typically involuntary, or not under conscious control, and may be found in blood vessels, the walls of hollow organs, and the urinary bladder. **Cardiac muscle** is involuntary and found in the heart, which helps propel blood throughout the body.

Nervous: Nervous tissue is unique in that it is able to coordinate information from sensory organs as well as communicate the proper behavioral responses. **Neurons,** or nerve cells, are the workhorses of the nervous system. They communicate via **action potentials** (electrical signals) and **neurotransmitters** (chemical signals).

Epithelial: Epithelial tissue covers the external surfaces of organs and lines many of the body's cavities. Epithelial tissue helps to protect the body from invasion by microbes (bacteria, viruses, parasites), fluid loss, and injury.

Epithelial cell shapes can be:

- Squamous: cells with a flat shape
- Cuboidal: cells with a cubed shape
- Columnar: cells shaped like a column

Epithelial cells can be arranged in four patterns:

- Simple: a type of epithelium composed solely from a single layer of cells
- Stratified: a type of epithelium composed of multiple layers of cells
- Pseudostratified: a type of epithelium that appears to be stratified but actually consists of only one layer of cells
- Transitional: a type of epithelium noted for its ability to expand and contract

Connective: Connective tissue supports and connects the tissues and organs of the body. Connective tissue is composed of cells dispersed throughout a matrix which can be gel, liquid, protein fibers, or salts. The primary protein fibers in the matrix are collagen (for strength), elastin (for flexibility), and reticulum (for support). Connective tissue can be categorized as either **loose** or **dense.** Examples of connective tissue include bones, cartilage, ligaments, tendons, blood, and adipose (fat) tissue.

Integumentary System

The **integumentary system** includes skin, hair, nails, oil glands, and sweat glands. The largest organ of the integumentary system (and of the body), the skin, acts as a barrier and protects the body from mechanical impact, variations in temperature, microorganisms, chemicals, and UV radiation from the sun. It regulates body temperature, peripheral circulation, and excretes waste through sweat. It also contains a large network of nerve cells that relay changes in the external environment to the brain.

Layers of Skin
Skin consists of three layers: the surface **epidermis**, the inner **dermis**, and the subcutaneous **hypodermis** that is below the dermis and contains a layer of fat and connective tissue, which are both important for insulation.

The whole epidermis is composed of epithelial cells that lack blood vessels. The outer epidermis is composed of dead cells, which surround the living cells underneath. The most inner epidermal tissue is a single layer of cells called the **stratum basale,** which is composed of rapidly dividing cells that push old cells to the skin's surface. When being pushed out, the cells' organelles disappear, and they start producing a protein called **keratin**, which eventually forms a tough waterproof layer. This outer layer sloughs off every four to five weeks. The **melanocytes** in the stratum basale produce the pigment melanin, which absorbs UV rays and protects the skin. Skin also produces vitamin D if exposed to sunlight.

The dermis underneath the epidermis contains supporting collagen fibers peppered with nerves, blood vessels, hair follicles, sweat glands, oil glands, and smooth muscles.

Skin's Involvement in Temperature Homeostasis
The skin has a thermoregulatory role in the human body that is controlled by a negative feedback loop. The control center of temperature regulation is the hypothalamus in the brain. When the hypothalamus is alerted by receptors from the dermis, it secretes hormones that activate effectors to keep internal temperature at a set point of 98.6°F (37°C). If the environment is too cold, the hypothalamus will initiate

a pathway that induces muscle shivering to release heat energy as well as constrict blood vessels to limit heat loss. In hot conditions, the hypothalamus will initiate a pathway that vasodilates blood vessels to increase heat loss and stimulate sweating for evaporative cooling. Evaporative cooling occurs when the hottest water particles evaporate and leave behind the coolest ones. This cools down the body.

Sebaceous Glands vs. Sweat Glands

The skin also contains oil glands, or **sebaceous glands**, and sweat glands that are **exocrine** because their substances are secreted through ducts. **Endocrine** glands secrete substances into the blood stream instead. Oil glands are attached to hair follicles. They secrete **sebum**, an oily substance that moisturizes the skin, protecting it from water loss. Sebum also keeps the skin elastic. Also, sebum's slight acidity provides a chemical defense against bacterial and fungal infections.

Sweat glands not attached to hair follicles are called **eccrine** glands. They are all over the body, and are the sweat glands responsible for thermoregulation. They also remove bodily waste by secreting water and electrolytes. Sweat glands attached to hair follicles are apocrine glands, and there are far fewer apocrine sweat glands than eccrine sweat glands in the body. **Apocrine** glands are only active post-puberty. They secrete a thicker, viscous substance that is attractive to bacteria, leading to the unpleasant smell in armpits, feet, and the groin. They are stimulated during stress and arousal.

Skeletal System

Axial Skeleton and Appendicular Skeleton

The skeletal system is composed of 206 bones interconnected by tough connective tissue called ligaments. The **axial skeleton** can be considered the north-south axis of the skeleton. It includes the spinal column, sternum, ribs, and skull. There are 80 bones in the axial skeleton, and 33 of them are vertebrae. The ribs make up 12 of the bones in the axial skeleton.

The remaining 126 bones are in the **appendicular skeleton**, which contains bones of the appendages like the collarbone (clavicle), shoulders (scapula), arms, hands, hips, legs, and feet. The arm bones consist of the upper humerus with the radius and ulna that attach to the hands. The wrists, hands, and fingers are composed of the carpals, metacarpals, and phalanges, respectively. The femur attaches to the hips. The patella or kneecap connects the femur to the fibula and tibia. The ankles, feet, and toes are composed of the tarsals, metatarsals, and phalanges, respectively.

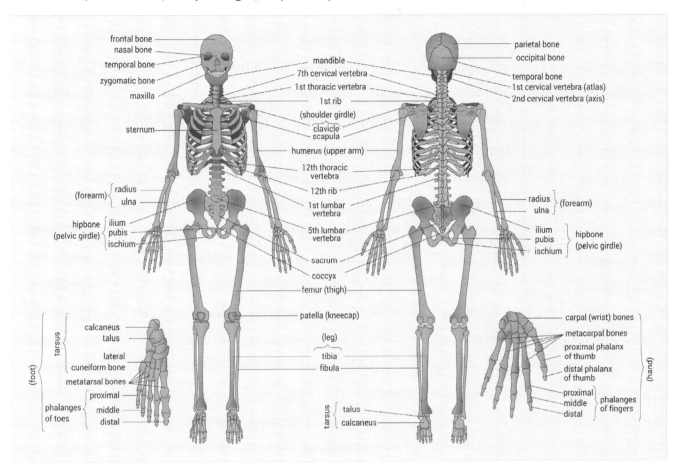

Functions of the Skeletal System

One of the skeletal system's most important functions is to protect vital internal organs. The skull protects the brain, the ribs protect the lungs and heart, the vertebrae protect the spinal column, and the pelvis protects the uterus and other reproductive organs. Yellow bone marrow stores lipids, or fats. Red bone marrow produces red and white blood cells as well as platelets in a process known as **hemopoiesis**. The bones themselves store the essential minerals calcium and phosphorus. The organization of the skeleton allows us to stand upright and acts as a foundation for organs and tissues to attach and maintain their location. This is similar to how the wooden frame of a house has room partitions to designate the type of room and floors that furniture can attach to.

The skeletal system and the muscular system are literally interconnected and allow for voluntary movement. Strong connective tissues called **tendons** attach bones to muscles. Most muscles work in opposing pairs and act as levers. For example, flexing the biceps brings the upper arm and lower arm closer together and flexing the triceps moves them apart. **Synovial joints** are movable joints, and they are rich with cartilage, connective tissue, and synovial fluid, which acts as a lubricant. The majority of joints are synovial joints, and they include hinge joints, like the one at the elbow, which permits flexion

149

and extension. joints are synovial joints, and they include hinge joints, like the one at the elbow, which allows for opening and closing.

The vertebrae are **cartilaginous joints**, which have spaces between them filled with cushion-like intervertebral discs that act as shock absorbers. The tight fit between the vertebrae and the intervertebral discs helps to protect the spinal cord inside by limiting the movement between two adjacent vertebrae. However, because there are so many vertebrae, the backbone as a whole is somewhat flexible.

Fibrous joints like those in the skull have fibrous tissue between the bones and no cavity between them. These are fixed joints that are immobile.

Compact and Spongy Bone

Osteoclasts, osteoblasts, and osteocytes are the three types of bone cells. **Osteoclasts** break down old bone, **osteoblasts** make new bone, and **osteocytes** are the mature functional bone cells. Bone is constantly regenerating due to the osteoblasts/osteoclasts that line all types of bones and the blood vessels inside them. The cells exist within a matrix of collagen fibers and minerals. The collagen fibers provide resistance to tension and the minerals provide resistance to compression. Because of the collagen and mineral matrix, bones have ample reinforcement to collectively support the entire human body.

Bones can be classified as any of the following:

- **Long bones** include tube-like rods like the arm and leg bones.
- **Short bones** are tube-like rods that are smaller than long bones like the fingers and toes.
- **Flat bones** are thin and flat like the ribs and breastbone.
- **Irregular bones**, like the vertebrae, are compact and don't fit into the other categories.

The outer tissue of the bone is surrounded by connective tissue known as **periosteum**. It appears shiny, smooth, and white. It protects the bone, anchors the bone to the connective tissue that surrounds muscles, and links the bone to the circulatory and nervous system. **Compact bone is underneath the periosteum and is made of a dense blend of tightly packed osteocytes. It serves as a mineral reservoir of calcium and phosphorus.** Compact bones have a **Haversian system** that is composed of embedded blood vessels, lymph vessels, and nerve bundles that span the interior of the bone from one end to the other. Branching from the central canal to the surface of the bone are the **canals of Volkmann,** which deliver materials to peripheral osteocytes. Concentric circles surround the central Haversian canal, and these **lamallae** have gaps between them called **lacunae** where osteocytes are embedded.

In contrast, **spongy bone** is very porous and more flexible than compact bone. It is at the ends of long bones and the central part of flat bones. It looks like a honeycomb, and the open spaces are connected by **trabeculae** which are beams of tissue that add support. They add strength without adding mass.

Cartilage is a very flexible connective tissue made of collagen and the flexible elastin. It has no blood vessels and obtains materials via diffusion. It is replaced by bone starting in infancy in a process called **ossification**.

Muscular System

The muscular system is responsible for involuntary and voluntary movement of the body. There are three types of muscle: skeletal, cardiac, and smooth.

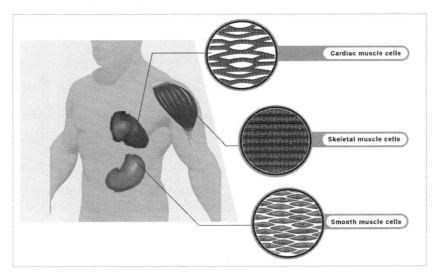

Skeletal Muscles

Skeletal muscles, or **voluntary muscles**, are attached to bones by tendons and are responsible for voluntary movement. The connecting tendons are made up of dense bands of connective tissue and have collagen fibers that firmly attach the muscle to the bone. Their fibers are actually woven into the coverings of the bone and muscle so that they can withstand pressure and tension. They usually work in opposing pairs like the biceps and triceps, for example. Muscles that work together are called **synergists.**

Skeletal muscles are made of bundles of long **fibers** that are composed of cells with many nuclei due to their length. These fibers contain **myofibrils,** and myofibrils are made of alternating **filaments.** The thicker myosin filaments are in between the smaller actin filaments in a unit called a **sarcomere**, and the overlapping regions of these filaments give the muscle its characteristic striated, or striped, appearance. Actin filaments are attached to exterior Z lines, myosin filaments are attached to a central M line, and when a muscle is at rest, there is a gap between the Z line and the myosin filaments. Only when the muscle contracts and the actin filaments slide over the myosin filaments does the myosin reach the Z line, as illustrated in the picture below. This **sliding-filament model of muscle contraction** is dependent on myosin molecules forming and breaking cross-bridges with actin in order to pull the actin filaments closer to the M line.

Skeletal muscles are controlled by the nervous system. Motor neurons connect to muscle fibers via neuromuscular junctions. Motor neurons must release the neurotransmitter **acetylcholine**, which releases calcium ions to stimulate myosin cross-bridging and contraction. As the acetylcholine stops being released, the contraction ends.

Smooth Muscles

Smooth muscles are responsible for involuntary movement, such as moving food through the digestive tract and moving blood through vessels. Their cells have only one nucleus and do not have striations because actin and myosin filaments do not have an organized arrangement like they do in skeletal muscles. Unlike skeletal muscle, smooth muscle doesn't rely on neuromuscular junctions for intercellular communication. Instead, they operate via gap junctions, which send impulses directly from cell to cell.

Cardiac Muscles

Cardiac muscle cells are found only in the heart where they control the heart's rhythm and blood pressure. Like skeletal muscle, cardiac muscle has striations, but cardiac muscle cells are smaller than skeletal muscle cells, so they typically have only one nucleus. Like smooth muscle, cardiac muscles do not require neurotransmitter release by motor neurons to function, and they instead operate via gap junctions.

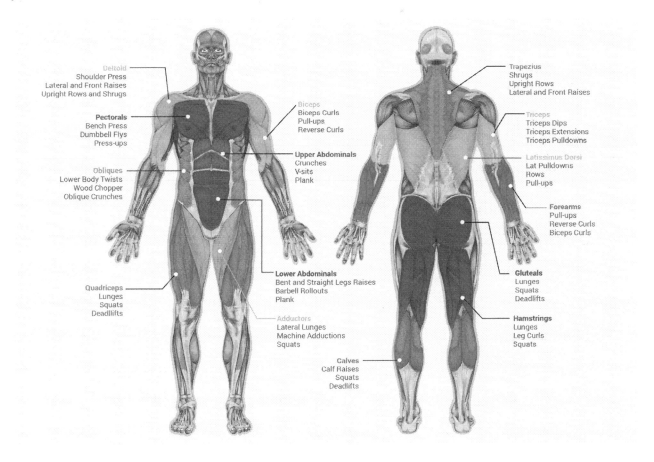

Nervous System

The human nervous system coordinates the body's response to stimuli from inside and outside the body. There are two major types of nervous system cells: neurons and neuroglia. **Neurons** are the workhorses of the nervous system and form a complex communication network that transmits electrical impulses termed **action potentials**, while **neuroglia** connect and support the neurons. Motor neurons use sodium and potassium pumps and channels in order to make action potentials occur.

Although some neurons monitor the senses, some control muscles, and some connect the brain to other neurons, all neurons have four common characteristics:

- **Dendrites:** These receive electrical signals from other neurons across small gaps called *synapses*.
- **Nerve cell body:** This is the hub of processing and protein manufacture for the neuron.
- **Axon:** This transmits the signal from the cell body to other neurons.
- **Terminals:** These bridge the neuron to dendrites of other neurons and deliver the signal via chemical messengers called **neurotransmitters.**

Here is an illustration of this:

There are two major divisions of the nervous system, central and peripheral:

Central Nervous System

The **central nervous system (CNS)** consists of the brain and spinal cord. Three layers of membranes called the meninges cover and separate the CNS from the rest of the body.

The major divisions of the brain are the forebrain, the midbrain, and the hindbrain.

The **forebrain** consists of the cerebrum, the thalamus and hypothalamus, and the rest of the limbic system. The **cerebrum** is the largest part of the brain, and its most well-documented part is the outer cerebral cortex. The cerebrum is divided into right and left hemispheres, and each cerebral cortex hemisphere has four discrete areas, or lobes: frontal, temporal, parietal, and occipital.

The **frontal lobe** governs duties such as voluntary movement, judgment, problem solving, and planning, while the other lobes are more sensory. The **temporal lobe** integrates hearing and language comprehension, the **parietal lobe** processes sensory input from the skin, and the **occipital lobe** processes visual input from the eyes. For completeness, the other two senses, smell and taste, are processed via the olfactory bulbs. The thalamus helps organize and coordinate all of this sensory input in a meaningful way for the brain to interpret.

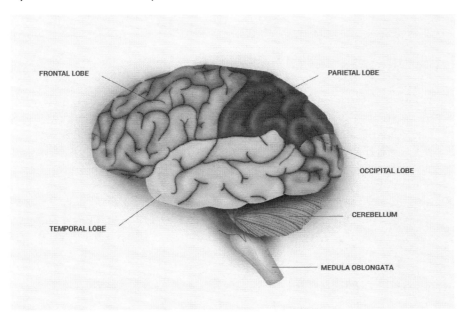

The **hypothalamus** controls the endocrine system and all of the hormones that govern long-term effects on the body. Each hemisphere of the limbic system includes a **hippocampus** (which plays a vital role in memory), an **amygdala** (which is involved with emotional responses like fear and anger), and other small bodies and nuclei associated with memory and pleasure.

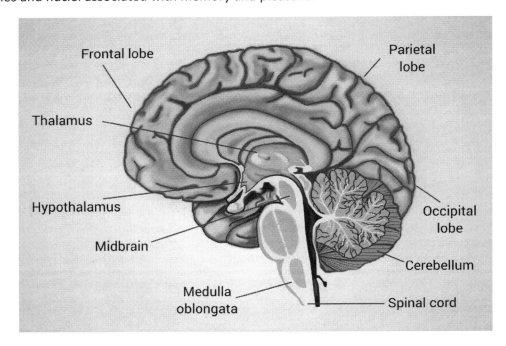

The **midbrain** is in charge of alertness, sleep/wake cycles, and temperature regulation, and it includes the **substantia nigra** which produces melatonin to regulate sleep patterns. The notable components of the **hindbrain** include the **medulla oblongata** and **cerebellum.** The medulla oblongata is located just above the spinal cord and is responsible for crucial involuntary functions such as breathing, swallowing, and the regulation of the heart rate and blood pressure. Together with other parts of the hindbrain, the midbrain and medulla oblongata form the **brain stem**. The brain stem connects the spinal cord to the rest of the brain. To the rear of the brain stem sits the cerebellum, which plays key roles in posture, balance, and muscular coordination. The spinal cord itself, which is encapsulated by the protective bony spinal column, carries sensory information to the brain and motor information to the body.

Peripheral Nervous System

The **peripheral nervous system (PNS)** includes all nervous tissue besides the brain and spinal cord. The PNS consists of the sets of cranial and spinal nerves and relays information between the CNS and the rest of the body. The PNS has two divisions: the autonomic nervous system and the somatic nervous system.

Autonomic Nervous System

The **autonomic nervous system (ANS)** governs involuntary, or reflexive, body functions. Ultimately, the autonomic nervous system controls functions such as breathing, heart rate, digestion, body temperature, and blood pressure.

The ANS is split between parasympathetic nerves and sympathetic nerves. These two nerve types are antagonistic and have opposite effects on the body. **Parasympathetic** nerves predominate resting conditions, and decrease heart rate, decrease breathing rate, prepare digestion, and allow urination and excretion. **Sympathetic** nerves, on the other hand, become active when a person is under stress or excited, and they increase heart rate, increase breathing rates, and inhibit digestion, urination, and excretion.

Somatic Nervous System and the Reflex Arc

The **somatic nervous system (SNS)** governs the conscious, or voluntary, control of skeletal muscles and their corresponding body movements. The SNS contains afferent and efferent neurons. **Afferent neurons carry sensory messages from the skeletal muscles, skin, or sensory organs to the CNS. Efferent neurons relay motor messages from the CNS to skeletal muscles, skin, or sensory organs.**

The SNS also has a role in involuntary movements called **reflexes**. A reflex is defined as an involuntary response to a stimulus. They are transmitted via what is termed a **reflex arc**, where a stimulus is sensed by an affector and its afferent neuron, interpreted and rerouted by an interneuron, and delivered to effector muscles by an efferent neuron where they respond to the initial stimulus. A reflex is able to bypass the brain by being rerouted through the spinal cord; the interneuron decides the proper course of action rather than the brain. The reflex arc results in an instantaneous, involuntary response. For example, a physician tapping on the knee produces an involuntary knee jerk referred to as the patellar tendon reflex.

Endocrine System

The **endocrine system** is made up of the ductless tissues and glands that secrete hormones directly into the bloodstream. It is similar to the nervous system in that it controls various functions of the body, but it does so via secretion of hormones in the bloodstream as opposed to nerve impulses. The endocrine system is also different because its effects last longer than that of the nervous system. Nerve impulses are immediate while hormone responses can last for minutes or even days.

The endocrine system works closely with the nervous system to regulate the physiological activities of the other systems of the body in order to maintain homeostasis. Hormone secretions are controlled by tight feedback loops that are generally regulated by the hypothalamus, the bridge between the nervous and endocrine systems. The hypothalamus receives sensory input via the nervous system and responds by stimulating or inhibiting the pituitary gland, which, in turn, stimulates or inhibits several other glands. The tight control is due to hormone secretions.

Hormones are chemicals that bind to specific target cells. Each hormone will only bind to a target cell that has a specific receptor that has the correct shape. For example, testosterone will not attach to skin cells because skin cells have no receptor that recognizes testosterone.

There are two types of hormones: steroid and protein. Steroid hormones are lipid, nonpolar substances, and most are able to diffuse across cell membranes. Once they do, they bind to a receptor that initiates a signal transduction cascade that affects gene expression. Non-steroid hormones bind to receptors on cell membranes that also initiate a signal transduction cascade that affects enzyme activity and chemical reactions.

Major Endocrine Glands

Hypothalamus: This gland is a part of the brain. It connects the nervous system to the endocrine system because it receives sensory information through nerves, and it sends instructions via hormones delivered to the pituitary.

157

Pituitary Gland: This gland is pea-sized and is found at the bottom of the hypothalamus. It has two lobes called the anterior and posterior lobes. It plays an important role in regulating other endocrine glands. For example, it secretes growth hormone, which regulates growth. Other hormones that are released by this gland control the reproductive system, childbirth, nursing, blood osmolarity, and metabolism.

The hormones and glands respond to each other via feedback loops, and a typical feedback loop is illustrated in the picture below. The hypothalamus and pituitary gland are master controllers of most of the other glands.

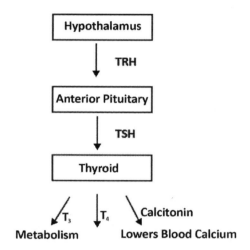

Thymus Gland: This gland is located in the chest cavity, embedded in connective tissue. It produces several hormones that are important for development and maintenance of T lymphocytes, which are important cells for immunity.

Adrenal Gland: One adrenal gland is attached to the top of each kidney. It produces epinephrine and norepinephrine which cause the "fight or flight" response in the face of danger or stress. These hormones raise heart rate, blood pressure, dilate bronchioles, and deliver blood to the muscles. All of these actions increase circulation and release glucose so that the body has an energy burst.

Pineal Gland: The pineal gland secretes melatonin, which is a hormone that regulates the body's circadian rhythm, which governs the natural wake-sleep cycle.

Testes and Ovaries: They secrete testosterone and both estrogen and progesterone, respectively. They are responsible for secondary sex characteristics, gamete development, and female hormones are important for embryonic development.

Thyroid Gland: This gland releases hormones like thyroxine and calcitonin. Thyroxine stimulates metabolism, and calcitonin monitors the amount of circulating calcium. Calcitonin signals the body to regulating calcium from bone reserves as well as kidney reabsorption of calcium.

Parathyroid Glands: These are four pea-sized glands located on the posterior surface of the thyroid. The main hormone that is secreted is called parathyroid hormone (PTH), which influences calcium levels like calcitonin, except it is antagonistic. PTH increases extracellular levels of calcium while calcitonin decreases it.

Pancreas: The pancreas is an organ that has both endocrine and exocrine functions. It functions outside of a typical feedback loop in that blood sugar seems to signal the pancreas itself. The endocrine functions are controlled by the pancreatic **islets of Langerhans**, which are groups of beta cells scattered throughout the gland that secrete insulin to lower blood sugar levels in the body. Neighboring alpha cells secrete glucagon to raise blood sugar. These complementary hormones keep blood sugar in check.

Cardiovascular System

The **cardiovascular system** (also called the **circulatory system**) is a network of organs and tubes that transport blood, hormones, nutrients, oxygen, and other gases to cells and tissues throughout the body. It is also known as the cardiovascular system. The major components of the circulatory system are the blood vessels, blood, and heart.

Blood Vessels

In the circulatory system, **blood vessels** are responsible for transporting blood throughout the body. The three major types of blood vessels in the circulatory system are arteries, veins, and capillaries. **Arteries** carry blood from the heart to the rest of the body. Veins carry blood from the body back to the heart. **Capillaries** connect arteries to veins and form networks that exchange materials between the blood and the cells.

In general, arteries are stronger and thicker than veins, as they withstand high pressures exerted by the blood as the heart pumps it through the body. Arteries control blood flow through either **vasoconstriction** (narrowing of the blood vessel's diameter) or **vasodilation** (widening of the blood vessel's diameter). The smallest arteries, which are farthest from the heart, are called **arterioles.** The blood in veins is under much lower pressures, so veins have valves to prevent the backflow of blood.

Most of the exchange between the blood and tissues takes place through the capillaries. There are three types of capillaries: continuous, fenestrated, and sinusoidal.

Continuous capillaries are made up of epithelial cells tightly connected together. As a result, they limit the types of materials that pass into and out of the blood. Continuous capillaries are the most common type of capillary. **Fenestrated capillaries** have openings that allow materials to be freely exchanged between the blood and tissues. They are commonly found in the digestive, endocrine, and urinary systems. **Sinusoidal capillaries** have larger openings and allow proteins and blood cells through. They are found primarily in the liver, bone marrow, and spleen.

Blood

Blood is vital to the human body. It is a liquid connective tissue that serves as a transport system for supplying cells with nutrients and carrying away their wastes. The average adult human has five to six quarts of blood circulating through their body. Approximately 55% of blood is plasma (the fluid portion), and the remaining 45% is composed of solid cells and cell parts. There are three major types of blood cells:

- Red blood cells, or **erythrocytes**, transport oxygen throughout the body. They contain a protein called **hemoglobin** that allows them to carry oxygen. The iron in the hemoglobin gives the cells and the blood their red colors.

- White blood cells, or **leukocytes**, are responsible for fighting infectious diseases and maintaining the immune system. Monocytes, lymphocytes (including B-cells and T-cells), neutrophils, basophils, and eosinophils compose the white blood cells. All are developed in bone marrow.

  - **Monocytes** eat and destroy invaders like bacteria and viruses.

  - **Lymphocytes** are responsible for antibody creation in the defense against invasive organisms and infections.

  - **Neutrophils**, the most abundant white blood cell, take out bacterial and fungal organisms. They are the first line of defense against infections.

  - **Basophils** and mast cells secrete histamine, the substance responsible for itching associated with allergic diseases.

  - **Eosinophils** target parasites and cancer cells, and are part of the body's allergic response. They have low phagocytic activity and primarily secrete destructive enzymes.

- **Platelets** are cell fragments that play a central role in the blood clotting process.

All blood cells in adults are produced in the bone marrow—red blood cells and most white blood cells are produced in the red marrow, and some white blood cells are produced in the yellow bone marrow.

Heart

The **heart** is a two-part, muscular pump that forcefully pushes blood throughout the human body. The human heart has four chambers—two upper atria and two lower ventricles separated by a partition called the septum. There is a pair on the left and a pair on the right. Anatomically, *left* and *right* correspond to the sides of the body that the patient themselves would refer to as left and right. Four valves help to section off the chambers from one another. Between the right atrium and ventricle, the three flaps of the **tricuspid valve** keep blood from backflowing from the ventricle to the atrium, similar to how the two flaps of the **mitral valve** work between the left atrium and ventricle. As these two valves lie between an atrium and a ventricle, they are referred to as **atrioventricular (AV) valves**. The other two valves are **semilunar (SL)** and control blood flow into the two great arteries leaving the ventricles.

160

The **pulmonary valve** connects the right ventricle to the pulmonary artery, while the **aortic valve** connects the left ventricle to the aorta.

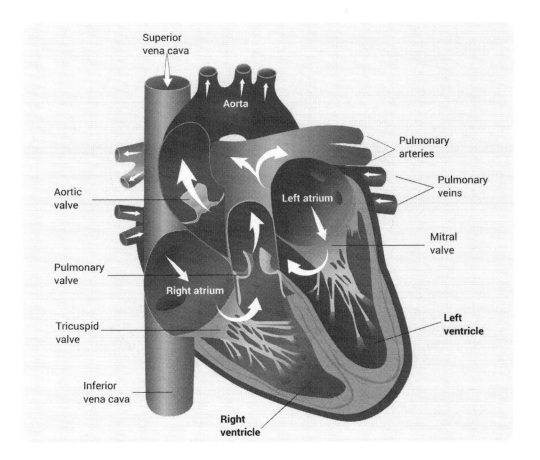

Cardiac Cycle

A **cardiac cycle** is one complete sequence of cardiac activity. The cardiac cycle represents the relaxation and contraction of the heart and can be divided into two phases: diastole and systole. **Diastole** is the phase during which the heart relaxes and fills with blood. It gives rise to the diastolic blood pressure (DBP), which is the bottom number of a blood pressure reading. **Systole** is the phase during which the heart contracts and discharges blood. It gives rise to the systolic blood pressure (SBP), which is the top number of a blood pressure reading. The heart's electrical conduction system coordinates the cardiac cycle.

Types of Circulation

Five major blood vessels manage blood flow to and from the heart: the superior and inferior venae cava, the aorta, the pulmonary artery, and the pulmonary vein. The superior vena cava is a large vein that drains blood from the head and the upper body. The **inferior vena cava** is a large vein that drains blood from the lower body. The **aorta** is the largest artery in the human body and carries blood from the heart to body tissues. The **pulmonary arteries** carry blood from the heart to the lungs. The **pulmonary veins** transport blood from the lungs to the heart.

In the human body, there are two types of circulation: pulmonary circulation and systemic circulation. **Pulmonary circulation** supplies blood to the lungs. Deoxygenated blood enters the right atrium of the heart and is routed through the tricuspid valve into the right ventricle. Deoxygenated blood then travels from the right ventricle of the heart through the pulmonary valve and into the pulmonary arteries. The pulmonary arteries carry the deoxygenated blood to the lungs. In the lungs, oxygen is absorbed, and carbon dioxide is released. The pulmonary veins carry oxygenated blood to the left atrium of the heart.

Systemic circulation supplies blood to all other parts of the body, except the lungs. Oxygenated blood flows from the left atrium of the heart through the mitral, or bicuspid, valve into the left ventricle of the heart. Oxygenated blood is then routed from the left ventricle of the heart through the aortic valve and into the aorta. The aorta delivers blood to the systemic arteries, which supply the body tissues. In the tissues, oxygen and nutrients are exchanged for carbon dioxide and other wastes. The deoxygenated blood along with carbon dioxide and wastes enter the systemic veins, where they are returned to the right atrium of the heart via the superior and inferior vena cava.

Respiratory System

The **respiratory system** enables breathing and supports the energy-making process in our cells. The respiratory system transports an essential reactant, oxygen, to cells so that they can produce energy in their mitochondria via cellular respiration. The respiratory system also removes carbon dioxide, a waste product of cellular respiration. This system is divided into the upper respiratory system and the lower respiratory system. The **upper system** comprises the nose, the nasal cavity and sinuses, and the pharynx. The **lower respiratory system** comprises the larynx (voice box), the trachea (windpipe), the small passageways leading to the lungs, and the lungs.

The pathway of oxygen to the bloodstream begins with the nose and the mouth. Upon inhalation, air enters the nose and mouth and passes into the sinuses where it gets warmed, filtered, and humidified. The throat, or the pharynx, allows the entry of both food and air; however, only air moves into the trachea, or windpipe, since the epiglottis covers the trachea during swallowing and prevents food from entering. The trachea contains mucus and cilia. The mucus traps many airborne pathogens while the cilia act as bristles that sweep the pathogens away toward the top of the trachea where they are either swallowed or coughed out.

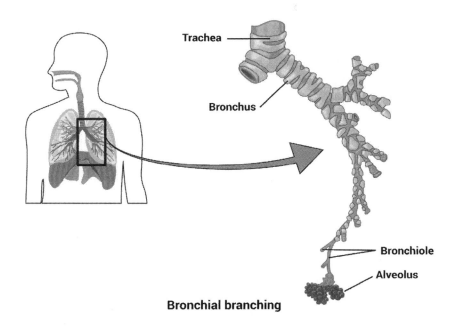

Bronchial branching

The **trachea** itself has two vocal cords at the top that make up the **larynx**. At its bottom, the trachea forks into two major **bronchi**—one for each lung. These bronchi continue to branch into smaller and smaller **bronchioles** before terminating in grape-like air sacs called **alveoli;** these alveoli are surrounded by capillaries and provide the body with an enormous amount of surface area to exchange oxygen and carbon dioxide gases, in a process called **external respiration**.

In total, the lungs contain about 1500 miles of airway passages. The right lung is divided into three lobes (superior, middle, and inferior), and the left lung is divided into two lobes (superior and inferior).

The left lung is smaller than the right lung, likely because it shares its space in the chest cavity with the heart.

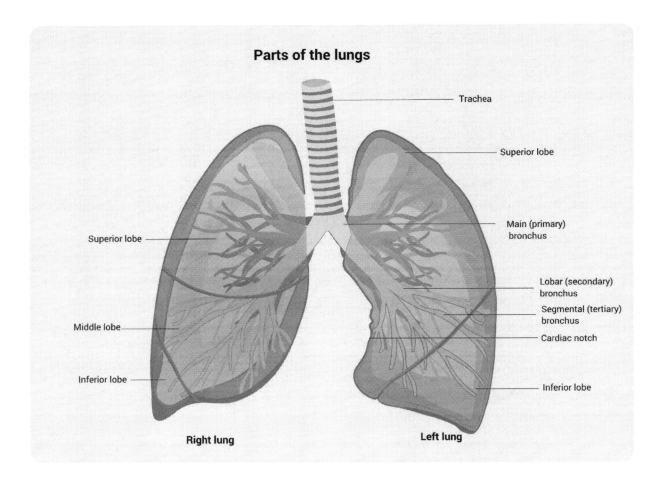

Parts of the lungs

Trachea

Superior lobe

Main (primary) bronchus

Lobar (secondary) bronchus

Segmental (tertiary) bronchus

Cardiac notch

Inferior lobe

Superior lobe

Middle lobe

Inferior lobe

Right lung

Left lung

A flat muscle underneath the lungs called the **diaphragm** controls breathing. When the diaphragm contracts, the volume of the chest cavity increases and indirectly decreases its air pressure. This decrease in air pressure creates a vacuum, and the lungs pull in air to fill the space. This process is called negative pressure breathing.

Upon **inhalation** or **inspiration,** oxygen in the alveoli diffuses into the capillaries to be carried by blood to cells throughout the body, in a process called **internal respiration**. A protein called hemoglobin in red blood cells easily bonds with oxygen, removing it from the blood and allowing more oxygen to diffuse in. This protein allows the blood to take in 60 times more oxygen than the body could without it, and this explains how oxygen can become so concentrated in blood even though it is only 21% of the atmosphere. While oxygen diffuses from the alveoli into the capillaries, carbon dioxide diffuses from the capillaries into the alveoli. When the diaphragm relaxes, the elastic lungs snap back to their original shape; this decreases the volume of the chest cavity and increases the air pressure until it is back to normal. This increased air pressure pushes the carbon dioxide waste from the alveoli through **exhalation** or **expiration.**

The autonomic nervous system controls breathing. The medulla oblongata gets feedback regarding the carbon dioxide levels in the blood and will send a message to the diaphragm that it is time for a contraction. While breathing can be voluntary, it is mostly under autonomic control.

Functions of the Respiratory System

The respiratory system has many functions. Most importantly, it provides a large area for gas exchange between the air and the circulating blood. It protects the delicate respiratory surfaces from environmental variations and defends them against pathogens. It is responsible for producing the sounds that the body makes for speaking and singing, as well as for non-verbal communication. It also helps regulate blood volume and blood pressure by releasing vasopressin, and it is a regulator of blood pH due to its control over carbon dioxide release, as the aqueous form of carbon dioxide is the chief buffering agent in blood. Erythrocytes use carbonic anhydrase to convert most carbon dioxide in the blood to bicarbonate ions.

Digestive System

The human body relies completely on the **digestive system** to meet its nutritional needs. After food and drink are ingested, the digestive system breaks them down into their component nutrients and absorbs them so that the circulatory system can transport them to other cells to use for growth, energy, and cell repair. These nutrients may be classified as proteins, lipids, carbohydrates, vitamins, and minerals.

The digestive system is thought of chiefly in two parts: the **digestive tract** (also called the **alimentary tract** or **gastrointestinal tract**) and the accessory digestive organs. The digestive tract is the pathway in which food is ingested, digested, absorbed, and excreted. It is composed of the mouth, pharynx, esophagus, stomach, small and large intestines, rectum, and anus. **Peristalsis**, or wave-like contractions of smooth muscle, moves food and wastes through the digestive tract. The accessory digestive organs are the salivary glands, liver, gallbladder, and pancreas.

Mouth and Stomach

The mouth is the entrance to the digestive system. Here, the mechanical and chemical digestion of the food begins. The food is chewed mechanically by the teeth and shaped into a **bolus** by the tongue so that it can be more easily swallowed by the esophagus. The food also becomes waterier and more pliable with the addition of saliva secreted from the salivary glands, the largest of which are the parotid glands. The glands also secrete **amylase** in the saliva, an enzyme which begins chemical digestion and breakdown of the carbohydrates and sugars in the food.

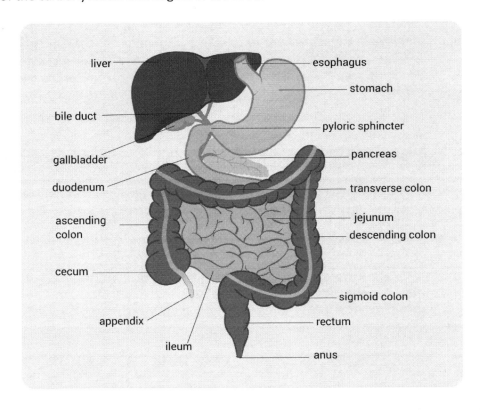

The food then moves through the pharynx and down the muscular esophagus to the stomach.

The stomach is a large, muscular sac-like organ at the distal end of the esophagus. Here, the bolus is subjected to more mechanical and chemical digestion. As it passes through the stomach, it is physically squeezed and crushed while additional secretions turn it into a watery nutrient-filled liquid that exits into the small intestine as **chyme.**

The stomach secretes a great many substances into the **lumen** of the digestive tract. Some cells produce gastrin, a hormone that prompts other cells in the stomach to secrete a gastric acid composed mostly of hydrochloric acid (HCl). The HCl is at such a high concentration and low pH that it denatures most proteins and degrades a lot of organic matter. The stomach also secretes mucous to form a protective film that keeps the corrosive acid from dissolving its own cells. Gaps in this mucous layer can lead to peptic ulcers. Finally, the stomach also uses digestive enzymes like proteases and lipases to break down proteins and fats; although there are some gastric lipases here, the stomach is most known for breaking down proteins.

166

Small Intestine

The chyme from the stomach enters the first part of the small intestine, the **duodenum,** through the **pyloric sphincter,** and its extreme acidity is partly neutralized by sodium bicarbonate secreted along with mucous. The presence of chyme in the duodenum triggers the secretion of the hormones secretin and cholecystokinin (CCK). Secretin acts on the pancreas to dump more sodium bicarbonate into the small intestine so that the pH is kept at a reasonable level, while CCK acts on the gallbladder to release the **bile** that it has been storing. Bile, a substance produced by the liver and stored in the gallbladder, helps to **emulsify** or dissolve fats and lipids.

Because of the bile (which aids in lipid absorption) and the secreted lipases (which break down fats), the duodenum is the chief site of fat digestion in the body. The duodenum also represents the last major site of chemical digestion in the digestive tract, as the other two sections of the small intestine (the **jejunum** and **ileum**) are instead heavily involved in absorption of nutrients.

The small intestine reaches 40 feet in length, and its cells are arranged in small finger-like projections called **villi.** This is due to its key role in the absorption of nearly all nutrients from the ingested and digested food, effectively transferring them from the lumen of the GI tract to the bloodstream, where they travel to the cells that need them. These nutrients include simple sugars like glucose from carbohydrates, amino acids from proteins, emulsified fats, electrolytes like sodium and potassium, minerals like iron and zinc, and vitamins like D and B12. Vitamin B12's absorption, though it takes place in the intestines, is actually aided by **intrinsic factor** that was released into the chyme back in the stomach.

Large Intestine

The leftover parts of food which remain unabsorbed or undigested in the lumen of the small intestine next travel through the **large intestine,** that may also be referred to as the **large bowel** or **colon.** The large intestine is mainly responsible for water absorption. As the chyme at this stage no longer has anything useful that can be absorbed by the body, it is now referred to as **waste,** and it is stored in the large intestine until it can be excreted from the body. Removing the liquid from the waste transforms it from liquid to solid stool, or **feces.**

This waste first passes from the small intestine to the **cecum,** a pouch that forms the first part of the large intestine. In herbivores, it provides a place for bacteria to digest cellulose, but in humans most of it is vestigial and is known as the appendix. From the cecum, waste next travels up the ascending colon, across the transverse colon, down the descending colon, and through the sigmoid colon to the rectum. The rectum is responsible for the final storage of waste before being expelled through the **anus.** The anal canal is a small portion of the rectum leading through to the anus and the outside of the body.

Pancreas

The **pancreas** has endocrine and exocrine functions. The endocrine function involves releasing the hormone insulin, which decreases blood sugar (glucose) levels, and glucagon, which increases blood sugar (glucose) levels, directly into the bloodstream. Both hormones are produced in the **islets of Langerhans,** insulin in the beta cells and glucagon in the alpha cells.

The exocrine function of the pancreas involves the secretion of inactive digestive enzymes (**zymogens**) from acinar cells into the main pancreatic duct. The main pancreatic duct joins the common bile duct, which empties into the small intestine (specifically the duodenum). The digestive enzymes are then activated and take part in the digestion of carbohydrates, proteins, and fats within chyme (the mixture of partially digested food and digestive juices).

Urinary System

The **urinary system** is made up of the kidneys, ureters, urinary bladder, and the urethra. It is the system responsible for removing waste products and balancing water and electrolyte concentrations in the blood. The urinary system has many important functions related to waste excretion. It regulates the concentrations of sodium, potassium, chloride, calcium, and other ions in the filtrate by controlling the amount of each that is reabsorbed during filtration. The reabsorption or secretion of hydrogen ions and bicarbonate contributes to the maintenance of blood pH. Certain kidney cells can detect any reductions in blood volume and pressure. If that happens, they secrete renin, which activates a hormone that causes increased reabsorption of sodium ions and water, raising volume and pressure. Under hypoxic conditions, kidney cells will secrete erythropoietin in order to stimulate red blood cell production. Kidney cells also synthesize **calcitriol**, which is a hormone derivative of vitamin D3 that aids in calcium ion absorption by the intestinal epithelium.

Under normal circumstances, humans have two functioning **kidneys** in the lower back and on either side of the spinal cord. They are the main organs that are responsible for filtering waste products out of the blood and regulating blood water and electrolyte levels. Blood enters the kidney through the renal artery, and urea and wastes are removed, while water and the acidity/alkalinity of the blood is adjusted. Toxic substances and drugs are also filtered. Blood exits through the renal vein, and the urine waste travels through the ureter to the bladder, where it is stored until it is eliminated through the urethra.

The kidneys have an outer **renal cortex** and an inner **renal medulla** that contain millions of tiny filtering units called **nephrons.** Nephrons have two parts: a glomerulus, which is the filter, and a tubule. The **glomerulus** is a network of capillaries covered by the **Bowman's capsule**, which is the entrance to the tubule. As blood enters the kidneys via the renal artery, the glomerulus allows for fluid and waste products to pass through it and enter the tubule. Blood cells and large molecules, such as proteins, do not pass through and remain in the blood.

The **filtrate** passes through the tubule, which has several parts. The proximal tubule comes first, and then the descending and ascending limbs of the loop of Henle dip into the medulla, followed by the distal tubule and collecting duct. The journey through the tubule involves a balancing act that regulates blood osmolarity, pH, and electrolytes exchange of materials between the tubule and the blood stream. The final product at the collecting tubule is called urine, and it is delivered to the bladder by the ureter. The most central part of the kidney is the **renal pelvis**, and it acts as a funnel by delivering the urine from the millions of the collecting tubules to the **ureters**. The filtered blood exits through the renal vein and is returned to circulation.

Here's a look at the genitourinary system:

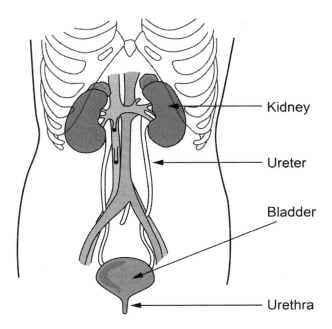

- Kidney
- Ureter
- Bladder
- Urethra

Here's a close up look at the kidney:

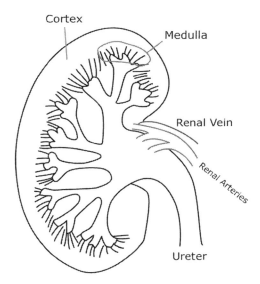

Cortex
Medulla
Renal Vein
Renal Arteries
Ureter

Waste Excretion

Once urine accumulates, it leaves the kidneys. The urine travels through the ureters into the **urinary bladder,** a muscular organ that is hollow and elastic. As more urine enters the urinary bladder, its walls stretch and become thinner so there is no significant difference in internal pressure. The urinary bladder stores the urine until the body is ready for urination, at which time the muscles contract and force the urine through the **urethra** and out of the body.

Reproductive System

The **reproductive system** is responsible for producing, storing, nourishing, and transporting functional reproductive cells, or gametes, in the human body. It includes the reproductive organs, also known as **gonads**, the reproductive tract, the accessory glands and organs that secrete fluids into the reproductive tract, and the **perineal structures**, which are the external genitalia.

Reproduction involves the passing of genes from one generation to the next, and that is accomplished through haploid gametes. Gametes have gone through meiosis and have 23 chromosomes, half the normal number. The male gamete is **sperm**, and the female gamete is an **egg** or **ovum.** When a sperm fertilizes an egg, they create a **zygote,** which is the first cell of a new organism. The zygote has a full set of 46 chromosomes because it received 23 from each parent. Because of gene shuffling during sperm and egg development, sperm and egg chromosome sets are all different, which results in the variety seen in humans.

Male Reproductive System

The entire male reproductive system is designed to generate sperm and produce semen that facilitate fertilization of eggs, the female gametes. The testes are the endocrine glands that secrete **testosterone**, a hormone that is important for secondary sex characteristics and sperm development, or **spermatogenesis.** Testosterone is in the androgen steroid-hormone family. The testes also produce and store 500 million spermatocytes, which are the male gametes, each day. Testes are housed in the **scrotum,** which is a sac that hangs outside the body so that spermatogenesis occurs at cooler and optimal conditions.

The **seminiferous tubules** within the testes produce spermatocytes, which after production travel to **epididymis** where they are stored as they mature. Then, the sperm move to the ejaculatory duct via the vas deferens. The ejaculatory duct contains more than just sperm. The **seminal vesicles** secrete an alkaline substance that will help sperm survive in the acidic vagina. The prostate gland secretes enzymes bathed in a milky white fluid that is important for thinning semen after ejaculation to increase its likelihood of reaching the egg. The **bulbourethral gland,** or **Cowper's gland,** secretes an alkaline fluid that lubricates the urethra prior to ejaculation to neutralize any acidic urine residue.

The sperm, along with all the exocrine secretions, are collectively called **semen.** Their destination is the vagina, and they can only get there if the penis is erect due to arousal and increased circulation. During sexual intercourse, ejaculation will forcefully expel the contents of the semen and effectively deliver the sperm to the egg. The muscular prostate gland is important for ejaculation. Each ejaculation releases 2 to 6 million sperm. Sperm has a whip-like flagellum tail that facilitates movement.

Female Reproductive System

The **vagina** is the passageway that sperm must travel through to reach an egg, the female gamete. Surrounding the vagina are the labia minor and labia major, both of which are folds that protect the urethra and the vaginal opening. The **clitoris** is rich in nerve-endings, making it sensitive and highly stimulated during sexual intercourse. It is above the vagina and urethra. An exocrine gland called the **Bartholin's glands** secretes a fluid during arousal that is important for lubrication.

The female gonads are the **ovaries.** Ovaries generally produce one immature gamete, an egg or oocyte, per month. They are also responsible for secreting the hormones **estrogen** and **progesterone.** Fertilization cannot happen unless the ejaculated sperm finds the egg, which is only available at certain times of the month. Eggs, or ova, develop in the ovaries in clusters surrounded by follicles, and after puberty, they are delivered to the uterus once a month via the **Fallopian tubes**.

The 28-day average journey of the egg to the uterus is called the menstrual cycle, and it is highly regulated by the endocrine system. The regulatory hormones Gonadotropin releasing hormone (GnRH), luteinizing hormone (LH), and follicle-stimulating hormone (FSH) orchestrate the menstrual cycle. Ovarian hormones estrogen and progesterone are also important in timing as well as for vascularization of the uterus in preparation for pregnancy. **Fertilization** usually happens around ovulation, which is when the egg is inside the fallopian tube. The resulting zygote travels down the tube and implants into the uterine wall. The uterus protects and nourishes the developing embryo for nine months until it is ready for the outside environment.

If the egg released is unfertilized, the uterine lining will slough off during **menstruation.** Should a fertilized egg, called a **zygote**, reach the uterus, it will embed itself into the uterine wall due to uterine vascularization that will deliver blood, nutrients, and antibodies to the developing embryo. The uterus is where the embryo will develop for the next nine months. **Mammary glands** are important female reproductive structures because they produce the milk provided for babies during **lactation**. Milk contains nutrients and antibodies that benefit the baby.

If you want to test your knowledge further on the anatomy and physiology section of the HESI exam, take our online practice quiz and the practice quiz on the next page.

testprepbooks.com/hesi-quiz

SCAN ME

Practice Quiz

1. What is the body plane that runs vertically through the body at right angles to the midline?
   a. Coronal
   b. Transverse
   c. Sagittal
   d. Superior

2. Which statement is true?
   a. Ligaments attach skeletal muscles to bone.
   b. Tendons connect bones at joints.
   c. Cartilage adds mechanical support to joints.
   d. Most veins deliver oxygenated blood to cells.

3. Which layer of skin contains sensory receptors and blood vessels?
   a. Epidermis
   b. Dermis
   c. Hypodermis
   d. Subcutaneous

4. What are concentric circles of bone tissue called?
   a. Lacunae
   b. Lamellae
   c. Trabeculae
   d. Diaphysis

5. When de-oxygenated blood first enters the heart, which of the following choices is in the correct order for its journey to the aorta?
   I. Tricuspid valve → Lungs → Mitral valve
   II. Mitral valve → Lungs → Tricuspid valve
   III. Right ventricle → Lungs → Left atrium
   IV. Left ventricle → Lungs → Right atrium
   a. I and III only
   b. I and IV only
   c. II and III only
   d. II and IV only

See answers on next page.

Answer Explanations

1. A: The coronal, or frontal, plane is a vertical plane positioned so that it divides the body into front (ventral) and back (dorsal) regions. The plane is positioned so that the face, kneecap, and toes are on the ventral side, and the vertebrae and heel are on the dorsal side. The coronal plane is one of three body planes. The other two are the transverse and sagittal planes. The transverse plane divides the anatomy into upper (cranial or head) and lower (caudal or tail) regions. The sagittal plane runs front/back perpendicular to the frontal plane and divides the anatomy into right and left regions.

2. C: Cartilage adds mechanical support to joints. It provides a flexible cushion that aids in mobility while offering support. The first two choices are switched—it is ligaments that connect bones at joints and tendons that attach skeletal muscles to bones. *D* is incorrect because arteries, not veins, deliver oxygenated blood.

3. B: The dermis is the skin layer that contains nerves, blood vessels, hair follicles, and glands. These structures are called skin appendages. These appendages are scattered throughout the connective tissue (elastin and collagen), and the connective tissue provides support to the outer layer, the epidermis. The epidermal surface is a thin layer (except feet and palms where it is thick) of continually-regenerating cells that don't have a blood supply of their own, which explains why superficial cuts don't bleed. The hypodermis is the subcutaneous layer underneath the dermis, and it is composed primarily of fat in order to provide insulation.

4. B: In the Haversian system found in compact bone, concentric layers of bone cells are called lamellae. Between the lamellae are lacunae, which are gaps filled with osteocytes. The Haversian canals on the outer regions of the bone contain capillaries and nerve fibers. Spongy (cancellous) bone is on the extremities of long bones, which makes sense because the ends are softer due to the motion at joints (providing flexibility and cushion). The middle of the bone between the two spongy regions is called the diaphysis region. Spongy bone is highly vascular and is the site of red bone marrow (the marrow that makes red blood cells). Long bones, on the other hand, are long, weight-bearing bones like the tibia or femur that contain yellow marrow in adulthood. Trabeculae is a dense, collagenous, rod-shaped tissue that add mechanical support to the spongy regions of bone. Muscular trabeculae can be found in the heart and are similar in that they offer physical reinforcement.

5. A: Carbon dioxide-rich blood is delivered from systemic circulation to the right atrium. It is pumped into the right ventricle. The tricuspid valve prevents backflow between the two chambers. From there, the pulmonary artery takes blood to the lungs where diffusion causes gas exchange. Then, oxygenated blood returns to the left atrium before getting pumped into the left ventricle. The mitral valve prevents the backflow of blood from the left ventricle to the atrium. Finally, blood is ejected from the left ventricle through the aorta to enter systemic circulation.

Physics

Nature of Motion

The measurement of an object's movement or change in position (x), over a change in time (t) is an object's **speed.** The **average speed** of an object is defined as the distance that the object travels divided by how long it takes the object to travel that distance.

$$Speed = \frac{distance}{time}$$

Distance is measured in meters, and time is measured in seconds. The standard scientific units for speed and velocity are meters/second (m/s):

$$\frac{meters}{second} = \frac{m}{s}$$

Units of miles/hour (mph) are also commonly used in America.

Velocity & Acceleration

Velocity
When the direction is included with the speed, it is referred to as the **velocity.** This is because velocity is the measure of the change in distance over the change in time.

For example, a car traveling east and another traveling west can have the same speed of 30 miles per hour (mph), but their velocities are different. If movement eastward is considered positive, then movement westward is negative. Thus, the eastbound car has a velocity of 30 mph while the westbound car has a velocity of -30 mph.

Another example where velocity and speed are different is with a car traveling around a bend in the road. The speed is constant along the road, but the direction (and therefore the velocity) changes continuously.

The fact that velocity has a *magnitude* (speed) and a direction makes it a **vector quantity**. A *vector* is an arrow pointing in the direction of motion, with its length proportional to its magnitude. A measurement such as speed is called a **scalar quantity** because it only has a numeric value without a particular direction.

A "change in position" refers to the difference in location of an object's starting point and an object's ending point. In science, this change is represented by the Greek letter Delta, Δ.

$$velocity\ (v) = \frac{\Delta x}{\Delta t}$$

Average velocity is calculated by averaging the beginning or initial velocity and the ending or final velocity of an object.

Acceleration

While an object's speed measures how fast the object's position will change in a certain amount of time, an object's **acceleration** measures how fast the object's speed will change in a certain amount of time. Acceleration can be thought of as the change in velocity or speed (Δv) divided by the change in the time (Δt).

$$acceleration\ (a) = \frac{\Delta v}{\Delta t}$$

Velocity is measured in meters/second and time is measured in seconds, so the standard unit for acceleration is meters/second^2 (m/s^2).

$$\frac{meters/second}{second} = \frac{meters}{second^2} = \frac{m}{s^2}$$

Acceleration is expressed by using both magnitude and direction, so it is a vector quantity like velocity. Acceleration is present when an object is slowing down, speeding up, or changing direction, since these represent instances where velocity is changing. This means that forces like friction and gravity accelerate objects and increase or decrease their velocities over time.

Projectile Motion

Projectile motion describes the way in which a projectile will move when the only force acting upon it is gravity. Since the force of Earth's gravity is nearly constant at sea level, its magnitude is approximated as a rate of 9.8 m/s^2. For projectile motion problems, the projectile is assumed to travel a curved path to the ground and ignore air resistance, wind speed, and other such complications.

Projectile motion has two components: horizontal and vertical. Without air resistance, there is no horizontal acceleration, so the horizontal velocity won't change. However, the vertical velocity will change because of gravity's acceleration on the projectile. A sample parabolic curve of projectile motion is shown below.

Projectile Path for a Bullet Fired Horizontally from a Hill (Ignoring Air Resistance)

Horizontal distance (d_x) is defined as the relationship between velocity (v_x) and time (t), where x is the movement along the horizontal plane (x-axis).

$$d_x = v_x t$$

Because of the force of gravity, the vertical velocity and position is continuously changing and thus more complicated to calculate. The following equations are different expressions of vertical motion:

$$v_f{}^2 = v_i{}^2 + 2ad$$

$$d = \frac{1}{2}at^2 + v_i t$$

$$v_f = v_i + at$$

These equations use v_f as the final velocity, v_i as the initial velocity, a as the acceleration, d as the horizontal distance traveled, and t as the time to describe functions of motion.

Newton's Laws of Motion

Sir Isaac Newton spent a great deal of time studying objects, forces, and how an object's motion responds to forces. Newton made great advancements by using mathematics to describe the motion of objects and to predict future motions of objects by applying his mathematical models to situations. Through his extensive research, Newton is credited for summarizing the basic laws of motion for objects here on Earth. These laws are as follows:

1. The law of inertia: An object in motion will remain in motion, unless acted upon by an outside force. An object at rest remains at rest, unless acted upon by an outside force. Simply put, **inertia** is the natural tendency of an object to continue along with what it is already doing; an outside force would have to act upon the object to make it change its course. This includes an object that is sitting still.

2. $F = ma$: The **force (F)** on an object is equal to the mass (m) multiplied by the acceleration (a) on that object. **Mass (m)** refers to the amount of a substance while acceleration (a) refers to a change in velocity over time.

   - In the case of a projectile falling to Earth's surface, the acceleration is due to gravity.

   - Multiplying an object's mass by its gravitational acceleration gives the special force that is called the object's **weight (W)**. Note that weight is a force and is a vector quantity while mass is in kilograms and is a scalar quantity, as it has no acceleration.

   - Forces are typically measured in **Newtons** (N), which are a derived SI unit equal to $1 \frac{\text{kg·m}}{\text{s}^2}$. You can find an object's weight in Newtons by multiplying its mass (in kilograms) by the acceleration of gravity (9.8 m/s^2 for Earth).

3. For every action, there is an equal and opposite reaction. This means that, if a book drops onto a desk, the book will exert a force on the desk due to hitting it, but the desk will also exert

an equal force on the book in the opposite direction. This is what sometimes causes fallen objects to bounce once or twice after hitting the ground.

A clear understanding of force is crucial to using Newton's laws of motion. **Forces** are anything acting upon an object either in motion or at rest; this includes friction and gravity. These forces can push or pull on a mass, and they have a magnitude and a direction. Forces are represented by a **vector,** which is the arrow lined up along the direction of the force with its tip at the point of application. The magnitude of the force is represented by the length of the vector. Large forces have long vector lengths.

Friction

Friction is a resistance to movement that always imparts a negative acceleration to an object. Because it accelerates an object in the opposite direction than it wants to go, friction will cause moving objects to slow down and eventually stop. Frictional force depends on several factors including the texture of the two surfaces and the amount of contact force pushing the surfaces together. There are four types of friction: static, sliding, rolling, and fluid friction. **Static friction** occurs between stationary objects, while **sliding friction** occurs when solid objects slide over each other. **Rolling friction** happens when a solid object rolls over another solid object, and **fluid friction** is a friction caused by an object moving through a fluid or through fluid layers. These 'fluids' can be either a gas or a liquid, so this also includes air resistance.

Rotation

Rotating and spinning objects have a special type of movement. A spinning top can move across a table, demonstrating linear motion, but it can also spin in place, demonstrating angular motion. Just as a car moves from place to place by changing its location, its velocity, and its acceleration, so too can a rotating object change its orientation, its angular velocity, and its angular acceleration.

For linear movement, the first thing that is described is the object's displacement. The **displacement** of the object is how far it moves from its starting location; this linear change in location is usually represented by the symbol Δx. However, for the angular movement of a simple solid like a sphere, the distance that its surface travels is not a good measure of its angular movement, since a large sphere would have to rotate a much smaller degree to move the same distance as a small sphere would. This angular distance is referred to as S, or the arc length.

A better measure of angular movement is the **angular displacement** θ, which is defined as the angle through which the object will rotate. Because there are a standard 360° in all circles, angular displacement can be used to compare angular movement between objects of different sizes, making it a much more versatile tool than the arc length. However, although a circle can be split up into 360 degrees, it can also be visualized as being split up into 2π **radians,** where radians is a unit similar to degrees that describes angles. The 2π is usually used in physics because a circle's circumference has a value of 2π times its radius, and radians is an easier unit to use than is degrees.

The angular displacement can be found by dividing the arc length that an object rotates through by the radius of the object's rotation. For example, if an object completes 1 full rotation, it has rotated through 360°. It has also traveled an arc length equal to its circumference, or $2\pi r$. Plugging this arc length S into

177

the equation below, it can be seen that the angular displacement is 2π, which is correct since it is equal to the $360°$ as discussed previously.

$$angular\ displacement\ (\theta) = \frac{S}{r}$$

The angular speed or **angular velocity, w,** is the measure of how quickly the object is rotating, and w is defined as the angular displacement that is accomplished in a certain amount of time, as shown below.

$$angular\ speed\ (\omega) = \frac{\Delta\theta}{\Delta t}$$

Similar to linear velocity, angular velocity may accelerate due to external forces, and this angular acceleration is given by the variable α. Its equation, the change in angular velocity over a change in time, is given below.

$$angular\ acceleration\ (\alpha) = \frac{\Delta\omega}{\Delta t}$$

When objects are exhibiting circular motion, they also demonstrate the **conservation of angular momentum,** meaning that the angular momentum of a system is always constant, regardless of the placement of the mass. **Rotational inertia** can be affected by how far the mass of the object is placed with respect to the center of rotation (**axis of rotation**). The larger the distance between the mass and the center of rotation, the slower the rotational velocity. Conversely, if the mass is closer to the center of rotation, the rotational velocity increases. A change in one affects the other, thus conserving the angular momentum. This holds true if no external forces act upon the system.

Uniform Circular Motion

Circular motion is similar in many ways to linear (straight line) motion; however, there are a few additional points to note. In uniform circular motion, a spinning object is always linearly accelerating because it is always changing direction. The force causing this constant acceleration on or around an axis is called the **centripetal force,** and it is often associated with centripetal acceleration. Centripetal force always pulls toward the axis of rotation; this means that the force will always pull towards the center of the rotation circle. The relationship between the velocity (v) of an object and the radius (r) of the circle is **centripetal acceleration**, and the equation is as follows:

$$centripetal\ acceleration\ (a_c) = \frac{v^2}{r}$$

According to Newton's law, force is the combination of two factors, mass and acceleration. This is demonstrated by centripetal force. Centripetal force is shown mathematically by using the mass of an object (m), the velocity (v), and the radius (r).

$$centripetal\ force\ (F_c) = \frac{mv^2}{r}$$

Kinetic Energy and Potential Energy

The two primary forms of energy are kinetic energy and potential energy. **Kinetic energy**, or KE, involves the energy of motion, and is easily found for Newtonian physics by an object's mass in kilograms and velocity in meters per second. Kinetic energy can be calculated using the following equation:

$$KE = \frac{1}{2}mv^2$$

Potential energy represents the energy possessed by an object by virtue of its position. In the classical example, an object's gravitational potential energy can be found as a simple function of its height or by what distance it drops. Potential energy, or PE, may be calculated using the following equation:

$$PE = mgh$$

Both kinetic energy and potential energy are scalar quantities measured in **Joules**. One Joule is the amount of energy that can push an object with 1 Newton of force for 1 meter, so it is also referred to as a Newton-meter. As mentioned previously, the **Law of Conservation of Energy** states that energy can neither be created nor destroyed. Therefore, potential and kinetic energy can be transformed into one another, depending on an object's speed and position.

Linear Momentum and Impulse

Motion creates something called **momentum.** This is a calculation of an object's mass multiplied by its velocity. Momentum can be described as the amount an object wants to continue moving along its current course. Momentum in a straight line is called linear momentum. Just as energy can be transferred and conserved, so too can momentum.

Changing the expression of Newton's second law of motion yields a new expression.

$$Force(F) = ma = m \times \frac{\Delta v}{\Delta t}$$

If both sides of the expression are multiplied by the change in time, the law produces the impulse equation.

$$F\Delta t = m\Delta v$$

This equation shows that the amount of force during a length of time creates an **impulse.** This means that if a force acts on an object during a given amount of time, it will have a determined impulse. However, if the same change in velocity happens over a longer amount of time, the required force is much smaller, due to the conservation of momentum.

$$p = mv$$

Linear momentum, p, is found by multiplying the mass of an object by its velocity. Since momentum, like mass and energy, is conserved, Newton's 2nd law can be restated for multiple objects. In this form, it can be used to understand the energy of objects that have interacted, since the conservation of momentum implies that the momentum before and after an interaction must be the same. This is best demonstrated in the case of elastic collision, where an object of mass m$_1$ with velocity v_1 collides with an object of mass m_2 with velocity v_2 and both object end with velocities v_1' and v_2', respectively.

$$m_1 v_1' + m_2 v_2' = m_1 v_1 + m_2 v_2$$

Universal Gravitation

Newton's **law of universal gravitation** addresses the universality of gravity. Gravity acts as a force at a distance and causes all bodies in the universe to attract each other.

The **force of gravity (F_g)** is proportional to the masses of two objects (m_1 and m_2) and inversely proportional to the square of the distance (r^2) between them. (G is the proportionality constant). This is shown in the following equation:

$$F_g = G \frac{m_1 m_2}{r^2}$$

All objects falling within the Earth's atmosphere are all affected by the force of gravity, so their rates of acceleration will be equal to 9.8 m/s^2, or gravity. Therefore, if two objects are dropped from the same height at the same time, they should hit the ground at the same time. This is irrespective of mass, since the previous kinetics equations don't include mass, so a bowling ball and a feather would theoretically fall at identical rates. Unfortunately, in the Earth's atmosphere, air resistance would slow the feather much more than the bowling ball, so the bowling ball would fall faster, but this effect can be minimized in a vacuum. In other words, without air resistance or other external forces acting on the objects, gravity will affect every object on the Earth with the same rate of acceleration.

Waves and Sound

Waves are periodic disturbances in a gas, liquid, or solid that are created as energy is transmitted. Each part of a wave has a different name and is used in different calculations. The four parts of a wave are the crest, the trough, the amplitude, and the wavelength. The **crest** is the highest point, while the **trough** is the lowest. The **amplitude** is the distance between a peak and the average of the wave; it is also the distance between a trough and the average of the wave, but an amplitude is always positive, since it is an absolute value. Finally, the distance between one wave and the exact same place on the next wave is the **wavelength.**

180

With amplitude and wavelength, it is possible to describe any wave, but an important question still remains unanswered: How fast is the wave traveling? A wave's speed can be shown as either its period or its frequency. A wave's period, T, is how long it takes for the wave to travel one wavelength, while a wave's frequency, f, is how many wavelengths are traveled in one second. These are inversely related, so they are reciprocals of each other, as shown below.

$$f = \frac{1}{T} \text{ and } T = \frac{1}{f}$$

The largest categories of waves are electromagnetic waves and mechanical waves. **Electromagnetic waves** can transmit energy through a vacuum and do not need a medium to travel through, examples of which are light, radio, microwaves, gamma rays, and other forms of electromagnetism. **Mechanical waves** can only transmit energy through another form of matter called a medium. The particles of the medium are shifted as the wave moves through the medium, and can be anything from solids to liquids to gasses. Examples of mechanical waves include auditory sounds heard by human ears in the air as well as percussive shocks like earthquakes.

There are two different forms of waves: transverse and longitudinal waves. **Transverse** waves are waves in which particles of the medium move in a direction perpendicular to the direction waves move, as in most electromagnetic waves. **Compression**, or longitudinal, waves are waves in which the particles of the medium move in a direction parallel to the direction the waves move, as in most mechanical waves. A good example of a longitudinal wave is sound. A good example of a longitudinal wave is sound. Waves travel within a medium at a speed that is determined by the wavelength (λ) and frequency (f) of the wave.

$$v = f\lambda$$

There is a proportional relationship between the amplitude of a wave and the potential energy in the wave. This means the taller the wave, the more stored energy it is transmitting.

Light

Light is an electromagnetic wave that is created by electric and magnetic interactions. Like other electromagnetic waves, light does not need a medium to travel. Light energy can be absorbed and changed into heat, reflected, or even transmitted.

A wave is reflected when it collides with a surface and bounces off, unharmed. The **law of reflection** shows that an **incident ray** (the wave that hits the surface) will bounce off the surface and become a reflected ray (the wave that leaves the surface). Because the wave doesn't lose any energy, the angle at which it hits the surface will be identical to the angle at which it leaves the surface, so the interaction produces identical waves. This is the definition of **reflection**.

On the other hand, a wave is refracted when a wave collides with a surface and bends, such as when the medium it is traveling through changes. Examples of **refraction** include the bending of light as it passes through a prism and sunlight passing through raindrops to create a rainbow.

To understand refraction, a 'normal' line is drawn perpendicular to the surface that the wave will hit. The angle created between the normal line and the incident ray is the angle of incidence, while the angle of reflection is the opposite and equal angle formed between the normal line and the reflected ray. The refraction of light depends on the varying speeds and densities of different media. As light

181

passes through different media, the wave will bend toward or away from the normal line, depending on the material it is transitioning to. **Snell's law** describes this behavior mathematically in the equation that follows:

$$n_1 \sin \theta_1 = n_2 \sin \theta_2$$

In this equation, n is the index of refraction and θ is the angle of refraction. The **index of refraction** determines the amount of light that bends or refracts when it encounters a medium. Materials that interact with and change the wave more will have higher indices of refraction, and any material's index of refraction can be found by the following equation.

$$n = \frac{c}{v_s}$$

Because the speed of light in a vacuum, c, is constant, it can be used to show how much a material will interact with a wave. The **refractive index, n,** shows how much the speed of light is changed when it travels through the material at a new velocity of v_s.

Optics

Spherical mirrors change the way light reflects. Lenses and curved mirrors are made to focus light in certain ways. There are several terms used to describe and define mirrors and lenses. The **principal axis** is a reference line that usually passes through the center of the curve of the mirror or lens. The **vertex, V,** is the point where the mirror is crossed by the principal axis. The sphere which contains the curve of the mirror has a center called the **center of curvature (C)**. The **focal point (F)** is halfway between the center of curvature and the vertex.

The **focal length (f)** is measured by how far the focal point is from the mirror. The following graphic shows a visual representation of these terms in a concave mirror.

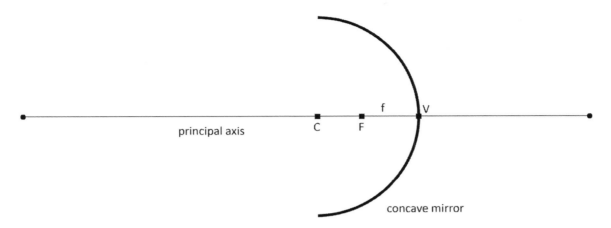

The focal lengths of concave mirrors are positive. Concave mirrors can produce images of various shapes and sizes as well as of different orientations based on the focal length of the mirror and the placement of the object. Convex mirrors differ from concave mirrors in that they have negative focal lengths. The other main difference is that convex mirrors always form images that are reduced in size and upright.

Lenses are pieces of transparent material molded to refract light rays to create an image. There are two types of lenses. Convex lenses, also called **converging lenses**, have positive focal lengths. Concave lenses, or **diverging lenses**, conversely have negative focal lengths. Images in convex lenses can look different depending on the focal length of the lens and where the object is located. Convex lenses only create images that are upright and smaller in size than the object.

Atomic Structure

All known matter is made of atoms. Atoms have a nucleus composed of **protons** (with a positive charge) and **neutrons** (with no net charge), which is surrounded by a cloud of **electrons** (with negative charges). Since protons have a positive charge and neutrons have a neutral charge, an atom's nucleus typically has an overall positive electrical charge, but because electrons orbiting the nucleus have an overall negative charge, an atom with equal numbers of protons and electrons is considered stable.

The properties of an atom vary with the number of electrons and their arrangement in shells around the nucleus. Electrons are organized into distributions of subshells called **electron configurations**. Subshells fill from the inside (closest to the nucleus) to the outside and are lettered starting with "k." The strength of the bond between the nucleus and the electron is called the **binding energy**. The binding energy is stronger for those shells located closer to the nucleus.

The number of electrons in each shell can be determined using the following equation using n for the shell number:

$$2n^2$$

The Nature of Electricity

The nature of electricity is based on the atoms of a given material, as objects develop electric charges when their atoms gain or lose electrons. The electrons that are in the furthest shell from an atom's nucleus are the most likely to interact, so they are specially termed **valence electrons**. If the electrons are tightly bound to their atoms, the material is an **insulator** because, like rubber, wood, and glass, the material prevents electrons from flowing freely. However, if the electrons are loosely bound to the atoms, the material is a **conductor** because, like iron and other metals, the electrons can flow freely throughout the material.

It is important to note that opposite charges attract each other, while like charges repel each other. Interestingly, the repulsive force between two electrons is equivalent to the attractive force between an electron and a proton (only in different directions). Coulomb described these repellant and attractive forces between two objects in his namesake law. This electrical **Coulomb force, F,** is determined by multiplying the charges of the two objects, q_1 and q_2, by a constant, k, and dividing by the distance they are from one another squared, r^2.

$$F = \frac{kq_1q_2}{r^2}$$

If the force is negative, then the objects attract each other because q_1 and q_2 are of opposite charges. If the force is positive, then the objects repel each other because q_1 and q_2 are of the same charge.

An electric charge naturally produces an electric field around itself. Electric fields can vary in strength and magnitude depending on the type of charge (positive or negative) that generates the field. The nature of electric fields can be tested using a test charge. Mathematically, the magnitude of an electric field (E) can be found using the following equation:

$$E = \frac{F}{q_o}$$

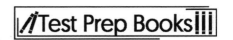

Where F is the force a test charge would undergo, and q_o is the magnitude of the test charge. Electric fields are vector quantities; this means they have both a magnitude and a direction. In the case of electric fields, it is the convention to define the direction of the field vector as the way a positive test charge would move when positioned in the electric field: towards a negative charge and away from other positive charges.

An **electric circuit** is usually comprised of circuit elements joined by a wire or other object that allows an electric charge to move along the path without interruption — this moving electric charge is called an electric **current.** However, constant electric currents may only exist in a complete circuit if there is a voltage difference in the circuit. **Voltage** is literally the distance that a circuit's electrical force could move one electron, but voltage can be visualized as how much energy a certain part of the circuit has available to push around electrons. Electrons will flow from regions of higher voltage to regions of lower voltage, so it is the difference in voltages between two parts of a circuit that makes a current actually flow.

In other words, voltage difference is the difference in potential energy between two places measured in **volts (V),** while a circuit is a closed path through which electrons can flow. Because every atom has positive charges that pull on electrons and resist their flow, most real circuits have a **resistance** level, measured in **ohms,** which is described as the opposition to the flow of electric charge. The amount of current that can flow through a circuit depends on the voltage difference and how well the wire resists the flow of electricity. **Ohm's law** gives us the relationship between voltage (V), current in amperes (I), and resistance in ohms (R).

$$V = I \times R$$

Series Circuits (A) and Parallel Circuits (B)
Practical circuits have numerous loads which can be hooked up "in series" (A) or "in parallel" (B), as shown below.

185

To determine the total voltage requirement for circuits with multiple component loads (in series or in parallel), it is necessary to find the equivalent resistance of the circuits.

Series circuits put resistors in a row or series so that current must flow from one to the other, while **parallel circuits** run resistors in parallel sections so that current can flow through one or the other. In a series circuit like the one in A, the voltage drops across each resistor, but the current is the same in all of them. The current must be the same across each resistor, as according to Ampere's law, the electrons in the current must continue flowing throughout the wire and not build up or disappear. In other words, the electrons going into the resistor must all go out so that the "flow in equals flow out."

The current through each resistor is the same, and the total voltage (V) equals the drop across R_1 plus the drop across R_2. The equivalent resistance is determined by solving Ohm's law for voltage:

$$V = V_1 + V_2 = IR_1 + IR_2 = I(R_1 + R_2) = IR_{eq}$$

Thus, in a series circuit, the equivalent resistance is equal to the sum of the component resistances, and this relation holds for any number of resistors in a series.

In a parallel circuit like the one in (B), the voltage is the same across each resistor because each is attached directly to the power source and the ground. The electric current is divided between the loads depending on their resistances, since it can flow through either of them, but not both. If the resistance is the same in both loads, then the same amount of current passes through each one. If the resistance is different in each load, then more current passes through the load with the lower resistance, since energy takes the path of least resistance.

The **equivalent resistance (R_{eq})** of the parallel circuit is determined by solving Ohm's law for the current through each resistor, setting it equal to the total current (R_t), and remembering that the voltages are all the same:

$$I_t = \frac{V}{R_{eq}} = \frac{V}{R_1} + \frac{V}{R_2} \quad \textbf{or} \quad \frac{1}{R_{eq}} = \frac{1}{R_1} + \frac{1}{R_2} \quad \textbf{so} \quad R_{eq} = \frac{1}{\frac{1}{R_1} + \frac{1}{R_2}}$$

In a parallel circuit, the equivalent resistance is equal to one over the sum of the reciprocals of the component resistances.

Magnetism and Electricity

Magnetism can occur naturally in certain types of materials like iron, nickel, and cobalt. If two straight rods are made from iron, they will usually have a naturally negative end (pole) and a positive end (pole). These charged poles react just like any charged item: opposite charges attract and like charges repel. They will attract each other when set up positive to negative, but if one rod is turned around, the two rods will repel each other due to the alignment of negative to negative and positive to positive.

Magnetic fields can also be created and amplified by using an electric current. The force of attraction between two magnetic fields is measured in **Teslas**. The relationship between magnetic forces and electrical forces can be explored by sending an electric current through a stretch of wire, which creates an electromagnetic force around the wire from the charge of the current, as long as the flow of electricity is sustained. This magnetic force can also attract and repel other items with magnetic properties. Depending upon the strength of the current in the wire, a smaller or larger magnetic force can be generated around this wire. As soon as the current is cut off, the magnetic force also stops. When a magnetic field produces an electric current, this is called an **electromagnetic induction**.

Practice Quiz

1. Velocity is a measure of which of the following?
   a. Speed with direction
   b. The change in speed over the change in time
   c. Acceleration with direction
   d. All of the above

2. Which of the following correctly lists the subatomic particles in an atom?
   a. Protons carry no charge in the nucleus, neutrons carry a negative charge in the nucleus, and electrons surround the nucleus in a cloud and carry a positive charge.
   b. Protons carry a positive charge in the nucleus, neutrons have no charge in the nucleus, and electrons have a negative charge and are found in a cloud surrounding the nucleus.
   c. Protons carry a positive charge in the nucleus, electrons have a negative charge in the nucleus, and neutrons have a negative charge and surround the nucleus in a cloud.
   d. Protons carry a positive charge, and they surround the nucleus in a cloud. The nucleus contains negatively charged electrons and neutrons, which carry no charge.

3. Which of the following equations is not an accurate representation of Ohm's Law?
   a. $V = I \times R$
   b. $R = \dfrac{V}{I}$
   c. $I = \dfrac{V}{R}$
   d. $V = \dfrac{R}{I}$

4. A football is kicked so that it leaves the punter's toe at a horizontal angle of 45 degrees. Ignoring any spin or tumbling, at what point is the upward vertical velocity of the football at a maximum?

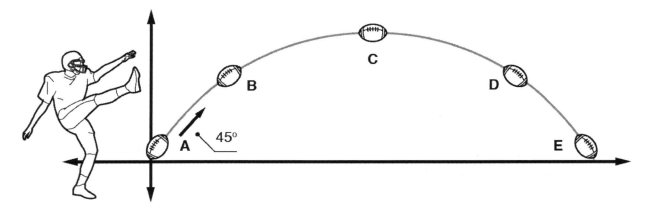

   a. At Point A
   b. At Point C
   c. At Points B and D
   d. At Points A and E

188

5. A cannonball is dropped from a height of 10 meters off of the ground. What is its approximate velocity just before it hits the ground?
   a. 9.81 m/s
   b. 14 m/s
   c. 32 m/s
   d. 1 m/s

6. The energy from electricity results from which of the following?
   a. The atomic structure of matter
   b. The ability to do work
   c. The neutrons in an atom
   d. Conductive materials like metals

7. Electric power can be measured in which of the following units?
   a. Volts
   b. Amperes
   c. Ohms
   d. Watts

8. Which of the following is true regarding series circuits?
   a. The voltage drops across each resistor, but the current is the same in all of them.
   b. The voltage is the same across each resistor, but the current drops after each of them.
   c. The voltage drops across each resistor, and the current drops in each of them.
   d. The voltage and current are the same across each of them in the series.

See answers on next page.

If you want to test your knowledge further on the
physics section of the HESI exam,
take our online practice quiz.

testprepbooks.com/hesi-quiz

SCAN ME

Answer Explanations

1. A: Velocity is a measure of speed with direction. To calculate velocity, find the distance covered and the time it took to cover that distance; change in position over the change in time. A standard measurement for velocity is in meters per second (m/s). The change in velocity over change in time is acceleration, while acceleration with direction has no specific name.

2. B: The structure of atoms is as follows: The central nucleus contains protons and neutrons. Protons have a positive charge (+1), and neutrons are neutral, so they do not carry a charge. Around the nucleus is a cloud, which contains electrons in rings called orbitals. Electrons are negatively charged (−1), and those in the outermost ring — farthest from the nucleus — tend to be easier to remove from the atom.

3. D: Ohm's Law describes the relation between voltage and amperage, where voltage is a measure of electromotive potential much like potential energy of motion in kinetics. Amperage measures the electric current or the flow rate of 1 coulomb of electrons in a second. The basic law is $V = I \times R$, but this can be manipulated in the following ways:

$$I = \frac{V}{R} \quad \text{or} \quad V = I \times R \quad \text{or} \quad R = \frac{V}{I}$$

4. A: The answer is that the upward velocity is at a maximum when it leaves the punter's toe. The acceleration due to gravity reduces the upward velocity every moment thereafter. The speed is the same at points A and E, but the velocity is different. At point E, the velocity has a maximum *negative* value.

5. B: The answer is 14 m/s. Remember that the cannonball at rest, y meters off the ground, has a potential energy of $PE = mgy$. As it falls, the potential energy is converted to kinetic energy until (at ground level) the kinetic energy is equal to the total original potential energy:

$$\frac{1}{2}mv^2 = mgy$$

Rearranged to solve for velocity, the equation is:

$$v = \sqrt{2gy}$$

This makes sense because all objects fall at the same rate, so the velocity *must* be independent of the mass; thus, Choice *D* is incorrect. Plugging the values into the equation, the result is 14 m/s. Remember, the way to figure this quickly is to have g equal to 10 m/s^2 rather than 9.81 m/s^2.

6. A: The physical structure of the atoms that compose matter lends itself to the production of electricity. The arrangement of the subatomic particles and the associated charges — mainly the negatively charged electrons in the cloud — are associated with the ability to create an electric current, which can be harnessed to do work.

7. D: The difference in potential between two separate points is a measure of volts. Amperes indicate the number of electrons that pass a specific point per second. Ohms measure the resistance to flow (essentially electrical friction). Watts are a measure of power or the rate at which electrical energy is used or converted into another type of energy. Watts are often converted to kilowatts or, when expressing power rates, kilowatt-hours.

8. B: When devices are connected in a series circuit, the voltage is the same across each device (or resistor) in the loop, but the current drops after each device. Recall that for lightbulbs connected in series, this is observed by a decrease in the brightness of each successive bulb. This is one of the disadvantages of a series circuit. In contrast, the current increases with the addition of each resistor in parallel circuits.

HESI A2 Practice Test #1

Mathematics

1. Which of the following is equivalent to the value of the digit 3 in the number 792.134?
    a. 3×10
    b. 3×100
    c. $\frac{3}{10}$
    d. $\frac{3}{100}$

2. Add $101,694 + 623$.
    a. 103,317
    b. 102,317
    c. 102,417
    d. 102,427

3. How will the number 847.89632 be written if rounded to the nearest hundredth?
    a. 847.90
    b. 900
    c. 847.89
    d. 847.896

4. What is the value of the sum of $\frac{1}{3}$ and $\frac{2}{5}$?
    a. $\frac{3}{8}$
    b. $\frac{11}{15}$
    c. $\frac{11}{30}$
    d. $\frac{4}{5}$

5. Add and express in reduced form $\frac{7}{12} + \frac{5}{9}$.
    a. $1\frac{5}{36}$
    b. $\frac{13}{9}$
    c. $\frac{41}{36}$
    d. $1\frac{4}{9}$

192

6. How will $\frac{4}{5}$ be written as a percent?

    a. 40%

    b. 125%

    c. 90%

    d. 80%

7. Subtract $7{,}236 - 978$.

    a. 6,268

    b. 5,258

    c. 6,358

    d. 6,258

8. What are all the factors of 12?

    a. 12, 24, 36

    b. 1, 2, 4, 6, 12

    c. 12, 24, 36, 48

    d. 1, 2, 3, 4, 6, 12

9. A construction company is building a new housing development with the property of each house measuring 30 feet wide. If the length of the street is zoned off at 345 feet, how many houses can be built on the street?

    a. 11

    b. 115

    c. 11.5

    d. 12

10. Subtract $653.4 - 59.38$.

    a. 595.92

    b. 594.11

    c. 594.02

    d. 593.92

11. Subtract and express in reduced form $\frac{19}{24} - \frac{1}{6}$.

    a. $\frac{5}{8}$

    b. $\frac{18}{6}$

    c. $\frac{15}{24}$

    d. $\frac{1}{3}$

12. If $-3(x + 4) = x + 8$, what is the value of x?

    a. $x = 4$

    b. $x = 2$

    c. $x = 5$

    d. $x = -5$

13. Multiply 346×13.
   a. 4,598
   b. 4,468
   c. 4,498
   d. 4,568

14. If $4x - 3 = 5$, what is the value of x?
   a. 1
   b. 2
   c. 3
   d. 4

15. A grocery store is selling individual bottles of water, and each bottle contains 750 milliliters of water. If 12 bottles are purchased, what conversion will correctly determine how many liters that customer will take home?
   a. 100 milliliters equals 1 liter
   b. 1,000 milliliters equals 1 liter
   c. 1,000 liters equals 1 milliliter
   d. 10 liters equals 1 milliliter

16. At the beginning of the day, Xavier has 20 apples. At lunch, he meets his sister Emma and gives her half of his apples. After lunch, he stops by his neighbor Jim's house and gives him 6 of his apples. He then uses $\frac{3}{4}$ of his remaining apples to make an apple pie for dessert at dinner. At the end of the day, how many apples does Xavier have left?
   a. 1
   b. 2
   c. 4
   d. 6

17. 12 is 40% of what number?
   a. 24
   b. 28
   c. 34
   d. 30

18. $3\frac{2}{3} - 1\frac{4}{5} =$

   a. $1\frac{13}{15}$

   b. $\frac{14}{15}$

   c. $2\frac{2}{3}$

   d. $\frac{4}{5}$

19. What is $\frac{660}{100}$ rounded to the nearest integer?

    a. 67

    b. 66

    c. 7

    d. 6

20. Which of the following is largest?

    a. -0.45

    b. -0.096

    c. -0.3

    d. -0.313

21. What is the value of b in this equation?

$$5b - 4 = 2b + 17$$

    a. 13

    b. 24

    c. 7

    d. 21

22. Katie works at a clothing company and sold 192 shirts over the weekend. One-third of the shirts that were sold were patterned and the rest were solid. Which mathematical expression would calculate the number of solid shirts Katie sold over the weekend?

    a. $192 \times \frac{1}{3}$

    b. $192 \div \frac{1}{3}$

    c. $192 \times (1 - \frac{1}{3})$

    d. $192 \div 3$

23. Arrange the following numbers from least to greatest value:

    $0.85, \frac{4}{5}, \frac{2}{3}, \frac{91}{100}$

    a. $0.85, \frac{4}{5}, \frac{2}{3}, \frac{91}{100}$

    b. $\frac{4}{5}, 0.85, \frac{91}{100}, \frac{2}{3}$

    c. $\frac{2}{3}, \frac{4}{5}, 0.85, \frac{91}{100}$

    d. $0.85, \frac{91}{100}, \frac{4}{5}, \frac{2}{3}$

24. Divide and reduce $\frac{5}{13} \div \frac{25}{169}$.

    a. $\frac{13}{5}$

    b. $\frac{65}{25}$

    c. $\frac{25}{65}$

    d. $\frac{5}{13}$

25. Express as a reduced mixed number $\frac{54}{15}$.

    a. $3\frac{3}{5}$

    b. $3\frac{1}{15}$

    c. $3\frac{3}{54}$

    d. $3\frac{1}{54}$

26. in the problem $5 \times 6 + 4 \div 2 - 1$, which operation should be completed first?

    a. Multiplication

    b. Addition

    c. Division

    d. Subtraction

27. Express as an improper fraction $8\frac{3}{7}$.

    a. $\frac{11}{7}$

    b. $\frac{21}{8}$

    c. $\frac{5}{3}$

    d. $\frac{59}{7}$

28. Express as an improper fraction $11\frac{5}{8}$.

    a. $\frac{55}{8}$

    b. $\frac{93}{8}$

    c. $\frac{16}{11}$

    d. $\frac{19}{5}$

29. Round to the nearest tenth: 8.067
   a. 8.07
   b. 8.1
   c. 8.00
   d. 8.11

30. When rounding 245.2678 to the nearest thousandth, which place value would be used to decide whether to round up or round down?
   a. Ten-thousandth
   b. Thousandth
   c. Hundredth
   d. Thousand

31. Carey bought 184 pounds of fertilizer to use on her lawn. Each segment of her lawn required $11\frac{1}{2}$ pounds of fertilizer to do a sufficient job. If a student were asked to determine how many segments could be fertilized with the amount purchased, what operation would be necessary to solve this problem?
   a. Multiplication
   b. Division
   c. Addition
   d. Subtraction

32. Which of the following is an equivalent measurement for 1.3 cm?
   a. 0.13 m
   b. 0.013 m
   c. 0.13 mm
   d. 0.013 mm

33. Alan currently weighs 200 pounds, but he wants to lose weight to get down to 175 pounds. What is this difference in kilograms? (1 pound is approximately equal to 0.45 kilograms.)
   a. 9 kg
   b. 11.25 kg
   c. 78.75 kg
   d. 90 kg

34. $\frac{14}{15} + \frac{3}{5} - \frac{1}{30} =$

   a. $\frac{19}{15}$

   b. $\frac{43}{30}$

   c. $\frac{4}{3}$

   d. $\frac{3}{2}$

197

35. Mo needs to buy enough material to cover the walls around the stage for a theater performance. If he needs 79 feet of wall covering, what is the minimum number of yards of material he should purchase if the material is sold only by whole yards?
    a. 23 yards
    b. 25 yards
    c. 26 yards
    d. 27 yards

36. Express 517 in Roman numerals.
    a. CXVII
    b. DCIIV
    c. DXVII
    d. VDVII

37. Convert 1500 hours into a 12-hour clock time.
    a. 3:00 p.m.
    b. 9:00 a.m.
    c. 3:00 a.m.
    d. 9:00 p.m.

38. $\frac{5}{3} \times \frac{7}{6} =$

    a. $\frac{3}{5}$

    b. $\frac{18}{3}$

    c. $\frac{45}{31}$

    d. $\frac{35}{18}$

39. Which common denominator would be used to evaluate $\frac{2}{3} + \frac{4}{5}$?
    a. 15
    b. 3
    c. 5
    d. 10

40. What time is 10:00am in military (24-hour clock) time?
    a. 0100 hours
    b. 1000 hours
    c. 1200 hours
    d. 0200 hours

41. 1 kilometer is how many centimeters?
    a. 100 cm
    b. 1,000 cm
    c. 10,000 cm
    d. 100,000 cm

42. What is the solution to $(2 \times 20) \div (7 + 1) + (6 \times 0.01) + (4 \times 0.001)$?
    a. 5.064
    b. 5.64
    c. 5.0064
    d. 48.064

43. The value of 6×12 is the same as:
    a. $2 \times 4 \times 4 \times 2$
    b. $7 \times 4 \times 3$
    c. $6 \times 6 \times 3$
    d. $3 \times 3 \times 4 \times 2$

44. A piggy bank contains 12 dollars' worth of nickels. A nickel weighs 5 grams, and the empty piggy bank weighs 1,050 grams. What is the total weight of the full piggy bank?
    a. 1,110 grams
    b. 1,200 grams
    c. 2,250 grams
    d. 2,200 grams

45. Last year, the New York City area received approximately $27\frac{3}{4}$ inches of snow. The Denver area received approximately 3 times as much snow as New York City. How much snow fell in Denver?

    a. 60 inches

    b. $27\frac{1}{4}$ inches

    c. $9\frac{1}{4}$ inches

    d. $83\frac{1}{4}$ inches

46. How many pints are in 15 gallons?
    a. 45 pts.
    b. 100 pts.
    c. 120 pts.
    d. 15 pts.

47. A patient has a temperature of 37.4 °C. What is this on the Fahrenheit scale?
    a. 99.23 °F
    b. 99.32 °F
    c. 98.32 °F
    d. 98.23 °F

48. What is the solution to the following problem in decimal form?

$$\frac{3}{5} \times \frac{7}{10} \div \frac{1}{2}$$

    a. 0.042
    b. 84%
    c. 0.84
    d. 0.42
    e. 42%

49. Twenty is 40% of what number?
    a. 60
    b. 8
    c. 200
    d. 70
    e. 50

50. Write the expression for six less than three times the sum of twice a number and one.
    a. $2x + 1 - 6$
    b. $3x + 1 - 6$
    c. $3(x + 1) - 6$
    d. $3(2x + 1) - 6$

51. After a 20% discount, Frank purchased a new refrigerator for $850. How much did he save from the original price?
    a. $170
    b. $212.50
    c. $105.75
    d. $200

52. Mom's car drove 72 miles in 90 minutes. How fast did she drive in feet per second?
    a. 0.8 feet per second
    b. 48.9 feet per second
    c. 0.009 feet per second
    d. 70.4 feet per second

53. $52.3 \times 10^{-3} =$
    a. 0.00523
    b. 0.0523
    c. 0.523
    d. 523

54. Jessica buys 10 cans of paint. Red paint costs $1 per can and blue paint costs $2 per can. In total, she spends $16. How many red cans did she buy?
    a. 2
    b. 3
    c. 4
    d. 5

55. A farmer owns two (non-adjacent) square plots of land, which he wishes to fence. The area of one is 1000 square feet, while the area of the other is 10 square feet. How much fencing does he need, in feet?

    a. 44

    b. $40\sqrt{10}$

    c. $440\sqrt{10}$

    d. $44\sqrt{10}$

Reading Comprehension

Questions 1-5 are based on the following passage:

This excerpt is an adaptation of Jonathan Swift's Gulliver's Travels into Several Remote Nations of the World.

My gentleness and good behaviour had gained so far on the emperor and his court, and indeed upon the army and people in general, that I began to conceive hopes of getting my liberty in a short time. I took all possible methods to cultivate this favourable disposition. The natives came, by degrees, to be less apprehensive of any danger from me. I would sometimes lie down, and let five or six of them dance on my hand; and at last the boys and girls would venture to come and play at hide-and-seek in my hair. I had now made a good progress in understanding and speaking the language. The emperor had a mind one day to entertain me with several of the country shows, wherein they exceed all nations I have known, both for dexterity and magnificence. I was diverted with none so much as that of the rope-dancers, performed upon a slender white thread, extended about two feet, and twelve inches from the ground. Upon which I shall desire liberty, with the reader's patience, to enlarge a little.

This diversion is only practised by those persons who are candidates for great employments, and high favour at court. They are trained in this art from their youth, and are not always of noble birth, or liberal education. When a great office is vacant, either by death or disgrace (which often happens,) five or six of those candidates petition the emperor to entertain his majesty and the court with a dance on the rope; and whoever jumps the highest, without falling, succeeds in the office. Very often the chief ministers themselves are commanded to show their skill, and to convince the emperor that they have not lost their faculty. Flimnap, the treasurer, is allowed to cut a caper on the straight rope, at least an inch higher than any other lord in the whole empire. I have seen him do the summerset several times together, upon a trencher fixed on a rope which is no thicker than a common packthread in England. My friend Reldresal, principal secretary for private affairs, is, in my opinion, if I am not partial, the second after the treasurer; the rest of the great officers are much upon a par.

1. Which of the following statements best summarizes the central purpose of this text?

    a. Gulliver details his fondness for the archaic yet interesting practices of his captors.

    b. Gulliver conjectures about the intentions of the aristocratic sector of society.

    c. Gulliver becomes acquainted with the people and practices of his new surroundings.

    d. Gulliver's differences cause him to become penitent around new acquaintances.

2. What is the word *principal* referring to in the following text?

My friend Reldresal, principal secretary for private affairs, is, in my opinion, if I am not partial, the second after the treasurer; the rest of the great officers are much upon a par.

a. Primary or chief
b. An acolyte
c. An individual who provides nurturing
d. One in a subordinate position

3. What can the reader infer from this passage?

I would sometimes lie down, and let five or six of them dance on my hand; and at last the boys and girls would venture to come and play at hide-and-seek in my hair.

a. The children tortured Gulliver.
b. Gulliver traveled because he wanted to meet new people.
c. Gulliver is considerably larger than the children who are playing around him.
d. Gulliver has a genuine love and enthusiasm for people of all sizes.

4. What is the significance of the word *mind* in the following passage?

The emperor had a mind one day to entertain me with several of the country shows, wherein they exceed all nations I have known, both for dexterity and magnificence.

a. The ability to think
b. A collective vote
c. A definitive decision
d. A mythological question

5. Which of the following assertions does NOT support the fact that games are a commonplace event in this culture?

a. My gentleness and good behavior . . . short time.
b. They are trained in this art from their youth . . . liberal education.
c. Very often the chief ministers themselves are commanded to show their skill . . . not lost their faculty.
d. Flimnap, the treasurer, is allowed to cut a caper on the straight rope . . . higher than any other lord in the whole empire.

6. As summer approaches, drowning incidents will increase. Drowning happens very quickly and silently. Most people assume that drowning is easy to spot, but a person who is drowning doesn't make noise or wave his arms. Instead, he will have his head back and his mouth open, with just his face out of the water. A person who is truly in danger of drowning is not able to wave his arms in the air or move much at all. Recognizing these signs of drowning can prevent tragedy.

The main purpose of this passage is to:

a. Explain the dangers of swimming
b. Show how to identify the signs of drowning
c. Explain how to be a lifeguard
d. Compare the signs of drowning

Questions 7–9 are based on the following passage:

This excerpt is an adaptation from "The 'Hatchery' of the Sun-Fish"--- *Scientific American,* #711

I have thought that an example of the intelligence (instinct?) of a class of fish which has come under my observation during my excursions into the Adirondack region of New York State might possibly be of interest to your readers, especially as I am not aware that any one except myself has noticed it, or, at least, has given it publicity.

The female sun-fish (called, I believe, in England, the roach or bream) makes a "hatchery" for her eggs in this wise. Selecting a spot near the banks of the numerous lakes in which this region abounds, and where the water is about 4 inches deep, and still, she builds, with her tail and snout, a circular embankment 3 inches in height and 2 thick. The circle, which is as perfect a one as could be formed with mathematical instruments, is usually a foot and a half in diameter; and at one side of this circular wall an opening is left by the fish of just sufficient width to admit her body.

The mother sun-fish, having now built or provided her "hatchery," deposits her spawn within the circular inclosure, and mounts guard at the entrance until the fry are hatched out and are sufficiently large to take charge of themselves. As the embankment, moreover, is built up to the surface of the water, no enemy can very easily obtain an entrance within the inclosure from the top; while there being only one entrance, the fish is able, with comparative ease, to keep out all intruders.

I have, as I say, noticed this beautiful instinct of the sun-fish for the perpetuity of her species more particularly in the lakes of this region; but doubtless the same habit is common to these fish in other waters.

7. What is the purpose of this passage?
   a. To show the effects of fish hatcheries on the Adirondack region
   b. To persuade the audience to study Ichthyology (fish science)
   c. To depict the sequence of mating among sun-fish
   d. To enlighten the audience on the habits of sun-fish and their hatcheries

8. How is the circle that keeps the larvae of the sun-fish made?
   a. It is formed with mathematical instruments.
   b. The sun-fish builds it with her tail and snout.
   c. It is provided to her as a "hatchery" by Mother Nature.
   d. The sun-fish builds it with her larvae.

9. The author included the third paragraph in the following passage to achieve which of the following effects?
   a. To complicate the subject matter
   b. To express a bias
   c. To insert a counterargument
   d. To conclude a sequence and add a final detail

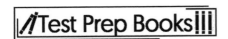

Questions 10–19 are based on the following passage:

In the quest to understand existence, modern philosophers must question if humans can fully comprehend the world. Classical western approaches to philosophy tend to hold that one can understand something, be it an event or object, by standing outside of the phenomena and observing it. It is then by unbiased observation that one can grasp the details of the world. This seems to hold true for many things. Scientists conduct experiments and record their findings, and thus many natural phenomena become comprehendible. However, several of these observations were possible because humans used tools in order to make these discoveries.

This may seem like an extraneous matter. After all, people invented things like microscopes and telescopes in order to enhance their capacity to view cells or the movement of stars. While humans are still capable of seeing things, the question remains if human beings have the capacity to fully observe and see the world in order to understand it. It would not be an impossible stretch to argue that what humans see through a microscope is not the exact thing itself, but a human interpretation of it.

This would seem to be the case in the "Business of the Holes" experiment conducted by Richard Feynman. To study the way electrons behave, Feynman set up a barrier with two holes and a plate. The plate was there to indicate how many times the electrons would pass through the hole(s). Rather than casually observe the electrons acting under normal circumstances, Feynman discovered that electrons behave in two totally different ways depending on whether or not they are observed. The electrons that were observed had passed through either one of the holes or were caught on the plate as particles. However, electrons that weren't observed acted as waves instead of particles and passed through both holes. This indicated that electrons have a dual nature. Electrons seen by the human eye act like particles, while unseen electrons act like waves of energy.

This dual nature of the electrons presents a conundrum. While humans now have a better understanding of electrons, the fact remains that people cannot entirely perceive how electrons behave without the use of instruments. We can only observe one of the mentioned behaviors, which only provides a partial understanding of the entire function of electrons. Therefore, we're forced to ask ourselves whether the world we observe is objective or if it is subjectively perceived by humans. Or, an alternative question: can man understand the world only through machines that will allow them to observe natural phenomena?

Both questions humble man's capacity to grasp the world. However, those ideas don't take into account that many phenomena have been proven by human beings without the use of machines, such as the discovery of gravity. Like all philosophical questions, whether man's reason and observation alone can understand the universe can be approached from many angles.

10. The word *extraneous* in paragraph two can be best interpreted as referring to which one of the following?
    a. Indispensable
    b. Bewildering
    c. Superfluous
    d. Exuberant

11. What is the author's motivation for writing the passage?
    a. Bring to light an alternative view on human perception by examining the role of technology in human understanding.
    b. Educate the reader on the latest astroparticle physics discovery and offer terms that may be unfamiliar to the reader.
    c. Argue that humans are totally blind to the realities of the world by presenting an experiment that proves that electrons are not what they seem on the surface.
    d. Reflect on opposing views of human understanding.

12. Which of the following most closely resembles the way in which paragraph four is structured?
    a. It offers one solution, questions the solution, and then ends with an alternative solution.
    b. It presents an inquiry, explains the detail of that inquiry, and then offers a solution.
    c. It presents a problem, explains the details of that problem, and then ends with more inquiry.
    d. It gives a definition, offers an explanation, and then ends with an inquiry.

13. For the classical approach to understanding to hold true, which of the following must be required?
    a. A telescope.
    b. The person observing must prove their theory beyond a doubt.
    c. Multiple witnesses present.
    d. The person observing must be unbiased.

14. Which best describes how the electrons in the experiment behaved like waves?
    a. The electrons moved up and down like actual waves.
    b. The electrons passed through both holes and then onto the plate.
    c. The electrons converted to photons upon touching the plate.
    d. Electrons were seen passing through one hole or the other.

15. The author mentions "gravity" in the last paragraph in order to do what?
    a. To show that different natural phenomena test man's ability to grasp the world.
    b. To prove that since man has not measured it with the use of tools or machines, humans cannot know the true nature of gravity.
    c. To demonstrate an example of natural phenomena humans discovered and understood without the use of tools or machines.
    d. To show an alternative solution to the nature of electrons that humans have not thought of yet.

16. Which situation best parallels the revelation of the dual nature of electrons discovered in Feynman's experiment?
    a. A man is born color-blind and grows up observing everything in lighter or darker shades. With the invention of special goggles he puts on, he discovers that there are other colors in addition to different shades.
    b. The coelacanth was thought to be extinct, but a live specimen was just recently discovered. There are now two living species of coelacanth known to man, and both are believed to be endangered.
    c. In the Middle Ages, blacksmiths added carbon to iron, thus inventing steel. The consequences of this important discovery would have its biggest effects during the industrial revolution.
    d. In order to better examine and treat broken bones, the x-ray machine was invented and put to use in hospitals and medical centers.

17. Which statement about technology would the author likely disagree with?
   a. Technology can help expand the field of human vision.
   b. Technology renders human observation irrelevant.
   c. Developing tools used in observation and research indicates growing understanding of our world itself.
   d. Studying certain phenomena necessitates the use of tools and machines.

18. As it is used in paragraph 4, the word *conundrum* most nearly means:
   a. platitude
   b. enigma
   c. solution
   d. hypothesis

19. What is the author's purpose in paragraph 3?
   a. To prove to the audience the thesis of the passage by providing evidence suggesting that electrons behave differently when observed by the human eye.
   b. To propose that the experiment conducted was not ethically done and to provide evidence that a new experiment should be conducted in order to reach the truth.
   c. To introduce the topic to the audience in a manner that puts it into a practical as well as historical understanding.
   d. To pose a question relating to the topic about whether humans fully observe phenomena in an objective or subjective sense.

Questions 20-24 are based on the following passage:

> The Middle Ages were a time of great superstition and theological debate. Many beliefs were developed and practiced, while some died out or were listed as heresy. Boethianism is a Medieval theological philosophy that attributes sin to gratification and righteousness with virtue and God's providence. Boethianism holds that sin, greed, and corruption are means to attain temporary pleasure, but that they inherently harm the person's soul as well as other human beings.
>
> In *The Canterbury Tales,* we observe more instances of bad actions punished than goodness being rewarded. This would appear to be some reflection of Boethianism. In the "Pardoner's Tale," all three thieves wind up dead, which is a result of their desire for wealth. Each wrong doer pays with their life, and they are unable to enjoy the wealth they worked to steal. Within his tales, Chaucer gives reprieve to people undergoing struggle, but also interweaves stories of contemptible individuals being cosmically punished for their wickedness. The thieves idolize physical wealth, which leads to their downfall. This same theme and ideological principle of Boethianism is repeated in the "Friar's Tale," whose summoner character attempts to gain further wealth by partnering with a demon. The summoner's refusal to repent for his avarice and corruption leads to the demon dragging his soul to Hell. Again, we see the theme of the individual who puts faith and morality aside in favor for a physical prize. The result, of course, is that the summoner loses everything.
>
> The examples of the righteous being rewarded tend to appear in a spiritual context within the *Canterbury Tales*. However, there are a few instances where we see

206

goodness resulting in physical reward. In the Prioress' Tale, we see corporal punishment for barbarism *and* a reward for goodness. The Jews are punished for their murder of the child, giving a sense of law and order (though racist) to the plot. While the boy does die, he is granted a lasting reward by being able to sing even after his death, a miracle that marks that the murdered youth led a pure life. Here, the miracle represents eternal favor with God.

Again, we see the theological philosophy of Boethianism in Chaucer's *The Canterbury Tales* through acts of sin and righteousness and the consequences that follow. When pleasures of the world are sought instead of God's favor, we see characters being punished in tragic ways. However, the absence of worldly lust has its own set of consequences for the characters seeking to obtain God's favor.

20. What would be a potential reward for living a good life, as described in Boethianism?
   a. A long life sustained by the good deeds one has done over a lifetime
   b. Wealth and fertility for oneself and the extension of one's family line
   c. Vengeance for those who have been persecuted by others who have a capacity for committing wrongdoing
   d. God's divine favor for one's righteousness

21. What might be the main reason why the author chose to discuss Boethianism through examining The Canterbury Tales?
   a. *The Canterbury Tales* is a well-known text.
   b. *The Canterbury Tales* is the only known fictional text that contains use of Boethianism.
   c. *The Canterbury Tales* presents a manuscript written in the medieval period that can help illustrate Boethianism through stories and show how people of the time might have responded to the idea.
   d. Within each individual tale in *The Canterbury Tales*, the reader can read about different levels of Boethianism and how each level leads to greater enlightenment.

22. What "ideological principle" is the author referring to in the middle of the second paragraph when talking about the "Friar's Tale"?
   a. The principle that the act of ravaging another's possessions is the same as ravaging one's soul.
   b. The principle that thieves who idolize physical wealth will be punished in an earthly sense as well as eternally.
   c. The principle that fraternization with a demon will result in one losing everything, including their life.
   d. The principle that a desire for material goods leads to moral malfeasance punishable by a higher being.

23. Which of the following words, if substituted for the word *avarice* in paragraph two, would LEAST change the meaning of the sentence?
   a. Perniciousness
   b. Pithiness
   c. Covetousness
   d. Precariousness

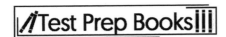
24. Based on the passage, what view does Boethianism take on desire?
    a. Desire does not exist in the context of Boethianism
    b. Desire is a virtue and should be welcomed
    c. Having desire is evidence of demonic possession
    d. Desire for pleasure can lead toward sin

25. Technology has been invading cars for the last several years, but there are some new high tech trends that are pretty amazing. It is now standard in many car models to have a rear-view camera, hands-free phone and text, and a touch screen digital display. Music can be streamed from a paired cell phone, and some displays can even be programmed with a personal photo. Sensors beep to indicate there is something in the driver's path when reversing and changing lanes. Rain-sensing windshield wipers and lights are automatic, leaving the driver with little to do but watch the road and enjoy the ride. The next wave of technology will include cars that automatically parallel park, and a self-driving car is on the horizon. These technological advances make it a good time to be a driver.

It can be concluded from this paragraph that:
    a. Technology will continue to influence how cars are made.
    b. Windshield wipers and lights are always automatic.
    c. It is standard to have a rear-view camera in all cars.
    d. Technology has reached its peak in cars.

Questions 26–35 are based upon the following passage:

"MANKIND being originally equals in the order of creation, the equality could only be destroyed by some subsequent circumstance; the distinctions of rich, and poor, may in a great measure be accounted for, and that without having recourse to the harsh ill sounding names of oppression and avarice. Oppression is often the consequence, but seldom or never the means of riches; and though avarice will preserve a man from being necessitously poor, it generally makes him too timorous to be wealthy.

But there is another and greater distinction for which no truly natural or religious reason can be assigned, and that is, the distinction of men into KINGS and SUBJECTS. Male and female are the distinctions of nature, good and bad the distinctions of heaven; but how a race of men came into the world so exalted above the rest, and distinguished like some new species, is worth enquiring into, and whether they are the means of happiness or of misery to mankind.

In the early ages of the world, according to the scripture chronology, there were no kings; the consequence of which was there were no wars; it is the pride of kings which throw mankind into confusion. Holland without a king hath enjoyed more peace for this last century than any of the monarchical governments in Europe. Antiquity favors the same remark; for the quiet and rural lives of the first patriarchs hath a happy something in them, which vanishes away when we come to the history of Jewish royalty.

Government by kings was first introduced into the world by the Heathens, from whom the children of Israel copied the custom. It was the most prosperous invention the Devil ever set on foot for the promotion of idolatry. The Heathens paid divine honors to their deceased kings, and the Christian world hath improved on the plan by doing the same to their living ones. How impious is the title of sacred majesty applied to a worm, who in the midst of his splendor is crumbling into dust!

As the exalting one man so greatly above the rest cannot be justified on the equal rights of nature, so neither can it be defended on the authority of scripture; for the will of the Almighty, as declared by Gideon and the prophet Samuel, expressly disapproves of government by kings. All anti-monarchical parts of scripture have been very smoothly glossed over in monarchical governments, but they undoubtedly merit the attention of countries, which have their governments yet to form. "Render unto Caesar the things which are Caesar's" is the scripture doctrine of courts, yet it is no support of monarchical government, for the Jews at that time were without a king, and in a state of vassalage to the Romans.

Near three thousand years passed away from the Mosaic account of the creation, till the Jews under a national delusion requested a king. Till then their form of government (except in extraordinary cases, where the Almighty interposed) was a kind of republic administered by a judge and the elders of the tribes. Kings they had none, and it was held sinful to acknowledge any being under that title but the Lord of Hosts. And when a man seriously reflects on the idolatrous homage which is paid to the persons of Kings, he need not wonder, that the Almighty ever jealous of his honor, should disapprove of a form of government which so impiously invades the prerogative of heaven.

Excerpt From: Thomas Paine. "Common Sense."

26. According to the passage, what role does avarice, or greed, play in poverty?
    a. It can make a man very wealthy.
    b. It is the consequence of wealth.
    c. Avarice can prevent a man from being poor, but too fearful to be very wealthy.
    d. Avarice is what drives a person to be very wealthy

27. Of these distinctions, which does the author believe to be beyond natural or religious reason?
    a. Good and bad
    b. Male and female
    c. Human and animal
    d. King and subjects

28. According to the passage, what are the Heathens responsible for?
    a. Government by kings
    b. Quiet and rural lives of patriarchs
    c. Paying divine honors to their living kings
    d. Equal rights of nature

29. Which of the following best states Paine's rationale for the denouncement of monarchy?
    a. It is against the laws of nature.
    b. It is against the equal rights of nature and is denounced in scripture.
    c. Despite scripture, a monarchal government is unlawful.
    d. Neither the law nor scripture denounce monarchy.

209

30. Based on the passage, what is the best definition of the word *idolatrous*?
    a. Worshipping heroes
    b. Being deceitful
    c. Sinfulness
    d. Engaging in illegal activities

31. What is the essential meaning of lines 41-44?
    And when a man seriously reflects on the idolatrous homage which is paid to the persons of Kings, he need not wonder, that the Almighty ever jealous of his honor, should disapprove of a form of government which so impiously invades the prerogative of heaven.

    a. God would disapprove of the irreverence of a monarchical government.
    b. With careful reflection, men should realize that heaven is not promised.
    c. God will punish those that follow a monarchical government.
    d. Belief in a monarchical government cannot coexist with belief in God.

32. Based on the passage, what is the best definition of the word *timorous* in the first paragraph?
    a. being full of fear
    b. a characteristic of shyness
    c. being able to see through someone
    d. being full of anger and hatred

33. The author's attitude toward the subject can best be described as:
    a. indifferent and fatigued
    b. impassioned and critical
    c. awed and enchanted
    d. enraged and sulky

34. The main purpose of the fourth paragraph is:
    a. To persuade the audience that heathens were more advanced than Christians.
    b. To explain how monarchs came into existence and how Christians adopted the same system.
    c. To describe the divination of English monarchs and how it is their birthright to be revered.
    d. To counteract the preceding paragraph by giving proof of the damage monarchs can cause.

35. In the last paragraph, what does the author mean by the "Mosaic account of creation"?
    a. The author means that creation is based on individuals composed of cells of two genetically different types.
    b. The author implies that the work of God is like a mosaic painting due to the various formations of creation.
    c. The author means that the kings of the past developed a system in which to maintain accounts of creation.
    d. The author implies that the recorded history of creation is a collection, collage, or pattern taken from various accounts of cultures.

Questions 36–45 are based on the following passages:

Passage I

Lethal force, or deadly force, is defined as the physical means to cause death or serious harm to another individual. The law holds that lethal force is only accepted when you or

210

another person are in immediate and unavoidable danger of death or severe bodily harm. For example, a person could be beating a weaker person in such a way that they are suffering severe enough trauma that could result in death or serious harm. This would be an instance where lethal force would be acceptable and possibly the only way to save that person from irrevocable damage.

Another example of when to use lethal force would be when someone enters your home with a deadly weapon. The intruder's presence and possession of the weapon indicate mal-intent and the ability to inflict death or severe injury to you and your loved ones. Again, lethal force can be used in this situation. Lethal force can also be applied to prevent the harm of another individual. If a woman is being brutally assaulted and is unable to fend off an attacker, lethal force can be used to defend her as a last-ditch effort. If she is in immediate jeopardy of rape, harm, and/or death, lethal force could be the only response that could effectively deter the assailant.

The key to understanding the concept of lethal force is the term *last resort*. Deadly force cannot be taken back; it should be used only to prevent severe harm or death. The law does distinguish whether the means of one's self-defense is fully warranted, or if the individual goes out of control in the process. If you continually attack the assailant after they are rendered incapacitated, this would be causing unnecessary harm, and the law can bring charges against you. Likewise, if you kill an attacker unnecessarily after defending yourself, you can be charged with murder. This would move lethal force beyond necessary defense, making it no longer a last resort but rather a use of excessive force.

Passage II

Assault is the unlawful attempt of one person to apply apprehension on another individual by an imminent threat or by initiating offensive contact. Assaults can vary, encompassing physical strikes, threatening body language, and even provocative language. In the case of the latter, even if a hand has not been laid, it is still considered an assault because of its threatening nature.

Let's look at an example: A homeowner is angered because his neighbor blows fallen leaves into his freshly mowed lawn. Irate, the homeowner gestures a fist to his fellow neighbor and threatens to bash his head in for littering on his lawn. The homeowner's physical motions and verbal threat heralds a physical threat against the other neighbor. These factors classify the homeowner's reaction as an assault. If the angry neighbor hits the threatening homeowner in retaliation, that would constitute an assault as well because he physically hit the homeowner.

Assault also centers on the involvement of weapons in a conflict. If someone fires a gun at another person, this could be interpreted as an assault unless the shooter acted in self-defense. If an individual drew a gun or a knife on someone with the intent to harm them, that would be considered assault. However, it's also considered an assault if someone simply aimed a weapon, loaded or not, at another person in a threatening manner.

211

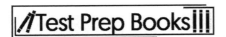

36. What is the purpose of the second passage?
    a. To inform the reader about what assault is and how it is committed
    b. To inform the reader about how assault is a minor example of lethal force
    c. To disprove the previous passage concerning lethal force
    d. The author is recounting an incident in which they were assaulted

37. Which of the following situations, according to the passages, would not constitute an illegal use of lethal force?
    a. A disgruntled cashier yells obscenities at a customer.
    b. A thief is seen running away with stolen cash.
    c. A man is attacked in an alley by another man with a knife.
    d. A woman punches another woman in a bar.

38. Given the information in the passages, which of the following must be true about assault?
    a. Assault charges are more severe than unnecessary use of force charges.
    b. There are various forms of assault.
    c. Smaller, weaker people cannot commit assaults.
    d. Assault is justified only as a last resort.

39. Which of the following, if true, would most seriously undermine the explanation proposed by the author of Passage I in the third paragraph?
    a. An instance of lethal force in self-defense is not absolutely absolved from blame. The law considers the necessary use of force at the time it is committed.
    b. An individual who uses lethal force under necessary defense is in direct compliance of the law under most circumstances.
    c. Lethal force in self-defense should be forgiven in all cases for the peace of mind of the primary victim.
    d. The use of lethal force is not evaluated on the intent of the user but rather the severity of the primary attack that warranted self-defense.

40. Based on the passages, what can be inferred about the relationship between assault and lethal force?
    a. An act of lethal force always leads to a type of assault.
    b. An assault will result in someone using lethal force.
    c. An assault with deadly intent can lead to an individual using lethal force to preserve their well-being.
    d. If someone uses self-defense in a conflict, it is called deadly force; if actions or threats are intended, it is called assault.

41. Which of the following best describes the way the passages are structured?
    a. Both passages open by defining a legal concept and then continue to describe situations that further explain the concept.
    b. Both passages begin with situations, introduce accepted definitions, and then cite legal ramifications.
    c. Passage I presents a long definition while the Passage II begins by showing an example of assault.
    d. Both cite specific legal doctrines, then proceed to explain the rulings.

42. What can be inferred about the role of intent in lethal force and assault?
    a. Intent is irrelevant. The law does not take intent into account.
    b. Intent is vital for determining the lawfulness of using lethal force.
    c. Intent is very important for determining both lethal force and assault; intent is examined in both parties and helps determine the severity of the issue.
    d. The intent of the assailant is the main focus for determining legal ramifications; it is used to determine if the defender was justified in using force to respond.

43. The author uses the example in the second paragraph of Passage II in order to do what?
    a. To demonstrate two different types of assault by showing how each specifically relates to the other
    b. To demonstrate a single example of two different types of assault, then adding in the third type of assault in the example's conclusion
    c. To prove that the definition of lethal force is altered when the victim in question is a homeowner and his property is threatened
    d. To suggest that verbal assault can be an exaggerated crime by the law and does not necessarily lead to physical violence

44. As it is used in the second passage, the word *apprehension* most nearly means:
    a. Pain
    b. Exhaustion
    c. Fear
    d. Honor

45. One of the main purposes of the last paragraph in the first passage is to state:
    a. How assault is different when used in the home versus when it is used out in public.
    b. A specific example of lethal force so that the audience will know what it looks like.
    c. Why police officers defend those who use lethal force but do not defend those who use assault.
    d. The concept of lethal force as a last resort and the point at which it can cross a line from defense to manslaughter.

46. In 1889, Jerome K. Jerome wrote a humorous account of a boating holiday. Originally intended as a chapter in a serious travel guide, the work became a prime example of a comic novel. Read the passage below, noting the word/words in italics. Answer the question that follows.

> I felt rather hurt about this at first; it seemed somehow to be a sort of slight. Why hadn't I got housemaid's knee? Why this invidious reservation? After a while, however, less grasping feelings prevailed. I reflected that I had every other known malady in the pharmacology, and I grew less selfish, and determined to do without housemaid's knee. Gout, in its most malignant stage, it would appear, had seized me without my being aware of it; and *zymosis* I had evidently been suffering with from boyhood. There were no more diseases after *zymosis*, so I concluded there was nothing else the matter with me.—Jerome K. Jerome, *Three Men in a Boat*

Which definition best fits the word *zymosis*?
    a. Discontent
    b. An infectious disease
    c. Poverty
    d. Bad luck

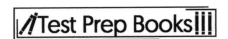

Questions 47–53 are based on the following passage:

As long ago as 1860 it was the proper thing to be born at home. At present, so I am told, the high gods of medicine have decreed that the first cries of the young shall be uttered upon the anesthetic air of a hospital, preferably a fashionable one. So young Mr. and Mrs. Roger Button were fifty years ahead of style when they decided, one day in the summer of 1860, that their first baby should be born in a hospital. Whether this anachronism had any bearing upon the astonishing history I am about to set down will never be known.

I shall tell you what occurred, and let you judge for yourself.

The Roger Buttons held an enviable position, both social and financial, in ante-bellum Baltimore. They were related to the This Family and the That Family, which, as every Southerner knew, entitled them to membership in that enormous peerage which largely populated the Confederacy. This was their first experience with the charming old custom of having babies— Mr. Button was naturally nervous. He hoped it would be a boy so that he could be sent to Yale College in Connecticut, at which institution Mr. Button himself had been known for four years by the somewhat obvious nickname of "Cuff."

On the September morning <u>consecrated</u> to the enormous event he arose nervously at six o'clock, dressed himself, adjusted an impeccable stock, and hurried forth through the streets of Baltimore to the hospital, to determine whether the darkness of the night had borne in new life upon its bosom.

When he was approximately a hundred yards from the Maryland Private Hospital for Ladies and Gentlemen he saw Doctor Keene, the family physician, descending the front steps, rubbing his hands together with a washing movement—as all doctors are required to do by the unwritten ethics of their profession.

Mr. Roger Button, the president of Roger Button & Co., Wholesale Hardware, began to run toward Doctor Keene with much less dignity than was expected from a Southern gentleman of that picturesque period. "Doctor Keene!" he called. "Oh, Doctor Keene!"

The doctor heard him, faced around, and stood waiting, a curious expression settling on his harsh, medicinal face as Mr. Button drew near.

"What happened?" demanded Mr. Button, as he came up in a gasping rush. "What was it? How is she? A boy? Who is it? What—"

"Talk sense!" said Doctor Keene sharply. He appeared somewhat irritated.

"Is the child born?" begged Mr. Button.

Doctor Keene frowned. "Why, yes, I suppose so—after a fashion." Again he threw a curious glance at Mr. Button.

From The Curious Case of Benjamin Button by F.S. Fitzgerald, 1922.

214

47. According to the passage, what major event is about to happen in this story?
    a. Mr. Button is about to go to a funeral.
    b. Mr. Button's wife is about to have a baby.
    c. Mr. Button is getting ready to go to the doctor's office.
    d. Mr. Button is about to go shopping for new clothes.

48. As it is used in the fourth paragraph, the word *consecrated* most nearly means:
    a. Numbed
    b. Chained
    c. Dedicated
    d. Moved

49. What does the author mean to do by adding the following statement?

    "rubbing his hands together with a washing movement—as all doctors are required to do by the unwritten ethics of their profession."

    a. Suggesting that Mr. Button is tired of the doctor.
    b. Trying to explain the detail of the doctor's profession.
    c. Hinting to readers that the doctor is an unethical man.
    d. Giving readers a visual picture of what the doctor is doing.

50. Which of the following best describes the development of this passage?
    a. It starts in the middle of a narrative in order to transition smoothly to a conclusion.
    b. It is a chronological narrative from beginning to end.
    c. The sequence of events is backwards—we go from future events to past events.
    d. To introduce the setting of the story and its characters.

51. As it is used in the first paragraph, the word *anachronism* most nearly means:
    a. Comparison
    b. Misplacement
    c. Aberration
    d. Amelioration

52. The main purpose of the first paragraph is:
    a. To explain the setting of the narrative and give information about the story.
    b. To present the thesis so that the audience can determine which points are valid later in the text.
    c. To introduce a counterargument so that the author can refute it in the next paragraph.
    d. To provide a description of the speaker's city and the building in which he works.

53. The end of the passage implies to the audience that:
    a. There is bad weather coming.
    b. The doctor thinks Mr. Button is annoying.
    c. The baby and the mother did not make it through labor.
    d. Something is unusual about the birth of the baby.

215

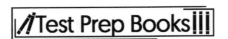

Use the passage below for questions 54 through 55:

<u>Caribbean Island Destinations</u>

Do you want to vacation at a Caribbean island destination? Who wouldn't want a tropical vacation? Visit one of the many Caribbean islands where visitors can swim in crystal blue waters, swim with dolphins, or enjoy family-friendly or adult-only resorts and activities. Every island offers a unique and picturesque vacation destination. Choose from these islands: Aruba, St. Lucia, Barbados, Anguilla, St. John, and so many more. A Caribbean island destination will be the best and most refreshing vacation ever . . . no regrets!

54. What is the topic of the passage?
   a. Caribbean island destinations
   b. Tropical vacation
   c. Resorts
   d. Activities

55. What is/are the supporting detail(s) of this passage?
   a. Cruising to the Caribbean
   b. Local events
   c. Family or adult-only resorts and activities
   d. All of the above

Vocabulary

1. What word meaning "on the opposite side" best fits in the following sentence:

   Although the patient's right knee had been hurting for a few months, he started experiencing _____ hip pain two weeks ago.

   a. Bilateral
   b. Ipsilateral
   c. Contralateral
   d. Alateral

2. Select the correct meaning of the underlined word in the following sentence:

   The patient's stomach appeared <u>distended</u>.

   a. Enlarged or expanded
   b. Sunken or concave
   c. Soft and flaccid
   d. Discolored or blotchy

3. What word meaning "rapidly or abruptly" best fits in the following sentence:

When the school group arrived, the noise level in the waiting room rose _____.

a. Concisely
b. Precipitously
c. Contingently
d. Preemptively

4. What word meaning "open" best fits in the following sentence:

After the obstruction was removed, the patient's bowel was _____.

a. Patent
b. Potent
c. Evident
d. Exude

5. What is the best definition of the word *amenorrhea*?
a. Excessive bleeding
b. Mental confusion
c. Loss of appetite
d. Absence of menstruation

6. Select the correct meaning of the underlined word in the following sentence:

After the trauma, new symptoms of the woman's <u>latent</u> infection emerged.

a. Chronic and debilitating
b. Acute but not necessarily severe
c. Present but not active or visible
d. Uncontrollable or volatile

7. What word meaning "obvious" best fits in the following sentence:

The patient's allergic reaction was _____, due to the widespread hives all over her extremities.

a. Obsolete
b. Covert
c. Overt
d. Colluded

217

8. Select the correct meaning of the underlined word in the following sentence:

The nurse reported that the patient experienced <u>dyspnea</u> and dizziness.

a. Difficulty breathing
b. Difficulty sleeping
c. Rapid pulse
d. Nasal discharge

9. Select the correct meaning of the underlined word in the following sentence:

The nurse explained the symptoms of the patient's <u>acute</u> illness and recommended increasing fluid intake.

a. Serious with a poor prognosis
b. Sudden or rapid onset
c. Debilitating and contagious
d. Chronic and slow to resolve

10. What word meaning "severe and harmful" best fits in the following sentence:

The patient was quarantined because the doctor was concerned he had a _____ disease.

a. Patent
b. Innocuous
c. Latent
d. Virulent

11. What is the best definition of the word *adverse*?
a. Unpredictable
b. Agitated
c. Undesirable
d. Progressive

12. What word meaning "so gradual that it's hardly apparent" best fits in the following sentence:

The nurse explained that atherosclerosis and coronary artery disease often have an _____ onset.

a. Precipitous
b. Insidious
c. Incipient
d. Paroxysmal

13. Select the correct meaning of the underlined word in the following sentence:

The graduate student noted that the common symptoms of the condition were malaise, weight loss, and <u>anuria</u>.

a. Lack of urine output
b. Excessive urine production
c. Memory loss
d. Lack of usual reflexes

14. What word meaning "closer to the trunk" best fits in the following sentence:

The knee is _____ to the ankle.

a. Dorsal
b. Distal
c. Proximal
d. Ventral

15. What word meaning "impenetrable" best fits in the following sentence:

Due to the contagious nature of the patient's infection, the nursing staff was told to don _____ masks and gloves.

a. Impotent
b. Hygienic
c. Impervious
d. Impending

16. Select the correct meaning of the underlined word in the following sentence:

The <u>etiology</u> of the disease is currently unknown.

a. Prognosis or outlook
b. Origin or cause
c. Mechanism of transmission
d. Incidence in the population

17. What word meaning "produced in the body" best fits in the following sentence:

Endorphins are touted as acting as _____ opioids, to help reduce pain.

a. Receptors
b. Synthetic
c. Exogenous
d. Endogenous

219

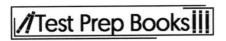
18. What word meaning "feverish" best fits in the following sentence:

The _____ baby was difficult to sooth.

   a. Febrile
   b. Futile
   c. Libel
   d. Liable

19. What is the best definition of the word *proliferated*?
   a. Multiplied or increased in number
   b. Responded to treatment
   c. Dwindled or decreased
   d. Expanded or grown in size

20. Select the correct meaning of the underlined word in the following sentence:

The <u>viscosity</u> of the patient's synovial fluid was abnormal.

   a. A fluid's cellular and nutrient profile
   b. A fluid's thickness or resistance to flow
   c. A fluid's color and transparency
   d. A fluid's sedimentation rate

21. What word meaning "on one's back" best fits in the following sentence:

The surgeon informed the patient that he would be _____ during the procedure.

   a. Prone
   b. Supine
   c. Dorsal
   d. Ventral

22. What is the best definition of the word *milieu*?
   a. Cytoplasm
   b. Organism
   c. Environment
   d. Autoclave

23. Select the correct meaning of the underlined word in the following sentence:

The prognosis was undetermined because of the <u>aberrant</u> nature of his illness.

   a. Overt
   b. Grave
   c. Radical
   d. Abnormal

220

24. What word meaning "wound with irregular borders" best fits in the following sentence:

    The rock climber got a serious _____ on his arm when the boulder moved.

    a. Incision
    b. Laceration
    c. Contusion
    d. Avulsion

25. Select the correct meaning of the underlined word in the following sentence:

    The patient's father had a history of chronic renal disease.

    a. Relating to the pancreas
    b. Relating to the liver
    c. Relating to the kidney
    d. Relating to hormones

26. Which word meaning "removal of necrotic tissue" best fits in the following sentence:

    The biker was hopeful that after his knee _____, he would be in less pain.

    a. Debridement
    b. Arthroscopy
    c. Distension
    d. Laparoscopy

27. Select the correct meaning of the underlined word in the following sentence:

    During her internship at the hospital, Cassandra got to triage a lot of patients.

    a. Diagnose or identify a problem
    b. Develop an effective treatment plan
    c. Evaluate and gather relevant medical history
    d. Sort based on problem severity

28. What word meaning "susceptible to" best fits in the following sentence:

    The malnourished child was _____ to rickets.

    a. Impended
    b. Invariable
    c. Prognosticated
    d. Predisposed

221

29. Which of the following words is most synonymous with the underlined word in the sentence below?

"I promise, I did not instigate the fight."

a. Begin
b. Ponder
c. Swim
d. Overwhelm

30. Select the correct meaning of the underlined word in the following sentence:

The nurse noted that the baby appeared indolent.

a. Underweight
b. Agitated
c. Lethargic
d. Alert

31. What word referring to "blood vessels that carry deoxygenated blood back to the heart" best fits in the following sentence:

The nurse was concerned about possible occlusions in the patient's _____.

a. Capillaries
b. Arteries
c. Ventricles
d. Veins

32. Select the correct meaning of the underlined word in the following sentence:

The medication had a buccal route of administration.

a. Under the tongue
b. In the rectum
c. Through the nasal cavity
d. Inside the cheek

33. What is the best definition of the word *instructor*?
a. Pupil
b. Teacher
c. Survivor
d. Dictator

34. What is the best definition of the word *expectorate*?
a. To cough out phlegm
b. To suppress a phlegm production
c. To stifle a cough
d. Yellowish or green sputum

222

35. What is the best definition of the word *residence*?
    a. Home
    b. Area
    c. Plan
    d. Resist

36. What is the best definition of the word *relinquish*?
    a. Stop repeatedly
    b. Give again
    c. Punish again
    d. Cease claim

37. What is the best definition of the word *germinate*?
    a. Lengthen
    b. Infect
    c. Develop
    d. Ail

38. What is the best definition of the word *indemnity?*
    a. Insurance
    b. Punishment
    c. Affinity
    d. Insolation

39. Select the correct meaning of the underlined word in the following sentence:

    Immediately after the holiday, staff interest grew <u>rampant</u>.

    a. Stagnant
    b. Mildly
    c. Unrestrained
    d. Wearily

40. Select the correct meaning of the underlined word in the following sentence:

    An increased pupil size is considered an <u>ominous</u> sign.

    a. Unequivocal
    b. Promising
    c. Auspicious
    d. Threatening

223

41. What word meaning "low blood sugar" best fits in the following sentence:

A patient with diabetes did not receive breakfast so the nurse was concerned he might have

_____.

a. Hypoglycemia
b. Ketoacidosis
c. Diabetic coma
d. Hyperglycemia

42. What is the best definition of the word *observed*?
a. Watched
b. Hunted
c. Scared
d. Sold

43. What word meaning "sleepy yet arousable to verbal stimuli" best fits in the following sentence:

The _____ patient was difficult to move to into the room.

a. Comatose
b. Delirious
c. Somnolent
d. Stuporous

44. What word meaning "coughing up blood" best fits in the following sentence:

A patient with tuberculosis should be monitored for _____.

a. Hematopoiesis
b. Hemoptysis
c. Hematemesis
d. Hematochezia

45. What is the best definition of the word *engorge*?
a. Nourish
b. Squeeze
c. Consume
d. Swell

46. What word meaning "mourning after loss" best fits in the following sentence:

The nurse referred the mother to _____ counseling.

a. Bereavement
b. Disposition
c. Depression
d. Belligerent

224

47. What word meaning "excessive thirst" best fits in the following sentence:

A common side effect of antispasmodics is _____.

   a. Anurea
   b. Polyploidy
   c. Polydipsia
   d. Polyurea

48. What is the best definition of the word *sentient*?
   a. Kind and genial
   b. Aging or dying
   c. Able to feel or perceive
   d. Nostalgic

49. Select the correct meaning of the underlined word in the following sentence:

The patient had a history of anxiety, emphysema, and a <u>peptic</u> ulcer.

   a. Relating to ingestion
   b. Relating to defecation
   c. Relating to digestion
   d. Relating to the pancreas

50. What word meaning "a muscle contraction that does not cause a change in muscle length" best fits in the following sentence:

The strength training protocol called for many _____ exercises.

   a. Isometric
   b. Isotonic
   c. Isokinetic
   d. Plyometric

51. What is the best definition of the word *nomad*?
   a. Munching
   b. Propose
   c. Wanderer
   d. Conscientious

52. What is the best definition of the word *perplexed*?
   a. Annoyed
   b. Vengeful
   c. Injured
   d. Confused

53. What is the best definition of the word *lyrical*?
   a. Whimsical
   b. Vague
   c. Fruitful
   d. Expressive

54. What is the best definition of the word *brevity*?
   a. Dullness
   b. Dangerous
   c. Brief
   d. Ancient

55. What is the best definition of the word *irate*?
   a. Angry
   b. Knowledgeable
   c. Tired
   d. Confused

Grammar

1. Select the best word for the blank in the following sentence:

   Tom couldn't decide which shirt to ___.

   a. ware
   b. where
   c. wear
   d. were

2. Identify the adjective clause in the following sentence.

   A boy who loves to ride bikes gets plenty of exercise.

   a. a boy who loves
   b. who loves to ride bikes
   c. to ride bikes
   d. gets plenty of exercise

3. Identify the adverbial clause in the following sentence.

   I want to work in the garden longer unless you are too tired.

   a. I want to work in the garden
   b. in the garden
   c. are too tired
   d. unless you are too tired

4. Identify the noun phrase in the following sentence.

The actor and actress rode in the long black limousine.

a. actor and actress
b. rode in the
c. the long black limousine
d. actress rode in

5. Armani got lost when she walked around Paris.

Rewrite, beginning with <u>Walking through Paris,</u> the next words will be:

a. you can get lost.
b. Armani found herself lost.
c. she should have gotten lost.
d. is about getting lost.

6. Which sentence does NOT include a gerund phrase?
a. Swimming several laps is a great way to get exercise.
b. The best way to swim quickly is using the flippers.
c. I can swim farther than the coach can in three minutes.
d. Learning to swim is not as difficult as you imagine it to be.

7. Which of the following sentences includes a nonessential appositive phrase?
a. Carrie Fisher, my second cousin, was an actress in the movie *Star Wars*.
b. The actor Harrison Ford also plays a lead role in *Star Wars*.
c. The movie *Star Wars* is about two hours long.
d. The movie *Star Wars* has become legendary.

8. Which of the following sentences highlights an absolute phrase?
a. One of my favorite activities is <u>going camping in the forest</u>.
b. <u>The fire crackling</u>, it is so exciting to be enveloped in nature.
c. The best drinks, <u>hot cocoa and coffee</u>, are served at campfires.
d. I love camping because it is the best experience <u>for school-age children</u>.

9. After his cat died, Phoenix buried the cat with her favorite toys in his backyard.

Rewrite, beginning with <u>Phoenix buried his cat</u> the next words will be:

a. in his backyard before she died.
b. after she died in the backyard.
c. with her favorite toys after she died.
d. after he buried her toys in the backyard.

227

10. While I was in the helicopter, I saw the sunset, and tears streamed down my face.

Rewrite, beginning with <u>Tears streamed down my face</u> the next words will be:

a. while I watched the helicopter fly into the sunset.
b. because the sunset flew up into the sky.
c. because the helicopter was facing the sunset.
d. when I saw the sunset from the helicopter.

For the next two questions, select the answer choice that best corrects the underlined portion of the sentence:

11. It is necessary for instructors to offer tutoring <u>to any students who need extra help in the class.</u>
    a. to any students who need extra help in the class.
    b. for any students that need extra help in the class.
    c. with any students who need extra help in the class.
    d. for any students needing any extra help in their class.

12. <u>Because many people</u> feel there are too many distractions to get any work done, I actually enjoy working from home.
    a. Because many people
    b. While many people
    c. Maybe many people
    d. With most people

Directions for questions 13-14: Rewrite the sentence in your head following the directions given below.

13. Student loan debt is at an all-time high, which is why many politicians are using this issue to gain the attention and votes of students, or anyone with student loan debt.

Rewrite, beginning with <u>Student loan debt is at an all-time high.</u> the next words will be which of the following:

a. because politicians want students' votes.
b. , so politicians are using the issue to gain votes.
c. , so voters are choosing politicians who care about this issue.
d. , and politicians want to do something about it.

14. Seasoned runners often advise new runners to get fitted for better quality running shoes because new runners often complain about minor injuries like sore knees or shin splints.

Rewrite, beginning with <u>Seasoned runners often advise new runners to get fitted for better quality running shoes.</u> the next words will be which of the following:

a. to help them avoid minor injuries.
b. because they know better.
c. , so they can run further.
d. to complain about running injuries.

15. What is the noun phrase in the following sentence?

Charlotte's new German shepherd puppy is energetic.

a. Puppy
b. Charlotte
c. German shepherd puppy
d. Charlotte's new German shepherd puppy

16. Which sentence shows grammatically correct parallelism?
a. He is the clown who inflated balloons and honked his nose.
b. He is the clown who inflated balloons and who honked his nose.
c. He is the clown that inflated balloons and who honked his nose.
d. He is the clown that inflated balloons and that honked his nose.

17. Which sentence shows grammatically correct parallelism?
a. My grandparents have been traveling and have been sightseeing.
b. My grandparents have been traveling and were sightseeing.
c. My grandparents were traveling and have been sightseeing.
d. My grandparents have been traveling and they're sightseeing.

18. Which sentence shows grammatically correct subordination?
a. The building was sturdy and solid; it crumbled during the earthquake.
b. The building was study and solid although it crumbled during the earthquake.
c. Although the building was sturdy and solid, it crumbled during the earthquake.
d. Despite being sturdy and solid, the building crumbled during the earthquake.

19. Which sentence is grammatically correct?
a. Every morning we would wake up, ate breakfast, and broke camp.
b. Every morning we would wake up, eat breakfast, and broke camp.
c. Every morning we would wake up, eat breakfast, and break camp.
d. Every morning we would wake up, ate breakfast, and break camp.

20. Polls show that more and more people in the US distrust the government and view it as dysfunctional and corrupt. Every election, the same people are voted back into office.

Which word or words would best link these sentences?

a. Not surprisingly,
b. Understandably,
c. And yet,
d. Therefore,

229

21. A student wants to rewrite the following sentence:

Entrepreneurs use their ideas to make money.

He wants to use the word *money* as a verb, but he isn't sure which word ending to use. What is the appropriate suffix to add to *money* to complete the following sentence?

Entrepreneurs _____ their ideas.

a. –ize
b. –ical
c. –en
d. –ful

22. Glorify, fortify, gentrify, acidify

Based on the preceding words, what is the correct meaning of the suffix *–fy*?

a. Marked by, given to
b. Doer, believer
c. Make, cause, cause to have
d. Process, state, rank

23. After a long day at work, Tracy had dinner with her family, and then took a walk to the park. What are the transitional words in the preceding sentence?
a. After, then
b. At, with, to
c. Had, took
d. A, the

24. Robert needed to find at least four sources for his final project, so he searched several library databases for reliable academic research.

Which words function as nouns in the preceding sentence?

a. Robert, sources, project, databases, research
b. Robert, sources, final, project, databases, academic, research
c. Robert, sources, project, he, library, databases, research
d. Sources, project, databases, research

25. Which sentence has a misplaced modifier?
a. The children love their cute and cuddly teddy bears.
b. Teddy bears are cute and cuddly; the children love them.
c. Cute and cuddly, the children love their teddy bears.
d. Cute and cuddly, the teddy bears are loved by many children.

26. Which of the following uses correct spelling?
    a. Jed was disatisfied with the acommodations at his hotel, so he requested another room.
    b. Jed was dissatisfied with the accommodations at his hotel, so he requested another room.
    c. Jed was dissatisfied with the accomodations at his hotel, so he requested another room.
    d. Jed was disatisfied with the accommodations at his hotel, so he requested another room.

27. Which example shows correct comma usage for dates?
    a. The due date for the final paper in the course is Monday, May 16, 2016.
    b. The due date for the final paper in the course is Monday, May 16 2016.
    c. The due date for the final project in the course is Monday, May, 16, 2016.
    d. The due date for the final project in the course is Monday May 16, 2016.

28. Which sentence shows grammatically correct parallelism?
    a. The puppies enjoy chewing and to play tug-o-war.
    b. The puppies enjoy to chew and playing tug-o-war.
    c. The puppies enjoy to chew and to play tug-o-war.
    d. The puppies enjoy chewing and playing tug-o-war.

29. At last night's company function, in honor of Mr. Robertson's retirement, several employees spoke kindly about his career achievements.

    In the preceding sentence, what part of speech is the word *function*?

    a. Adjective
    b. Adverb
    c. Verb
    d. Noun

30. Which of the examples uses the correct plural form?
    a. Tomatos
    b. Analysis
    c. Cacti
    d. Criterion

31. Which of the following examples uses correct punctuation?
    a. The moderator asked the candidates, "Is each of you prepared to discuss your position on global warming?".
    b. The moderator asked the candidates, "Is each of you prepared to discuss your position on global warming?"
    c. The moderator asked the candidates, 'Is each of you prepared to discuss your position on global warming?'
    d. The moderator asked the candidates, "Is each of you prepared to discuss your position on global warming"?

32. Select the best word for the blank in the following sentence.

    Garth _____ many pets that he cares for.

    a. has
    b. had
    c. have
    d. haves

33. In which of the following sentences does the word *part* function as an adjective?
    a. The part Brian was asked to play required many hours of research.
    b. She parts ways with the woodsman at the end of the book.
    c. The entire team played a part in the success of the project.
    d. Ronaldo is part Irish on his mother's side of the family.

34. All of Shannon's family and friends helped her to celebrate her 50th birthday at Café Sorrento. Which of the following is the complete subject of the preceding sentence?
    a. Family and friends
    b. All
    c. All of Shannon's family and friends
    d. Shannon's family and friends

35. Which of the following sentences uses second person point of view?
    a. I don't want to make plans for the weekend before I see my work schedule.
    b. She had to miss the last three yoga classes due to illness.
    c. Pluto is no longer considered a planet because it is not gravitationally dominant.
    d. Be sure to turn off all of the lights before locking up for the night.

36. As the tour group approached the bottom of Chichen Itza, the prodigious Mayan pyramid, they became nervous about climbing its distant peak.

    Based on the context of the sentence, which of the following words shows the correct meaning of the word *prodigious*?

    a. Very large
    b. Famous
    c. Very old
    d. Fancy

37. Which of the following sentences correctly uses a hyphen?
    a. Last-year, many of the players felt unsure of the coach's methods.
    b. Some of the furniture she selected seemed a bit over - the - top for the space.
    c. Henry is a beagle-mix and is ready for adoption this weekend.
    d. Geena works to maintain a good relationship with her ex-husband to the benefit of their children.

38. Which of the following examples correctly uses quotation marks?
    a. "A Wrinkle in Time" was one of my favorite novels as a child.
    b. Though he is famous for his roles in films like "The Great Gatsby" and "Titanic," Leonardo DiCaprio has never won an Oscar.
    c. Sylvia Plath's poem, "Daddy" will be the subject of this week's group discussion.
    d. "The New York Times" reported that many fans are disappointed in some of the trades made by the Yankees this off-season.

39. Which of the following sentences shows correct word usage?
    a. It's often been said that work is better then rest.
    b. Its often been said that work is better then rest.
    c. It's often been said that work is better than rest.
    d. Its often been said that work is better than rest.

Directions for questions 40-41: Rewrite the sentence in your head following the directions given below. Keep in mind that your new sentence should be well written and should have essentially the same meaning as the original sentence.

40. There are many risks in firefighting, including smoke inhalation, exposure to hazardous materials, and oxygen deprivation, so firefighters are outfitted with many items that could save their lives, including a self-contained breathing apparatus.

Rewrite, beginning with <u>so firefighters</u>

the next words will be which of the following:
    a. are exposed to lots of dangerous situations.
    b. need to be very careful on the job.
    c. wear life-saving protective gear.
    d. have very risky jobs.

41. Though social media sites like Facebook, Instagram, and Snapchat have become increasingly popular, experts warn that teen users are exposing themselves to many dangers such as cyberbullying and predators.

Rewrite, beginning with <u>experts warn that</u>

The next words will be which of the following?
    a. Facebook is dangerous.
    b. they are growing in popularity.
    c. teens are using them too much.
    d. they can be dangerous for teens.

42. While studying vocabulary, a student notices that the words *circumference*, *circumnavigate*, and *circumstance* all begin with the prefix *circum–*. The student uses her knowledge of affixes to infer that all of these words share what related meaning?
    a. Around, surrounding
    b. Travel, transport
    c. Size, measurement
    d. Area, location

233

Directions for questions 43 – 50: Select the best version of the underlined part of the sentence. If there is no mistake, choose Correct as is.

43. <u>Those are also memories that my siblings and me</u> have now shared with our own children.
    a. Those are also memories that I and my siblings
    b. Those are also memories that me and my siblings
    c. Those are also memories that my siblings and I
    d. *Correct as is*

44. Ginger was born and raised <u>in Maywood of Chicago, Illinois in 1955.</u>
    a. in Chicago, Illinois of Maywood in 1955.
    b. in Maywood, of Chicago, Illinois in 1955.
    c. in Maywood of Chicago, Illinois, in 1955.
    d. *Correct as is*

45. Virginia was attracted to the <u>Committee's approach</u> toward the new legislature.
    a. Committies' approach
    b. Committees approach
    c. Committees' approach
    d. *Correct as is*

46. Franz went to a high school five minutes from his <u>house. He</u> played in the marching band.
    a. Franz went to a high school five minutes from his house and played in the marching band.
    b. Franz went to a high school five minutes from his house but played in the marching band.
    c. Franz went to a high school five minutes from his house, he played in the marching band.
    d. *Correct as is*

47. After school, the news team <u>was held by a press conference</u> that shed light on the parking lot issues.
    a. holds a press conference
    b. held a press conference
    c. holding a press conference
    d. *Correct as is*

48. <u>In 2015; seven years later,</u> it was finally revealed that their dog, Bear, was part Husky.
    a. In 2015. Seven years later,
    b. In 2015, seven years later,
    c. In 2015 seven years later,
    d. *Correct as is*

49. Last week, my teacher shared this information <u>with me "One day these rules won't matter, but what's inside your head and heart will."</u>
    a. with me. "One day these rules won't matter, but what's inside your head and heart will."
    b. with me: "One day these rules won't matter, but what's inside your head and heart will."
    c. with me: "One day these rules won't matter, but what's inside your head and heart will".
    d. *Correct as is*

50. Society <u>raising it's children to be</u> decent human beings with something valuable to contribute to the world.
    a. raising its children to be
    b. raises its children to be
    c. raising its' children to be
    d. *Correct as is*

Directions for questions 51-55: Rewrite the sentence in your head following the directions given below. Keep in mind that your new sentence should be well written and should have essentially the same meaning as the original sentence.

51. I won't go to the party unless some of my friends go.

Rewrite, beginning with <u>I will go the party</u>. The next words will be

    a. if I want to.
    b. if my friends go.
    c. since a couple of my friends are going.
    d. unless people I know go.

52. He had a broken leg before the car accident, so it took him a long time to recover.

Rewrite, beginning with <u>He took a long time to recover from the car accident</u>. The next words will be

    a. from his two broken legs.
    b. after he broke his leg.
    c. because he already had a broken leg.
    d. since he broke his leg again afterward.

53. We had a party the day after Halloween to celebrate my birthday.

Rewrite, beginning with <u>It was my birthday</u>. The next words will be

    a. , so we celebrated with a party the day after Halloween.
    b. the day of Halloween so we celebrated with a party.
    c. , and we celebrated with a Halloween party the day after.
    d. a few days before Halloween, so we threw a party.

54. Over time, certain traits develop in animals that enable them to thrive in these environments.

Rewrite, beginning with <u>Animals thrive in these environments</u>. The next words will be

    a. over a certain amount of time with changing traits.
    b. which contain traits that allow animals to thrive.
    c. and animals have changing traits over time.
    d. due to certain traits in them that develop over time.

55. I've sat through many lectures and always come away learning something.

Rewrite, beginning with <u>I have always learned something</u>. The next words will be

235

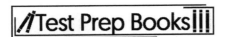

a. from the many lectures I've sat through.
b. when I sit through lectures.
c. and have sat through many lectures.
d. from going away to many lectures.

Biology

1. Which is true regarding DNA?
    a. It is the genetic code.
    b. It provides energy.
    c. It is single-stranded.
    d. All of the above.

2. Which is the cellular organelle used to tag, package, and ship out proteins destined for other cells or locations?
    a. The Golgi apparatus
    b. The lysosome
    c. The centrioles
    d. The mitochondria

3. How do cellulose and starch differ?
    a. Cellulose and starch are proteins with different R groups.
    b. Cellulose is a polysaccharide made up of glucose molecules and starch is a polysaccharide made up of galactose molecules.
    c. Cellulose and starch are both polysaccharides made up of glucose molecules, but they are connected with different types of bonds.
    d. Cellulose and starch are the same molecule, but cellulose is made by plants and starch is made by animals.

4. Esther is left-handed. Hand dominance is a genetic factor. If being right-handed is a dominant trait over being left-handed, which of the following cannot be true about Esther's parents?
    a. Her parents are both right-handed.
    b. Her parents are both left-handed.
    c. Only one parent is right-handed.
    d. All of the above can be true.

5. What is the probability of $AaBbCcDd \times AAbbccDD$ having a child with genotype $AAbbccDD$?
    a. 1/2
    b. 1/4
    c. 1/8
    d. 1/16

6. Which statement regarding meiosis is correct?
    a. Meiosis produces four diploid cells.
    b. Meiosis contains two cellular divisions separated by interphase II.
    c. Meiosis produces cells with two sets of chromosomes.
    d. Crossing over occurs in the prophase of meiosis I.

236

7. What molecule serves as the hereditary material for prokaryotic and eukaryotic cells?
    a. Proteins
    b. Carbohydrates
    c. Lipids
    d. DNA

8. What is a product of photosynthesis?
    a. Water
    b. Sunlight
    c. Oxygen
    d. Carbon Dioxide

9. What is cellular respiration?
    a. Making high-energy sugars
    b. Breathing
    c. Breaking down food to release energy
    d. Sweating

10. Which one of the following can perform photosynthesis?
    a. Mold
    b. Ant
    c. Mushroom
    d. Algae

11. Which taxonomic system is commonly used to describe the hierarchy of similar organisms today?
    a. Aristotle system
    b. Linnaean system
    c. Cesalpino system
    d. Darwin system

12. What is the Latin specific name for humans?
    a. *Homo sapiens*
    b. *Homo erectus*
    c. *Canis familiaris*
    d. *Homo habilis*

13. What organelles have two layers of membranes?
    a. Nucleus, chloroplast, mitochondria
    b. Nucleus, Golgi apparatus, mitochondria
    c. ER, chloroplast, lysosome
    d. Chloroplast, lysosome, ER

14. When human cells divide by meiosis, how many chromosomes do the resulting cells contain?
    a. 96
    b. 54
    c. 46
    d. 23

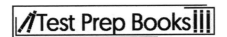

15. Which is an organelle found in a plant cell but not an animal cell?
    a. Mitochondria
    b. Chloroplast
    c. Golgi body
    d. Nucleus

16. Which of the following correctly expresses the molecular investment for each molecule of G3P produced by the Calvin cycle?
    a. 6 ATP molecules and 9 NADP+ molecules are invested for each molecule of G3P that is produced.
    b. 9 ATP molecules and 6 NADP+ molecules are invested for each molecule of G3P that is produced.
    c. 6 ATP molecules and 9 NADPH molecules are invested for each molecule of G3P that is produced.
    d. 9 ATP molecules and 6 NADPH molecules are invested for each molecule of G3P that is produced.

17. What are the net products of anaerobic glycolysis?
    a. 2 pyruvate molecules, 2 NADH molecules, and 2 ATP molecules
    b. 2 pyruvate molecules, 2 NADH molecules, and 4 ATP molecules
    c. 2 pyruvate molecules, 2 NAD+ molecules, and 2 ATP molecules
    d. 2 pyruvate molecules, 2 NAD+ molecules, and 4 ATP molecules

18. Which of the following correctly states the relationship between the glucose molecules that initially enter into glycolysis and the number of rounds of the citric acid cycle that can be completed?
    a. One round of the citric acid cycle can be completed for each glucose molecule that enters glycolysis.
    b. One round of the citric acid cycle can be completed for every 2 glucose molecules that enter glycolysis.
    c. Two rounds of the citric acid cycle can be completed for each glucose molecule that enters glycolysis.
    d. One round of the citric acid cycle can be completed for every 4 glucose molecule that enter glycolysis.

19. What are the two steps of oxidative phosphorylation?
    a. Electron Transport Chain and Citric Acid Cycle
    b. Krebs Cycle and Electron Transport Chain
    c. Proton Pump and Facilitated Diffusion
    d. Electron Transport Chain and Chemiosmosis

20. Where is the nucleolus located in both plant and animal cells?
    a. Near the chloroplast
    b. Inside the mitochondria
    c. Inside the nucleus
    d. Attached to the cell membrane

21. In which organelle do eukaryotes carry out aerobic respiration?
    a. Golgi apparatus
    b. Nucleus
    c. Mitochondrion
    d. Cytosol

22. What kind of energy do plants use in photosynthesis to create chemical energy?
    a. Light
    b. Electric
    c. Nuclear
    d. Cellular

23. What type of biological molecule includes monosaccharides?
    a. Protein
    b. Carbohydrate
    c. Nucleic acid
    d. Lipid

24. What are the molecular "energy" investments necessary for every G3P molecule produced by the Calvin cycle?
    a. 9 ATP molecules and 6 NADPH molecules
    b. 9 ATP molecules and 6 NADP$^+$ molecules
    c. 6 ATP molecules and 9 NADP$^+$ molecules
    d. 6 ATP molecules and 9 NADPH molecules

25. What does the cell membrane do?
    a. Builds proteins
    b. Breaks down large molecules
    c. Contains the cell's DNA
    d. Controls which molecules are allowed in and out of the cell

26. Describe the synthesis of the lagging strand of DNA.
    a. DNA polymerases synthesize DNA continuously after initially attaching to a primase.
    b. DNA polymerases synthesize DNA discontinuously in pieces called Okazaki fragments after initially attaching to primases.
    c. DNA polymerases synthesize DNA discontinuously in pieces called Okazaki fragments after initially attaching to RNA primers.
    d. DNA polymerases synthesize DNA discontinuously in pieces called Okazaki fragments which are joined together in the end by a DNA helicase.

Questions 27–30 pertain to the passage:

> Greenhouses are glass structures that people grow plants in. They allow plants to survive and grow even in the cold winter months by providing light and trapping warm air inside. Light is allowed in through the clear glass walls and roof. Warm air comes in as sunlight through the glass roof. The sunlight is converted into heat, or infrared energy, by the surfaces inside the greenhouse. This heat energy then takes longer to pass back through the glass surfaces and causes the interior of the greenhouse to feel warmer than the outside climate.
>
> Plants may grow better inside a greenhouse versus outside for several reasons. There is more control of the temperature and humidity of the environment inside the greenhouse. The carbon dioxide produced by plants is trapped inside the greenhouse and can increase the rate of photosynthesis of the plants. There are also fewer pests and diseases inside the greenhouse.

Figure 1 below shows how a greenhouse works.

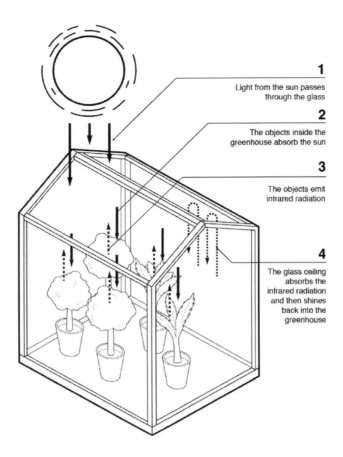

1
Light from the sun passes through the glass

2
The objects inside the greenhouse absorb the sun

3
The objects emit infrared radiation

4
The glass ceiling absorbs the infrared radiation and then shines back into the greenhouse

Scientist A wants to compare how a tomato plant grows inside a greenhouse versus outside a greenhouse.

Figure 2 below shows a graph of her results over 3 months.

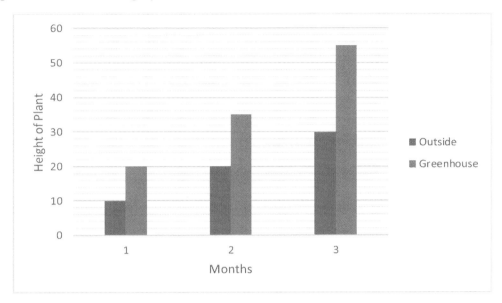

27. Looking at Figure 1, what gets trapped inside the greenhouse that helps plants grow?
    a. Short-wavelength IR
    b. Long-wavelength IR
    c. Cold air
    d. Water

28. Which plant grew taller from Scientist A's experiment?
    a. Outside
    b. Both grew to the same height.
    c. They both remained the same height for 3 months.
    d. Greenhouse

29. What gets converted to heat inside a greenhouse?
    a. Water
    b. Sunlight
    c. Plants
    d. Oxygen

30. What type of wavelength moves through the greenhouse glass easily according to Figure 1?
    a. Short-wavelength IR
    b. Oxygen
    c. Carbon dioxide
    d. Long-wavelength IR

Chemistry

1. How many centimeters is 0.78 kilometers?
   - a. 7.8 cm
   - b. 0.078 cm
   - c. 78,000 cm
   - d. 780 cm

2. Which of the following correctly matches a category of protein with a physiologic example?
   - a. Keratin is a structural protein
   - b. Antigens are hormonal proteins
   - c. Channel proteins are marker proteins
   - d. Actin is a transport protein

3. Most catalysts found in biological systems are which of the following?
   - a. Special lipids called cofactors.
   - b. Special proteins called enzymes.
   - c. Special lipids called enzymes.
   - d. Special proteins called cofactors.

4. Which statement is true regarding atomic structure?
   - a. Protons orbit around a nucleus.
   - b. Neutrons have a positive charge.
   - c. Electrons are in the nucleus.
   - d. Protons have a positive charge.

5. The acceleration of a falling object due to gravity has been proven to be 9.8 m/s^2. A scientist drops a cactus four times and measures the acceleration with an accelerometer and gets the following results: 9.79 m/s^2, 9.81 m/s^2, 9.80 m/s^2, and 9.78 m/s^2. Which of the following accurately describes the measurements?
   - a. They're both accurate and precise.
   - b. They're accurate but not precise.
   - c. They're precise but not accurate.
   - d. They're neither accurate nor precise.

6. Which is NOT a disaccharide?
   - a. Sucrose
   - b. Lactose
   - c. Maltose
   - d. Mannose

7. How many mL of a 12.0 M stock solution of HCl should be added to water to create 250 mL of a 1.50 M solution of HCl?
   - a. 31.2 mL
   - b. 30.3 mL
   - c. 31.35 mL
   - d. 31.3 mL

8. If a reading is above the curve on a solubility curve, the solvent is considered to be which of the following?
    a. Unsaturated
    b. Supersaturated
    c. Stable
    d. Saturated

9. Which of the following correctly lists the maximum number of electrons that the first three orbitals can accommodate?
    a. 2, 4, 8
    b. 1, 4. 8
    c. 2, 2, 8
    d. 2, 8, 8

10. Which of the following is true regarding ionic bonds?
    a. The metallic substance usually transfers an electron to the nonmetal.
    b. The metallic substance often has a high electron affinity.
    c. The ionic substances formed have low melting and boiling points because of the relatively weak bonds.
    d. The formation of ionic bonds is an endothermic reaction.

11. What is the most electronegative element?
    a. Hydrogen
    b. Fluorine
    c. Oxygen
    d. Chlorine

12. In covalent bonding, how does the number of electrons involved in bonding affect bond length?
    a. The more electrons shared, the longer the bond.
    b. The more electrons shared, the shorter the bond.
    c. The more electrons transferred, the longer the bond.
    d. The more electrons transferred, the shorter the bond.

13. Which is the metric prefix for 10^{-3}?
    a. Milli
    b. Centi
    c. Micro
    d. Deci

14. Which of the following statements is true regarding Lewis structures for metallic compounds?
    a. Lewis structures are most accurate for metallic compounds because of the natural way electrons in metallic substances arrange themselves in rather predictable, geometric arrangements.
    b. Lewis structures are not common for metallic compounds because of the free-roaming ability of the electrons.
    c. A Lewis symbol for an element entering a metallic bond can have dots on just the bonded side of the compound, for a maximum of two dots.
    d. Lewis structures help visualize the electrons in metallic compounds more easily than in covalent structures, where the electron sharing cannot be depicted well.

243

15. What is ionization energy?
    a. One-half the distance between the nuclei of atoms of the same element.
    b. A measurement of the tendency of an atom to form a chemical bond.
    c. The amount of energy needed to remove a valence electron from a gas or ion.
    d. The ability or tendency of an atom to accept an electron into its valence shell.

16. For gaseous reactants, how does decreasing the pressure in the system affect the reaction rate?
    a. The reaction rate increases because the frequency of collisions increases.
    b. The reaction rate increases because the frequency of collisions decreases.
    c. The reaction rate decreases because the frequency of collisions increases.
    d. The reaction rate decreases because the frequency of collisions decreases.

17. What can be said about the reaction described by the following generic chemical equation?
$$aA\ (s)+bB\ (aq) \leftrightarrow cC\ (s)+dD\ (aq)$$

    a. The reaction is in static equilibrium.
    b. The reaction is in dynamic equilibrium.
    c. The reaction is in heterogenous equilibrium.
    d. The reaction is in homogenous equilibrium.

18. Based on collision theory, what is the effect of temperature on the rate of chemical reaction?
    a. Increasing the temperature slows the reaction.
    b. Decreasing the temperature speeds up the reaction.
    c. Increasing the temperature speeds up the reaction.
    d. Collision theory and temperature are unrelated.

19. Burning a piece of paper is what type of change?
    a. Chemical change
    b. Physical change
    c. Sedimentary change
    d. Potential change

20. Which of the following is true?
    a. A base acts as a proton donor in a chemical equation.
    b. A base is an electron-pair acceptor in a chemical equation.
    c. An acid increases the concentration of H^+ ions when it is dissolved in water.
    d. An acid increases the concentration of OH^- ions when it is dissolved in water.

21. Which of the following is a synthesis reaction?
    a. $2NO+O_2 \rightarrow 2NO_2$
    b. $H_2CO_3 \rightarrow H_2O+CO_2$
    c. $Mg+2HCl \rightarrow MgCl_2+H_2$
    d. $Zn+2\ HCl \rightarrow ZnCl_2+H_2$

22. What type of reaction is $CH_4+2O_2 \rightarrow CO_2+2H_2O$?
    a. Substitution Reaction
    b. Combustion Reaction
    c. Redox Reaction
    d. Acid-Base Reaction

23. What is the percent yield for the reaction that produces 45 grams of CaO if 65 grams were expected out of the reaction $CaCO_3 \rightarrow CaO + CO_2$?
 a. 6.9%
 b. 69%
 c. 144%
 d. 14.4%

24. Which of the following statements is true?
 a. When an atom, ion, or molecule loses its electrons and becomes more positively charged, it has been reduced.
 b. When an atom, ion, or molecule loses its electrons and becomes more positively charged, it has been oxidized.
 c. When an atom, ion, or molecule loses its electrons and becomes more negatively charged, it has been oxidized.
 d. When an atom, ion, or molecule loses its electrons and becomes more negatively charged, it has been reduced.

25. Which of the following correctly shows a conjugate acid paired with its conjugate base?
 a. H_2SO_4 (acid) and HSO_4^- (conjugate base)
 b. HSO_4^- (acid) and H_2SO_4 (conjugate base)
 c. H_2SO_4 (acid) and HSO_4^+ (conjugate base)
 d. HSO_4^+ (acid) and H_2SO_4 (conjugate base)

26. Ice is a crystalline solid made up of repeating units of water molecules. Which choice does NOT describe a property of an ice cube?
 a. Has an exact melting point
 b. Breaks across a plane
 c. Becomes soft before it melts
 d. Bonds break at the same time when it melts

27. What is the molecular formula for the molecule represented in the following Lewis diagram?

 a. CH_3-H_2O
 b. CH_3
 c. CH_3O
 d. CH_3OH

28. What type of solid is a semiconductor such as silicon?
    a. Metallic solid
    b. Neutral solid
    c. Ionic solid
    d. Covalent network solid

29. What type of reaction occurs when fossil fuels react with oxygen gas?
    a. Combustion
    b. Combination
    c. Vaporization
    d. Solidification

30. Which coefficient would fill in the blank in the following equation to correctly balance the chemical reaction between iron oxide and carbon monoxide: $FeO_3 + 3CO \rightarrow Fe + \_\_CO_2$?
    a. 1
    b. 3
    c. 2
    d. 6

Anatomy and Physiology

1. Eosinophils are best described as which of the following?
    a. A type of leukocyte that secretes histamine, which stimulates the inflammatory response.
    b. The most abundant type of leukocyte that secretes substances that are toxic to pathogens.
    c. A type of leukocyte found under mucous membranes that defends against multicellular parasites.
    d. A type of circulating leukocyte that is aggressive and has high phagocytic activity.

2. Which of the following is one of the functions of the stratum basale layer of the epidermis?
    a. Repelling water
    b. Protecting against UV rays
    c. Producing keratin
    d. Producing oil to lubricate and protect the skin

3. Tendons connect what?
    a. Muscle to muscle
    b. Bone to bone
    c. Muscle to bone
    d. Muscle to ligament

4. How does cartilage obtain nutrients?
    a. A network of fine capillaries
    b. An extensive network of internal vasculature
    c. Carrier proteins
    d. Diffusion

5. In terms of levels of organization in the body, the next level up from cells is which of the following? In other words, groups of cells are arranged into which of the following?
   a. Organ systems
   b. Atoms
   c. Organs
   d. Tissues

6. Which of the following is NOT one of the functions of sebum?
   a. Protecting the skin from water loss
   b. Moisturizing the skin
   c. Helping with thermoregulation by assisting with evaporative cooling
   d. Providing a chemical defense against bacterial and fungal infections

7. Which of the following statements accurately describes the basics of the sliding filament model of muscle contraction?
   a. Myosin filaments form and break cross-bridges with actin in order to pull the actin filaments closer to the M line.
   b. Actin filaments form and break cross-bridges with myosin in order to pull the myosin filaments closer to the M line.
   c. Myosin filaments form and break cross-bridges with actin in order to pull the actin filaments closer to the Z line.
   d. Actin filaments form and break cross-bridges with myosin in order to pull the myosin filaments closer to the Z line.

8. What is one of the characteristics of transitional epithelial tissue that differentiates it from other types of epithelial tissue?
   a. It is composed solely from a single layer of cells.
   b. It appears to be stratified but actually consists of only one layer of cells.
   c. It helps protect the body from invasions of microbes like bacteria and parasites.
   d. It can expand and contract.

9. What structures are made by the body's white blood cells that fight bacterial infections?
   a. Antibodies
   b. Antibiotics
   c. Vaccines
   d. Red blood cells

10. Which blood component is chiefly responsible for oxygen transport?
   a. Platelets
   b. Red blood cells
   c. White blood cells
   d. Plasma cells

11. Which of the following is NOT a bone of the axial skeleton?
   a. Sternum
   b. Mandible
   c. Ilium
   d. Atlas

12. Where does sperm maturation take place in the male reproductive system?
    a. Seminal vesicles
    b. Prostate gland
    c. Epididymis
    d. Vas Deferens

13. Which hormone in the female reproductive system is responsible for progesterone production?
    a. FSH
    b. LH
    c. hCG
    d. Estrogen

14. Which epithelial tissue comprises the cell layer found in a capillary bed?
    a. Squamous
    b. Cuboidal
    c. Columnar
    d. Stratified

15. When considering anatomical direction, what is the position of the clavicle to the humerus?
    a. Lateral
    b. Medial
    c. Distal
    d. Inferior

16. What is the body plane that runs vertically through the body at right angles to the midline?
    a. Coronal
    b. Transverse
    c. Sagittal
    d. Superior

17. Which statement is true?
    a. Ligaments attach skeletal muscles to bone.
    b. Tendons connect bones at joints.
    c. Cartilage adds mechanical support to joints.
    d. Most veins deliver oxygenated blood to cells.

18. Which layer of skin contains sensory receptors and blood vessels?
    a. Epidermis
    b. Dermis
    c. Hypodermis
    d. Subcutaneous

19. Receptors in the dermis help the body maintain homeostasis by relaying messages to what area of the brain?
    a. The cerebellum
    b. The brain stem
    c. The pituitary gland
    d. The hypothalamus

20. The radius and ulna are to the humerus what the tibia and fibula are to the _____.
    a. Mandible
    b. Femur
    c. Scapula
    d. Carpal

21. What are concentric circles of bone tissue called?
    a. Lacunae
    b. Lamellae
    c. Trabeculae
    d. Diaphysis

22. When de-oxygenated blood first enters the heart, which of the following choices is in the correct order for its journey to the aorta?
    I. Tricuspid valve → Lungs → Mitral valve
    II. Mitral valve → Lungs → Tricuspid valve
    III. Right ventricle → Lungs → Left atrium
    IV. Left ventricle → Lungs → Right atrium

    a. I and III only
    b. I and IV only
    c. II and III only
    d. II and IV only

23. Which characteristics are true for skeletal muscle?
    I. Contain sarcomeres
    II. Have multiple nuclei
    III. Are branched

    a. I only
    b. I and II only
    c. I, II, and III only
    d. II and III only

24. Which is the simplest nerve pathway that bypasses the brain?
    a. Autonomic
    b. Reflex arc
    c. Somatic
    d. Sympathetic

25. Using anatomical terms, what is the relationship of the sternum relative to the deltoid?
    a. Medial
    b. Lateral
    c. Superficial
    d. Posterior

26. Which of the following areas of the body has the highest density of sweat glands?
    a. Upper back
    b. Arms
    c. Soles of feet/palms
    d. Head

27. Which statement is NOT true regarding brain structure?
    a. The corpus collosum connects the hemispheres.
    b. Broca and Wernicke's areas are associated with speech and language.
    c. The cerebellum is important for long-term memory storage.
    d. The brainstem is responsible for involuntary movement.

28. Which is the first event to happen in a primary immune response?
    a. Macrophages ingest pathogens and present their antigens.
    b. Neutrophils aggregate and act as cytotoxic, nonspecific killers of pathogens.
    c. B lymphocytes make pathogen-specific antibodies.
    d. Helper T cells secrete interleukins to activate pathogen-fighting cells.

29. Which of the following is not considered to be a primary function of the proprioceptive system?
    a. Provide awareness of position and kinesthesia within the surroundings
    b. Produce coordinated reflexes to maintain muscle tone and balance
    c. Provide peripheral feedback information to the central nervous system to help modify movements and motor response
    d. Provide cushioning to joints during impact

30. Which of the following correctly explains the order of how muscle spindles sense the rate and magnitude of increasing muscle tension as the muscle lengthens?
    a. The muscle spindle is stretched, sensory neurons in the spindle are activated, an impulse is sent to the spinal cord, motor neurons that innervate extrafusal fibers are signaled to relax
    b. The muscle spindle is stretched, motor neurons in the spindle are activated, an impulse is sent to the spinal cord, sensory neurons that innervate extrafusal fibers are signaled to relax
    c. Sensory neurons in the spindle are activated, the muscle spindle is stretched, an impulse is sent to the spinal cord, motor neurons that innervate extrafusal fibers are signaled to relax
    d. The muscle spindle is stretched, sensory neurons in the spindle are activated, an impulse is sent to the spinal cord, sensory neurons that innervate intrafusal fibers are signaled to relax

Physics

1. Circular motion occurs around what?
    a. The center of mass
    b. The center of matter
    c. An elliptical
    d. An axis

250

2. Which of the following is true of an object at rest on Earth?
   a. It has no forces acting upon it.
   b. It has no gravity acting upon it.
   c. It is in transition.
   d. It is in equilibrium.

3. Which statement is true regarding electrostatic charges?
   a. Like charges attract.
   b. Like charges repel.
   c. Like charges are neutral.
   d. Like charges neither attract nor repel.

4. Which is not a form of energy?
   a. Light
   b. Sound
   c. Heat
   d. Mass

5. Which of the following is a vector quantity?
   a. Mass
   b. Length
   c. Velocity
   d. Speed

6. Why would a pencil appear to bend at the water line in a glass of water?
   a. The wood of the pencil becomes warped from being in the water.
   b. It appears to bend because of the refraction of light traveling from air to water.
   c. The pencil temporarily bends because of its immersion into separate mediums.
   d. The reflection of the light from water to a human's pupil creates the illusion of a warping object.

7. What is the current when a 3.0 V battery is wired across a lightbulb that has a resistance of 6.0 ohms?
   a. 0.5 A
   b. 18.0 A
   c. 0.5 J
   d. 18.0 J

8. The law of the conservation of energy states which of the following?
   a. Energy should be stored in power cells for future use.
   b. Energy will replenish itself once exhausted.
   c. Energy cannot be created or destroyed.
   d. Energy should be saved because it can run out.

9. Running electricity through a wire generates which of the following?
   a. A gravitational field
   b. A frictional field
   c. An acoustic field
   d. A magnetic field

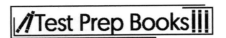

10. Which of the following depicts a form of potential energy?
    a. The light given off by a lamp
    b. The gravitational pull of a black hole
    c. The heat from a microwaved burrito
    d. The motion of a pendulum

11. A car is traveling at a constant velocity of 25 m/s. How long does it take the car to travel 45 kilometers in a straight line?
    a. 1 hour
    b. 3600 seconds
    c. 1800 seconds
    d. 900 seconds

12. A ship is traveling due east at a speed of 1 m/s against a current flowing due west at a speed of 0.5 m/s. How far has the ship travelled from its point of departure after two hours?
    a. 1.8 kilometers west of its point of departure
    b. 3.6 kilometers west of its point of departure
    c. 1.8 kilometers east of its point of departure
    d. 3.6 kilometers east of its point of departure

13. A car is driving along a straight stretch of highway at a constant speed of 60 km/hour when the driver slams the gas pedal to the floor, reaching a speed of 132 km/hour in 10 seconds. What's the average acceleration of the car after the engine is floored?
    a. 1 m/s^2
    b. 2 m/s^2
    c. 3 m/s^2
    d. 4 m/s^2

14. A spaceship with a mass of 100,000 kilograms is far away from any planet. To accelerate the craft at the rate of 0.5 m/sec^2, what is the rocket thrust?
    a. 98.1 N
    b. 25,000 N
    c. 50,000 N
    d. 75,000 N

15. The gravitational acceleration on Earth averages 9.81 m/s^2. An astronaut weighs 1962 N on Earth. The diameter of Earth is six times the diameter of its moon. What's the mass of the astronaut on Earth's moon?
    a. 100 kilograms
    b. 200 kilograms
    c. 300 kilograms
    d. 400 kilograms

16. A football is kicked so that it leaves the punter's toe at a horizontal angle of 45 degrees. Ignoring any spin or tumbling, at what point is the upward vertical velocity of the football at a maximum?

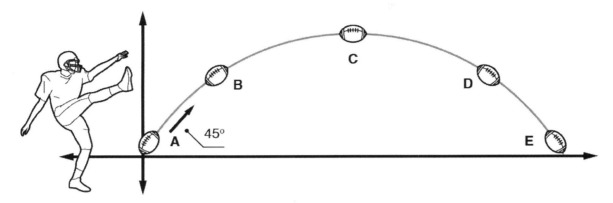

 a. At Point A
 b. At Point C
 c. At Points B and D
 d. At Points A and E

17. The skater is shown spinning in Figure (a), then bringing in her arms in Figure (b). Which sequence accurately describes what happens to her angular velocity?

(a)   **(b)**

 a. Her angular velocity decreases from (a) to (b)
 b. Her angular velocity doesn't change from (a) to (b)
 c. Her angular velocity increases from (a) to (b)
 d. It's not possible to determine what happens to her angular velocity if her weight is unknown.

18. A cannonball is dropped from a height of 10 meters off of the ground. What is its approximate velocity just before it hits the ground?
   a. 9.81 m/s
   b. 14 m/s
   c. 32 m/s
   d. It can't be determined without knowing the cannonball's mass

19. The pendulum is held at point A, and then released to swing to the right. At what point does the pendulum have the greatest kinetic energy?

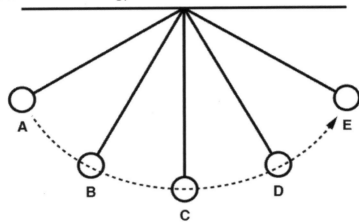

   a. At Point B
   b. At Point C
   c. At Point D
   d. At Point E

20. Which statement is true of the total energy of the pendulum?

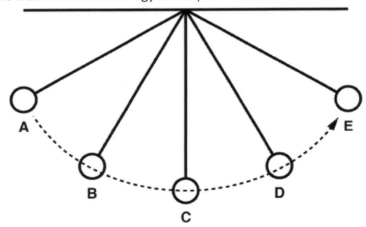

   a. Its total energy is at a maximum and equal at Points A and E.
   b. Its total energy is at a maximum at Point C.
   c. Its total energy is the same at Points A, B, C, D, and E.
   d. The total energy can't be determined without knowing the pendulum's mass.

Answer Explanations #1

Mathematics

1. D: $\dfrac{3}{100}$

Each digit to the left of the decimal point represents a higher multiple of 10 and each digit to the right of the decimal point represents a quotient of a higher multiple of 10 for the divisor. The first digit to the right of the decimal point is equal to the value divided by 10. The second digit to the right of the decimal point is equal to the value divided by (10 × 10), or the value divided by 100.

2. B: 102,317

Set up the problem and add each column, starting on the far right (ones). Add, carrying anything over 9 into the next column to the left. Solve from right to left.

3. A: 847.90

The hundredths place value is located two digits to the right of the decimal point (the digit 9 in the original number). The digit to the right of the place value is examined to decide whether to round up or keep the digit. In this case, the digit 6 is 5 or greater so the hundredth place is rounded up. When rounding up, if the digit to be increased is a 9, the digit to its left is increased by one and the digit in the desired place value is made a zero. Therefore, the number is rounded to 847.90.

4. B: $\dfrac{11}{15}$

Fractions must have like denominators to be added. We are trying to add a fraction with a denominator of 3 to a fraction with a denominator of 5, so we have to convert both fractions to their respective equivalent fractions that have a common denominator. The common denominator is the least common multiple (LCM) of the two original denominators. In this case, the LCM is 15, so both fractions should be changed to equivalent fractions with a denominator of 15.

To determine the numerator of the new fraction, the old numerator is multiplied by the same number by which the old denominator is multiplied to obtain the new denominator.

For the fraction $\dfrac{1}{3}$, 3 multiplied by 5 will produce 15.

Therefore, the numerator is multiplied by 5 to produce the new numerator:

$$\frac{1 \times 5}{3 \times 5} = \frac{5}{15}$$

For the fraction $\dfrac{2}{5}$, multiplying both the numerator and denominator by 3 produces $\dfrac{6}{15}$. When fractions have like denominators, they are added by adding the numerators and keeping the denominator the same:

$$\frac{5}{15} + \frac{6}{15} = \frac{11}{15}$$

255

5. A: $1\frac{5}{36}$

Set up the problem and find a common denominator for both fractions.

$$\frac{7}{12}+\frac{5}{9}$$

Multiply each fraction to convert to a common denominator.

$$\frac{7}{12}\times\frac{3}{3}+\frac{5}{9}\times\frac{4}{4}$$

Once over the same denominator, add across the top. The total is over the common denominator.

$$\frac{21+20}{36}=\frac{41}{36}$$

Convert to a mixed number.

$$\frac{41}{36}=1\frac{5}{36}$$

6. D: 80%

To convert a fraction to a percent, the fraction is first converted to a decimal. To do so, the numerator is divided by the denominator: $4 \div 5 = 0.8$. To convert a decimal to a percent, the number is multiplied by 100:

$$0.8 \times 100 = 80\%$$

7. D: 6,258

Set up the problem, with the larger number on top. Begin subtracting with the far-right column (ones). Borrow 10 from the column to the left when necessary.

8. D: 1, 2, 3, 4, 6, 12

A given number divides evenly by each of its factors to produce an integer (no decimals). The number 5, 7, 8, 9, 10, 11 (and their opposites) do not divide evenly into 12. Therefore, these numbers are not factors.

9. A: 11

To determine the number of houses that can fit on the street, the length of the street is divided by the width of each house: $345 \div 30 = 11.5$. Although the mathematical calculation of 11.5 is correct, this answer is not reasonable. Half of a house cannot be built, so the company will need to either build 11 or 12 houses. Since the width of 12 houses (360 feet) will extend past the length of the street, only 11 houses can be built.

10. C: 594.02

Set up the problem, with the larger number on top and numbers lined up at the decimal. Insert 0 in any blank spots to the right of the decimal as placeholders. Begin subtracting with the far-right column. Borrow 10 from the column to the left when necessary.

11. A: $\frac{5}{8}$

Set up the problem and find a common denominator for both fractions.

$$\frac{19}{24} - \frac{1}{6}$$

Multiply the second fraction to convert to a common denominator.

$$\frac{19}{24} - \frac{1}{6} \times \frac{4}{4}$$

Once over the same denominator, subtract across the top.

$$\frac{19 - 4}{24} = \frac{15}{24}$$

Reduce by dividing the numerator and denominator by a common factor (3).

$$\frac{15}{24} = \frac{5}{8}$$

12. D: $x = -5$

When solving a linear equation, distribution is performed if necessary: $-3(x + 4) \rightarrow -3x - 12 = x + 8$. This means that any like terms on the same side of the equation are combined.

The equation is manipulated to get the variable on one side. In this case, subtracting x from both sides produces:

$$-4x - 12 = 8$$

The variable is isolated using inverse operations to undo addition/subtraction. Adding 12 to both sides produces $-4x = 20$.

The variable is isolated using inverse operations to undo multiplication/division. Remember if dividing by a negative number, the sign is flipped. In this case, dividing by -4 on both sides produces $x = -5$.

13. C: 4,498

Line up the numbers (the number with the most digits on top) to multiply. Begin with the left column on top and the left column on bottom.

Move one column left on top and multiply by the far-right column on the bottom. Remember to carry over after you multiply.

Starting on the far-right column, on top, repeat this pattern for the next number left on the bottom. Write the answers below the first line of answers. Remember to begin with a zero placeholder.

Continue the pattern.

Add the answer rows together, making sure they are still lined up correctly.

14. B: Add 3 to both sides to get $4x = 8$. Then divide both sides by 4 to get $x = 2$.

15. B: $12 \times 750 = 9,000$

Therefore, there are 9,000 milliliters of water, which must be converted to liters. 1,000 milliliters equals 1 liter; therefore, 9 liters of water are purchased.

16. A: This problem can be solved using basic arithmetic. Xavier starts with 20 apples, then gives his sister half, so 20 divided by 2.

$$\frac{20}{2} = 10$$

He then gives his neighbor 6, so 6 is subtracted from 10.

$$10 - 6 = 4$$

Lastly, he uses $\frac{3}{4}$ of his apples to make an apple pie, so to find remaining apples, the first step is to subtract $\frac{3}{4}$ from one and then multiply the difference by 4.

$$\left(1 - \frac{3}{4}\right) \times 4 = ?$$

$$\left(\frac{4}{4} - \frac{3}{4}\right) \times 4 = ?$$

$$\left(\frac{1}{4}\right) \times 4 = 1$$

17. D: 40% is $\frac{4}{10}$. The number itself must be $\frac{10}{4}$ of 12, or $\frac{10}{4} \times 12 = 10 \times 3 = 30$.

18. A: Convert these numbers to improper fractions: $\frac{11}{3} - \frac{9}{5}$. Take 15 as a common denominator:

$$\frac{11}{3} - \frac{9}{5} = \frac{55}{15} - \frac{27}{15} = \frac{28}{15} = 1\frac{13}{15}$$

19. C: Dividing by 100 means shifting the decimal point of the numerator to the left by 2. The result is 6.6 and rounds to 7.

20. B: Because these decimals are all negative, the number that is the largest will be the number whose absolute value is the smallest, as that will be the negative number with the least value. Thus, it will be the "least negative" (closest to zero). To figure out which number has the smallest absolute value, look at the first non-zero digits. The first non-zero digit in Choice *B* is in the hundredths place. The other three all have non-zero digits in the tenths place, so Choice *B* is closest to zero; thus, it is the largest of the four negative numbers.

21. C: To solve for the value of b, isolate the variable b on one side of the equation.

Start by moving the lower value of -4 to the other side by adding 4 to both sides:

$$5b - 4 = 2b + 17$$

$$5b - 4 + 4 = 2b + 17 + 4$$

$$5b = 2b + 21$$

Then subtract $2b$ from both sides:

$$5b - 2b = 2b + 21 - 2b$$

$$3b = 21$$

Then divide both sides by 3 to get the value of b:

$$\frac{3b}{3} = \frac{21}{3}$$

$$b = 7$$

22. C: $\frac{1}{3}$ of the shirts sold were patterned. Therefore, $1 - \frac{1}{3} = \frac{2}{3}$ of the shirts sold were solid. Anytime "of" a quantity appears in a word problem, multiplication should be used.

Therefore:

$$192 \times \frac{2}{3} = \frac{192 \times 2}{3} = \frac{384}{3} = 128 \text{ solid shirts were sold}$$

The entire expression is $192 \times \left(1 - \frac{1}{3}\right)$.

23. C: The first step is to depict each number using decimals.

$$\frac{91}{100} = 0.91$$

Dividing the numerator by denominator of $\frac{4}{5}$ to convert it to a decimal yields 0.80, while $\frac{2}{3}$ becomes 0.66 recurring. Rearrange each expression in ascending order, as found in Choice *C*.

24. A: 13/5

Set up the division problem.

$$\frac{5}{13} \div \frac{25}{169}$$

259

Flip the second fraction and multiply.

$$\frac{5}{13} \times \frac{169}{25}$$

Simplify and reduce with cross multiplication.

$$\frac{1}{1} \times \frac{13}{5}$$

Multiply across the top and across the bottom to solve.

$$\frac{1 \times 13}{1 \times 5} = \frac{13}{5}$$

25. A: $3\frac{3}{5}$. Divide 54 by 15:

$$15\overline{)54}$$
$$\underline{-45}$$
$$9$$

The result is $3\frac{9}{15}$. Reduce the remainder for the final answer, $3\frac{3}{5}$.

26. A: Using the order of operations, multiplication and division are computed first from left to right. Multiplication is on the left; therefore, multiplication should be performed first.

27. D: $\frac{59}{7}$

The original number was $8\frac{3}{7}$. Multiply the denominator by the whole number portion. Add the numerator and put the total over the original denominator.

$$\frac{(8 \times 7) + 3}{7} = \frac{59}{7}$$

28. B: $\frac{93}{8}$

The original number was $11\frac{5}{8}$. Multiply the denominator by the whole number portion. Add the numerator and put the total over the original denominator.

$$\frac{(8 \times 11) + 5}{8} = \frac{93}{8}$$

29. B: 8.1

To round 8.067 to the nearest tenths, use the digit in the hundredths.

6 in the hundredths is greater than 5, so round up in the tenths.

$$8.\underline{0}67$$

260

0 becomes a 1.

8.1

30. A: The place value to the right of the thousandth place, which would be the ten-thousandth place, is what gets used. The value in the thousandth place is 7. The number in the place value to its right is greater than 4, so the 7 gets bumped up to 8. Everything to its right turns to a zero, to get 245.2680. The zero is dropped because it is part of the decimal.

31. B: This is a division problem because the original amount needs to be split up into equal amounts. The mixed number $11\frac{1}{2}$ should be converted to an improper fraction first:

$$11\frac{1}{2} = \frac{(11 \times 2) + 1}{2} = \frac{23}{2}$$

Carey needs to determine how many times $\frac{23}{2}$ goes into 184. This is a division problem:

$$184 \div \frac{23}{2} = ?$$

The fraction can be flipped, and the problem turns into the multiplication:

$$184 \times \frac{2}{23} = \frac{368}{23}$$

This improper fraction can be simplified into 16 because $368 \div 23 = 16$. The answer is 16 lawn segments.

32. B: 100 cm is equal to 1 m. 1.3 divided by 100 is 0.013. Therefore, 1.3 cm is equal to 0.013 m. Because 1 cm is equal to 10 mm, 1.3 cm is equal to 13 mm.

33. B: Using the conversion rate, the projected weight loss of 25 pounds is multiplied by 0.45 kg/lb to get the amount in kilograms (11.25 kg).

34. D: Start by taking a common denominator of 30.

$$\frac{14}{15} = \frac{28}{30}$$

$$\frac{3}{5} = \frac{18}{30}$$

$$\frac{1}{30} = \frac{1}{30}$$

Add and subtract the numerators for the next step.

$$\frac{28}{30} + \frac{18}{30} - \frac{1}{30} = \frac{28 + 18 - 1}{30} = \frac{45}{30} = \frac{3}{2}$$

In the last step the 15 is factored out from the numerator and denominator.

261

35. D: In order to solve this problem, the number of feet in a yard must be established. There are 3 feet in every yard. The equation to calculate the minimum number of yards is $79 \div 3 = 26\frac{1}{3}$.

If the material is sold only by whole yards, then Mo would need to round up to the next whole yard in order to cover the extra $\frac{1}{3}$ yard. Therefore, the answer is 27 yards. None of the other choices meets the minimum whole yard requirement.

36. C: DXVII

Break down the number into parts.

$517 = 500 + 10 + 5 + 2$

500 is represented by D or $500 = D$

10 is represented by X or $10 = X$

5 is represented by V or $5 = V$

2 is represented by II.

Combine the Roman numerals.

DXVii

37. A: 3:00 p.m. Since military time starts with 0100 at 1:00 a.m., add 14 to get to 1500 hours, or 3:00 p.m.

38. D: To take the product of two fractions, just multiply the numerators and denominators.

$$\frac{5}{3} \times \frac{7}{6} = \frac{5 \times 7}{3 \times 6} = \frac{35}{18}$$

The numerator and denominator have no common factors, so this is simplified completely.

39. A: A common denominator must be found. The least common denominator is 15 because it has both 5 and 3 as factors. The fractions must be rewritten using 15 as the denominator.

40. B: 1000 hours. Anything before noon converts over from its a.m. value.

41. D: 100,000.0 cm. To convert from kilometers to centimeters, move the decimal 5 places to the right.

$$1.0 \text{ Km} = 100,000.0 \text{ cm}$$

262

42. A: Operations within the parentheses must be completed first. Then, division is completed. Finally, addition is the last operation to complete. When adding decimals, digits within each place value are added together. Therefore, the expression is evaluated as:

$$(2 \times 20) \div (7 + 1) + (6 \times 0.01) + (4 \times 0.001)$$

$$40 \div 8 + 0.06 + 0.004$$

$$5 + 0.06 + 0.004 = 5.064$$

43. D: By grouping the four numbers in the answer into factors of the two numbers of the question (6 and 12), it can be determined that:

$$(3 \times 2) \times (4 \times 3) = 6 \times 12$$

Alternatively, each of the answer choices could multiplied out and compared to the original value. 6×12 has a value of 72. The answer choices respectively have values of 64, 84, 108, and 72, so answer D is the correct choice.

44. C: A dollar contains 20 nickels. Therefore, if there are 12 dollars' worth of nickels, there are $12 \times 20 = 240$ nickels. Each nickel weighs 5 grams. Therefore, the weight of the nickels is $240 \times 5 = 1,200$ grams. Adding in the weight of the empty piggy bank, the filled bank weighs 2,250 grams.

45. D: To find Denver's total snowfall, 3 must be multiplied times $27\frac{3}{4}$. In order to easily do this, the mixed number should be converted into an improper fraction.

$$27\frac{3}{4} = \frac{27 \times 4 + 3}{4} = \frac{111}{4}$$

Therefore, Denver had approximately $\frac{3 \times 111}{4} = \frac{333}{4}$ inches of snow. The improper fraction can be converted back into a mixed number through division.

$$\frac{333}{4} = 83\frac{1}{4} \text{ inches}$$

46. C: 120 pts

List out and set up equivalencies.

$$8 \text{ pts} = 1 \text{ gal}$$

Set up the equivalencies with the initial values.

$$\frac{15 \text{ gal}}{1} \times \frac{8 \text{ pts}}{1 \text{ gal}}$$

Cross-cancel units then multiply across the top and the bottom.

$$\frac{15 \times 8 \text{ pts}}{1} = 120 \text{ pts}$$

263

47. B: 99.32 °F

Set up the equation for converting Celsius to Fahrenheit.

$$°F = \frac{9}{5} \times °C + 32$$

Fill in the givens.

$$°F = \frac{9}{5} \times 37.4 + 32$$

Solve the equation in in parentheses. Multiply, then add.

$$°F = 67.32 + 32$$

$$°F = 99.32 \ °F$$

48. C: The first step in solving this problem is expressing the result in fraction form. Separate this problem first by solving the division operation of the last two fractions. When dividing one fraction by another, invert or flip the second fraction and then multiply the numerator and denominator.

$$\frac{7}{10} \times \frac{2}{1} = \frac{14}{10}$$

Next, multiply the first fraction with this value:

$$\frac{3}{5} \times \frac{14}{10} = \frac{42}{50}$$

In this instance, you can find the decimal form by converting the fraction into $\frac{x}{100}$, where x is the number from which the final decimal is found. Multiply both the numerator and denominator by 2 to get the fraction as an expression of $\frac{x}{100}$.

$$\frac{42}{50} \times \frac{2}{2} = \frac{84}{100}$$

In decimal form, this would be expressed as 0.84.

49. E: Setting up a proportion is the easiest way to represent this situation. The proportion becomes $\frac{20}{x} = \frac{40}{100}$, where cross-multiplication can be used to solve for x. The answer can also be found by observing the two fractions as equivalent, knowing that twenty is half of forty, and fifty is half of one-hundred.

50. D: The expression is three times the sum of twice a number and 1, which is $3(2x + 1)$. Then, 6 is subtracted from this expression.

51. B: Since $850 is the price *after* a 20% discount, $850 represents 80% of the original price. To determine the original price, set up a proportion with the ratio of the sale price (850) to original price (unknown) equal to the ratio of sale percentage (where x represents the unknown original price):

$$\frac{850}{x} = \frac{80}{100}$$

To solve a proportion, cross multiply and set the products equal to each other:

$$(850)(100) = (80)(x)$$

Multiplying each side results in the equation:

$$85,000 = 80x$$

To solve for x, divide both sides by 80:

$$\frac{85,000}{80} = \frac{80x}{80}$$

$$x = 1,062.5$$

Remember that x represents the original price. Subtracting the sale price from the original price ($1,062.50 − $850) indicates that Frank saved $212.50.

52. D: This problem can be solved by using unit conversion. The initial units are miles per minute. The final units need to be feet per second. Converting miles to feet uses the equivalence statement 1 mi = 5,280 ft. Converting minutes to seconds uses the equivalence statement 1 min = 60 s. Setting up the ratios to convert the units is shown in the following equation:

$$\frac{72 \text{ mi}}{90 \text{ min}} \times \frac{1 \text{ min}}{60 \text{ s}} \times \frac{5,280 \text{ ft}}{1 \text{ mi}} = 70.4 \frac{\text{ft}}{\text{s}}$$

The initial units cancel out, and the new units are left.

53. B: Multiplying by 10^{-3} means moving the decimal point three places to the left, putting in zeroes as necessary.

54. C: We are trying to find x, the number of red cans. The equation can be set up like this:

$$x + 2(10 - x) = 16$$

The left x is actually multiplied by $1, the price per red can. Since we know Jessica bought 10 total cans, $10 - x$ is the number blue cans that she bought. We multiply the number of blue cans by $2, the price per blue can.

That should all equal $16, the total amount of money that Jessica spent. Working that out gives us:

$$x + 20 - 2x = 16$$

$$20 - x = 16$$

$$x = 4$$

55. D: The first field has an area of 1000 feet, so the length of one side is $\sqrt{1000} = 10\sqrt{10}$. Since there are four sides to a square, the total perimeter is $40\sqrt{10}$. The second square has an area of 10 square feet, so the length of one side is $\sqrt{10}$, and the total perimeter is $4\sqrt{10}$. Adding these together gives:

$$40\sqrt{10} + 4\sqrt{10} = (40 + 4)\sqrt{10} = 44\sqrt{10}$$

Reading Comprehension

1. C: Gulliver becomes acquainted with the people and practices of his new surroundings. Choice *C* is the correct answer because it most extensively summarizes the entire passage. While Choices *A* and *B* are reasonable possibilities, they reference portions of Gulliver's experiences, not the whole. Choice *D* is incorrect because Gulliver doesn't express repentance or sorrow in this particular passage.

2. A: Principal refers to *chief* or *primary* within the context of this text. Choice *A* is the answer that most closely aligns with this definition. Choices *B* and *D* make reference to a helper or followers while Choice *C* doesn't meet the description of Reldresal from the passage.

3. C: One can reasonably infer that Gulliver is considerably larger than the children who were playing around him because multiple children could fit into his hand. Choice *B* is incorrect because there is no indication of stress in Gulliver's tone. Choices *A* and *D* aren't the best answer because though Gulliver seems fond of his new acquaintances, he didn't travel there with the intentions of meeting new people or to express a definite love for them in this particular portion of the text.

4. C: The emperor made a *definitive decision* to expose Gulliver to their native customs. In this instance, the word *mind* was not related to a vote, question, or cognitive ability.

5. A: Choice *A* is correct. This assertion does *not* support the fact that games are a commonplace event in this culture because it mentions conduct, not games. Choices *B, C,* and *D* are incorrect because these do support the fact that games were a commonplace event.

6. B: The point of this passage is to show what drowning looks like. Choice *A* is incorrect because while drowning is a danger of swimming, the passage doesn't include any other dangers. The passage is not intended for lifeguards specifically, but for a general audience, so Choice *C* is incorrect. There are a few signs of drowning, but the passage does not compare them; thus, Choice *D* is incorrect.

7. D: To enlighten the audience on the habits of sun-fish and their hatcheries. Choice *A* is incorrect because although the Adirondack region is mentioned in the text, there is no cause or effect relationships between the region and fish hatcheries depicted here. Choice *B* is incorrect because the text does not have an agenda, but rather is meant to inform the audience. Finally, Choice *C* is incorrect because the text says nothing of how sun-fish mate.

8. B: The sun-fish builds it with her tail and snout. The text explains this in the second paragraph: "she builds, with her tail and snout, a circular embankment 3 inches in height and 2 thick." Choice *A* is used in the text as a simile.

9. D: To conclude a sequence and add a final detail. The concluding sequence is expressed in the phrase "[t]he mother sun-fish, having now built or provided her 'hatchery.'" The final detail is the way in which the sun-fish guards the "inclosure." Choices *A, B,* and *C* are incorrect.

10. C: *Extraneous* most nearly means *superfluous,* or *trivial.* Choice *A, indispensable,* is incorrect because it means the opposite of *extraneous.* Choice *B, bewildering,* means *confusing* and is not relevant to the context of the sentence. Finally, Choice *D* is incorrect because although the prefix of the word is the same, ex-, the word exuberant means elated or enthusiastic, and is irrelevant to the context of the sentence.

11. A: Bring to light an alternative view on human perception by examining the role of technology in human understanding. This is a challenging question because the author's purpose is somewhat open-ended. The author concludes by stating that the questions regarding human perception and observation can be approached from many angles. Thus, they do not seem to be attempting to prove one thing or another. Choice *B* is incorrect because we cannot know for certain whether the electron experiment is the latest discovery in astroparticle physics because no date is given. Choice *C* is a broad generalization that does not reflect accurately on the writer's views. While the author does appear to reflect on opposing views of human understanding (Choice *D*), the best answer is Choice *A.*

12. C: It presents a problem, explains the details of that problem, and then ends with more inquiry. The beginning of this paragraph literally "presents a conundrum," explains the problem of partial understanding, and then ends with more questions, or inquiry. There is no solution offered in this paragraph, making Choices *A* and *B* incorrect. Choice *D* is incorrect because the paragraph does not begin with a definition.

13. D: Looking back in the text, the author describes that classical philosophy holds that understanding can be reached by careful observation. This will not work if they are overly invested or biased in their pursuit. Choices *A* and *C* are in no way related and are completely unnecessary. A specific theory is not necessary to understanding, according to classical philosophy mentioned by the author. Again, the key to understanding is observing the phenomena outside of it, without bias or predisposition. Thus, Choice *B* is wrong.

14. B: The electrons passed through both holes and then onto the plate. Choices *A* and *C* are incorrect because such movement is not mentioned at all in the text. In the passage, the author says that electrons that were physically observed appeared to pass through one hole or another. Remember, the electrons that were observed doing this were described as acting like particles. Therefore, Choice *D* is incorrect. Recall that the plate actually recorded electrons passing through both holes simultaneously and hitting the plate. This behavior, the electron activity that wasn't seen by humans, was characteristic of waves. Thus, Choice *B* is the correct answer.

15. C: The author mentions "gravity" to demonstrate an example of natural phenomena humans discovered and understood without the use of tools or machines. Choice *A* mirrors the language in the beginning of the paragraph but is incorrect in its intent. Choice *B* is incorrect; the paragraph mentions nothing of "not knowing the true nature of gravity." Choice *D* is incorrect as well. There is no mention of an "alternative solution" in this paragraph.

16. A: The important thing to keep in mind is that we must choose a scenario that best parallels, or is most similar to, the discovery of the experiment mentioned in the passage. The important aspects of the experiment can be summed up like so: humans directly observed one behavior of electrons and then through analyzing a tool (the plate that recorded electron hits), discovered that there was another electron behavior that could not be physically seen by human eyes. This summary best parallels the scenario in Choice *A*. Like Feynman, the colorblind person can observe one aspect of the world but through the special goggles (a tool), he is able to see a natural phenomenon that he could not physically see on his own. While Choice *D* is compelling, the x-ray helps humans see the broken bone, but it does not necessarily reveal that the bone is broken in the first place. The other choices do not parallel the scenario in question. Therefore, Choice *A* is the best choice.

17. B: The author would not agree that technology renders human observation irrelevant. Choice *A* is incorrect because much of the passage discusses how technology helps humans observe what cannot be seen with the naked eye; therefore, the author would agree with this statement. This line of reasoning is also why the author would agree with Choice *D*, making it incorrect as well. As indicated in the second paragraph, the author seems to think that humans create inventions and tools with the goal of studying phenomena more precisely. This indicates increased understanding as people recognize limitations and develop items to help bypass the limitations and learn. Therefore, Choice *C* is incorrect as well. Again, the author doesn't attempt to disprove or dismiss classical philosophy.

18. B: The word *conundrum* most nearly means *enigma*, which is a mystery or riddle. *Platitude* means a banal or overused saying. *Solution* is incorrect here; and *hypothesis* implies a theory or assumption, so this is also incorrect.

19. A: To prove to the audience the thesis of the passage by providing evidence suggesting that electrons behave differently when observed by the human eye. The thesis' best evidence is found in this paragraph because of the experiment depicting how electrons behave in a dual nature. Choice *B* is incorrect; the paragraph mentions nothing about the experiment being unethical. Choice *C* is incorrect; this is characteristic of the first paragraph. Choice *D* is incorrect; this is more characteristic of the second paragraph.

20. D: The author explains that Boethianism is a Medieval theological philosophy that attributes sin to temporary pleasure and righteousness with virtue and God's providence. Besides Choice *D*, the choices listed are all physical things. While these could still be divine rewards, Boethianism holds that the true reward for being virtuous is in God's favor. It is also stressed in the article that physical pleasures cannot be taken into the afterlife. Therefore, the best choice is *D*, God's favor.

21. C: *The Canterbury Tales* presents a manuscript written in the medieval period that can help illustrate Boethianism through stories and show how people of the time might have responded to the idea. Choices *A* and *B* are generalized statements, and we have no evidence to support Choice *B*. Choice *D* is very compelling, but it looks at Boethianism in a way that the author does not. The author does not mention "different levels of Boethianism" when discussing the tales, only that the concept appears differently in different tales. Boethianism also doesn't focus on enlightenment.

22. D: The author is referring to the principle that a desire for material goods leads to moral malfeasance punishable by a higher being. Choice *A* is incorrect; while the text does mention thieves ravaging others' possessions, it is only meant as an example and not as the principle itself. Choice *B* is incorrect for the same reason as *A*. Choice *C* is mentioned in the text and is part of the example that proves the principle, and also not the principle itself.

23. C: The word *avarice* most nearly means *covetousness*, or extremely desirous of money or wealth. Choice *A* means *evil* or *mischief* and does not relate to the context of the sentence. Choice *B* is also incorrect, because *pithiness* means *shortness* or *conciseness*. Choice *D* is close because *precariousness* means dangerous or instability, which goes well with the context. However, we are told of the summoner's specific characteristic of greed, which makes Choice *C* the best answer.

24. D: Desire for pleasure can lead toward sin. Boethianism acknowledges desire as something that leads out of holiness, so Choice *A* is incorrect. Choice *B* is incorrect because in the passage, Boethianism is depicted as being wary of desire and anything that binds people to the physical world. Choice *C* can be eliminated because the author never says that desire indicates demonic possession.

25. A: The passage discusses recent technological advances in cars and suggests that this trend will continue in the future with self-driving cars. Choice *B* and *C* are not true, so these are both incorrect. Choice *D* is also incorrect because the passage suggests continuing growth in technology, not a peak.

26. C: In lines 6 and 7, it is stated that avarice can prevent a man from being necessitously poor, but too timorous, or fearful, to achieve real wealth. According to the passage, avarice does not tend to make a person very wealthy. The passage states that oppression, not avarice, is the consequence of wealth. The passage does not state that avarice drives a person's desire to be wealthy.

27. D: Paine believes that the distinction that is beyond a natural or religious reason is between king and subjects. He states that the distinction between good and bad is made in heaven. The distinction between male and female is natural. He does not mention anything about the distinction between humans and animals.

28. A: The passage states that the Heathens were the first to introduce government by kings into the world. The quiet lives of patriarchs came before the Heathens introduced this type of government. It was Christians, not Heathens, who paid divine honors to living kings. Heathens honored deceased kings. Equal rights of nature are mentioned in the paragraph, but not in relation to the Heathens.

29. B: Paine asserts that a monarchy is against the equal rights of nature and cites several parts of scripture that also denounce it. He doesn't say it is against the laws of nature. Because he uses scripture to further his argument, it is not despite scripture that he denounces the monarchy. Paine addresses the law by saying the courts also do not support a monarchical government.

30. A: To be *idolatrous* is to worship idols or heroes, in this case, kings. It is not defined as being deceitful. While idolatry is considered a sin, it is an example of a sin, not a synonym for it. Idolatry may have been considered illegal in some cultures, but it is not a definition for the term.

31. A: The essential meaning of the passage is that the Almighty, God, would disapprove of this type of government. While heaven is mentioned, it is done so to suggest that the monarchical government is irreverent, not that heaven isn't promised. God's disapproval is mentioned, not his punishment. The passage refers to the Jewish monarchy, which required both belief in God and kings.

32. A: The word *timorous* means being full of fear. The author concludes that extreme greed (avarice) makes people too afraid to be prosperous.

33. B: The author's attitude is closest to Choice *B,* impassioned and critical. Choice *A* is incorrect; the author is not indifferent or fatigued—on the contrary, there is a lot of energy and some underlying passion in the writing. Choice *C* is incorrect; the word *enchanted* means delighted, and the author is more critical and concerned of a monarchial government than enchanted with it. Choice *D* is not the best answer; although the author is passionate and critical of a monarchy, there is more logic than anger coming from the words.

34. B: To explain how monarchs came into existence and how Christians adapted to this way of government. Choice *A* is incorrect; the author does not agree that heathens were more advanced than Christians in this paragraph, it only explains the catalyst of the monarchial systems. Choice *C* is incorrect; the author would in fact disagree with the divination of the English monarchs. Choice *D* is incorrect; the paragraph *does* believe that monarchs cause damage, but the paragraph does not act as a counterargument to the one preceding it.

35. D: The author implies that the recorded history of creation is a collection, collage, or pattern taken from various accounts of cultures. Choice *A* is incorrect; there is no talk of cells or biology in the paragraph. Since "mosaic" modifies the word "account," we know that it is the account of creation that is mosaic, not creation itself, which makes Choice *B* incorrect. Choice *C* is also incorrect; the paragraph does not mention kings developing a system of recording accounts of creation.

36. A: The purpose is to inform the reader about what assault is and how it is committed. Choice *B* is incorrect because the passage does not state that assault is a lesser form of lethal force, only that an assault can use lethal force, or alternatively, lethal force can be utilized to counter a dangerous assault. Choice *C* is incorrect because the passage is informative and does not have a set agenda. Finally, Choice *D* is incorrect because although the author uses an example in order to explain assault, it is not indicated that this is the author's personal account.

37. C: If the man being attacked in an alley by another man with a knife used self-defense by lethal force, it would not be considered illegal. The presence of a deadly weapon indicates mal-intent and because the individual is isolated in an alley, lethal force in self-defense may be the only way to preserve his life. Choices *A* and *B* can be ruled out because in these situations, no one is in danger of immediate death or bodily harm by someone else. Choice *D* is an assault and does exhibit intent to harm, but this situation isn't severe enough to merit lethal force; there is no intent to kill.

38. B: As discussed in the second passage, there are several forms of assault, like assault with a deadly weapon, verbal assault, or threatening posture or language. Choice *A* is incorrect because the author does mention what the charges are on assaults; therefore, we cannot assume that they are more or less than unnecessary use of force charges. Choice *C* is incorrect because anyone is capable of assault; the author does not state that one group of people cannot commit assault. Choice *D* is incorrect because assault is never justified. Self-defense resulting in lethal force can be justified.

39. D: The use of lethal force is not evaluated on the intent of the user, but rather on the severity of the primary attack that warranted self-defense. This statement most undermines the last part of the passage because it directly contradicts how the law evaluates the use of lethal force. Choices *A* and *B* are stated in the paragraph, so they do not undermine the explanation from the author. Choice *C* does not necessarily undermine the passage, but it does not support the passage either. It is more of an opinion that does not offer strength or weakness to the explanation.

40. C: An assault with deadly intent can lead to an individual using lethal force to preserve their well-being. Choice *C* is correct because it clearly establishes what both assault and lethal force are and gives the specific way in which the two concepts meet. Choice *A* is incorrect because lethal force doesn't necessarily result in assault. This is also why Choice *B* is incorrect. Not all assaults would necessarily be life-threatening to the point where lethal force is needed for self-defense. Choice *D* is compelling but ultimately too vague; the statement touches on aspects of the two ideas but fails to present the concrete way in which the two are connected to each other.

41. A: Both passages open by defining a legal concept and then continue to describe situations in order to further explain the concept. Choice *D* is incorrect because while the passages utilize examples to help explain the concepts discussed, the author doesn't indicate that they are specific court cases. It's also clear that the passages don't open with examples, but instead, they begin by defining the terms addressed in each passage. This eliminates Choice *B*, and ultimately reveals Choice *A* to be the correct answer. Choice *A* accurately outlines the way both passages are structured. Because the passages follow a nearly identical structure, the Choice *C* can easily be ruled out.

42. C: Intent is very important for determining both lethal force and assault; intent is examined in both parties and helps determine the severity of the issue. Choices *A* and *B* are incorrect because it is clear in both passages that intent is a prevailing theme in both lethal force and assault. Choice *D* is compelling, but if a person uses lethal force to defend himself or herself, the intent of the defender is also examined in order to help determine if there was excessive force used. Choice *C* is correct because it states that intent is important for determining both lethal force and assault, and that intent is used to gauge the severity of the issues. Remember, just as lethal force can escalate to excessive use of force, there are different kinds of assault. Intent dictates several different forms of assault.

43. B: The example is used to demonstrate a single example of two different types of assault, then adding in a third type of assault to the example's conclusion. The example mainly provides an instance of "threatening body language" and "provocative language" with the homeowner gesturing threats to his neighbor. It ends the example by adding a third type of assault: physical strikes. This example is used to show the variant nature of assaults. Choice *A* is incorrect because it doesn't mention the "physical strike" assault at the end and is not specific enough. Choice *C* is incorrect because the example does not say anything about the definition of lethal force or how it might be altered. Choice *D* is incorrect, as the example mentions nothing about cause and effect.

44. C: The word *apprehension* most nearly means fear. The passage indicates that "assault is the unlawful attempt of one person to apply fear/anxiety on another individual by an imminent threat." The creation of fear in another individual seems to be a property of assault.

45. D: Choice *D* is the best answer, "The concept of lethal force as a last resort and the point at which it can cross a line from defense to manslaughter." The last paragraph of the first passage states what the term "last resort" means and how it's distinguished in the eyes of the law.

46. B: The correct answer is an infectious disease. By reading and understanding the context of the passage, all other options can be eliminated since the author restates zymosis as disease.

47. B: Mr. Button's wife is about to have a baby. The passage begins by giving the reader information about traditional birthing situations. Then, we are told that Mr. and Mrs. Button decide to go against tradition to have their baby in a hospital. The next few passages are dedicated to letting the reader know how Mr. Button dresses and goes to the hospital to welcome his new baby. There is a doctor in this excerpt, as Choice *C* indicates, and Mr. Button does put on clothes, as Choice *D* indicates. However, Mr. Button is not going to the doctor's office nor is he about to go shopping for new clothes.

48. C: Dedicated. Mr. Button is dedicated to the task before him. Choice *A*, numbed, Choice *B*, chained, and Choice *D*, moved, all could grammatically fit in the sentence. However, they are not synonyms with *consecrated* like Choice *C* is.

49. D: Giving readers a visual picture of what the doctor is doing. The author describes a visual image—the doctor rubbing his hands together—first and foremost. The author may be trying to make a comment about the profession; however, the author does not "explain the detail of the doctor's profession" as Choice *B* suggests.

50. D: To introduce the setting of the story and its characters. We know we are being introduced to the setting because we are given the year in the very first paragraph along with the season: "one day in the summer of 1860." This is a classic structure of an introduction of the setting. We are also getting a long explanation of Mr. Button, what his work is, who is related to him, and what his life is like in the third paragraph.

51. B: The word *anachronism* most nearly means misplacement. Choice *A*, comparison, is an analogy or similarity to something. Choice *C*, *aberration*, means abnormality. Choice *D*, *amelioration*, means improvement.

52. A: To explain the setting of the narrative and give information about the story. The setting of a narrative is the time and place. We see from the first paragraph that the year is 1860. We also can discern that it is summer, and Mr. and Mrs. Button are about to have a baby. This tells us both the setting and information about the story.

53. D: Something is unusual about the birth of the baby. The word "curious" is thrown in at the end twice, which tells us the doctor is suspicious about something having to do with the birth of the baby, since that is the most recent event to happen. Mr. Button is acting like a father who is expecting a baby, and the doctor seems confused about something.

54. A: The topic of the passage is Caribbean island destinations. The *topic* of the passage can be described in a one- or two-word phrase. Remember, when paraphrasing a passage, it is important to include the topic. Paraphrasing is when one puts a passage into their own words.

55. C: Family or adult-only resorts and activities are supporting details in this passage. *Supporting details* are details that help readers better understand the main idea. They answer questions such as who, what, where, when, why, or how. In this question, cruises and local events are not discussed in the passage, whereas family and adult-only resorts and activities support the main idea.

Vocabulary

1. C: Contralateral. As a prefix, *contra-* means opposite or against. In this case, *contralateral* means on the opposite side of the body.

2. A: Enlarged or expanded. A *distended* stomach or other organ is bloated or swollen because of internal pressure.

3. B: Precipitously. *Concisely* means in a few words or efficiently worded, *contingently* refers to something that will occur only if something else happens first, and *preemptively* means something taken as a precaution or measure against an anticipated risk or problem, often as a way to try and prevent it.

4. A: Patent. In a medical context, a *patent* vessel is unobstructed and open. An atherosclerotic vessel with deposited plaques would probably not be *patent.*

5. D: Absence of menstruation. The prefix *a-* means "not" or "anti." *Menses* is the menstrual cycle, and the suffix *-rhea* means "flow." Therefore, *amenorrhea* is the absence of a menstrual period.

6. C: Present but not active or visible. A *latent* disease is present but not detectable in a symptomatic way. It may be dormant, but has to potential to become symptomatic in the future with discernable manifestations for the patient.

7. C: Overt. *Obsolete* means outdated or no longer produced or used, *covert* means not outwardly acknowledged or shown, and to *collude* is to conspire.

8. A: Difficulty breathing. The prefix *dys-* means dysfunctional or abnormal. *-Pnea* in a medical context refers to respiration and breathing. Sleep apnea is a breathing disorder that can occur during sleep.

9. B: Sudden or rapid onset. An *acute* illness is the opposite of a *chronic* one, which is a disease that the patient has had for a long time. A sinus infection is an acute illness, while multiple sclerosis is a chronic one.

10. D: Virulent. *Patent* means open, *innocuous* means harmless, and *latent* means dormant.

11. C: Undesirable. An adverse reaction to a medication is an undesirable side effect or consequence of taking the drug.

12. B: Insidious. *Precipitous* means rapid or steep, *incipient* means emergent or at an initial state, and *paroxysmal* means a sudden intensification or recurrence of symptoms, as in a paroxysmal attack of a muscle spasm in the lumbar spine.

13. A: Lack of urine output. Again, the prefixes *a-* or *an-* mean "without" or "not," and *-uria* refers to urine.

14. C: Proximal. *Distal* is the opposite of proximal. Distal means further from the trunk (usually down an extremity).

15. C: Impervious. *Impotent,* in the medical context, means unable to achieve sexual arousal (for a man). In general, the word means powerless. *Hygienic* means sanitary. *Impending* means imminent.

16. B: Origin or cause. Some diseases have an unknown etiology.

17. D: Endogenous. The prefix *endo-* means "within" or "containing," and *-genous* means originating in or producing. The prefix *exo-* means the "outside."

Test Prep Books!!!

18. A: Febrile. *Futile* means pointless, *libel* is printed defamation of someone's character, and *liable* means responsible, especially in a legal sense.

19. A: Multiplied or increased in number. Given the right conditions, bacterial cells *proliferate* rapidly.

20. B: A fluid's thickness or resistance to flow. A viscous fluid is in contrast to a runny one. For example, honey is more viscous than water.

21. B: Supine. *Prone* is the position on one's stomach.

22. C: Environment. For example, the internal *milieu* usually refers to interstitial fluid.

23. D: Abnormal. *Overt* means outwardly demonstrative, *grave* means severe or serious, and *radical* means revolutionary or progressive.

24. B: Laceration. An *incision* is a more precise cut, as in one made by a surgeon using a scalpel during surgery. A *contusion* is a bruise and an *avulsion* is a type of fracture where a piece of the bone is ripped off.

25. C: Relating to the kidney. The renal blood vessels serve the kidneys.

26. A: Debridement. An *arthroscopy* is a type of surgical procedure on a joint using a camera and small scope, *distension* is swelling or bloating, and a *laparoscopy* is a surgical procedure that involves the insertion of a fiberoptic instrument.

27. D: Sort based on problem severity. Patients entering the ER need to be triaged so that they are treated in order of urgency.

28. D: Predisposed. *Predisposed* means inclined to a specific condition or action.

29. A: *Instigate* refers to initiating or bringing about an action. While instigating something can be overwhelming, *overwhelm* describes the action, not what the action is. None of these choices match this except for *begin*, which is synonymous with instigate.

30. C: Lethargic. *Indolent* can also mean lazy or aversive to activity.

31. D: Veins. Arteries bring blood from the heart to the tissues and veins return the blood to the heart from the tissues.

32. D: Inside the cheek. An example of a medication with a buccal route of administration is nitroglycerine in the treatment of angina.

33. B: Teacher. *Pupil* means student.

34. A: To cough out phlegm. Someone with pneumonia may *expectorate* in the sink.

35. A: Home. Like the word *reside,* which means to inhabit, a *residence* is where someone lives.

36. D: To *relinquish* something is to give up claim to it. For example, a spouse trying to be more considerate may relinquish the TV remote so that their partner can choose a show.

37. C: To *germinate* is to develop or come into existence. A novel marketing idea might germinate at a business lunch. In a botany context, it also means to sprout or bud.

38. A: Insurance. *Indemnity* is an insurance or other security or safeguard against a financial burden or loss.

39. C: Unrestrained. *Stagnant* means still or unchanging, like a body of water with no active flow.

40. D: Threatening. Choices *B* and *C, promising* and *auspicious,* are antonyms of *ominous.*

41. A: Hypoglycemia. *Hypo-* means "below" or "beneath," and *glycemia* comes from glucose, so it refers to blood sugar.

42. A: Watched. To *observe* is to watch or examine with one's eyes.

43. C: Somnolent. Someone *comatose* is unresponsive to stimuli. Someone *delirious* is either ecstatic or mentally disturbed and seeing illusions.

44. B: Hemoptysis. The suffix *-ptysis* means spitting of matter.

45. D: Swell. A tissue that is *engorged* is swollen with fluid. For example, a new mom will have breasts engorged with milk to nurture her baby.

46. A: Bereavement. *Disposition* is someone's personality or affect, *depression* is a state of a low mood, and *belligerent* means aggressive and hostile.

47. C: Polydipsia. *Poly-* means "many" or "multiple" and the suffix *-dipsia* refers to thrist.

48. C: Able to feel or perceive. A *sentient* being is living and able to perceive or feel something and respond.

49. C: Relating to digestion. *Peptic* comes from *pepsin,* which is a stomach enzyme that helps degrade proteins.

50. A: Isometric. The prefix *iso-* means "same" and *-metric* refers to length.

51. C: Nomadic tribes are those who, throughout history and even today, prefer to wander their lands instead of settling in any specific place. *Wanderer* best describes these people.

52. D: *Perplexed* means baffled or puzzled, which are synonymous with *confused.*

53. D: *Lyrical* is used to refer to something being poetic or song-like, characterized by showing enormous imagination and description. While the context of lyrical can be playful or even whimsical, the best choice is *expressive*, since whatever emotion lyrical may be used to convey in context will be expressive in nature.

54. C: *Brevity* literally means brief or concise. Note the similar beginnings of *brevity* and *brief*—from the Latin "brevis," meaning brief.

55. A: *Irate* means being in a state of anger. Clearly this is a negative word that can be paired with another word in kind. The closest word to match this is obviously *angry*. Research would also reveal that irate comes from the Latin "ira," which means anger.

Grammar

1. C: While all of these words are spelled similarly and sound the same, the correct answer is Choice *C*, *wear*, which means to cover or equip. We *wear* clothes. Choice *A*, *ware*, refers to an item that is created or manufactured. Choice *B* is incorrect because *where* asks for a specific location. Choice *D*, *were*, is the second person plural version of *to be*, so it is completely irrelevant to the sentence.

2. B: The clause *who loves to ride bikes* is a restrictive adjective clause modifying the noun *boy*. Choice *A* is incorrect because *a boy who loves* is a phrase not a clause. Choice *C* is incorrect because *to ride bikes* is an infinitive phrase and does not have a subject. Choice *D* is incorrect because *gets plenty of exercise* is not a clause; it has no subject.

3. D: The adverbial clause *unless you are too tired* modifies the verb *want*. Choice *A* is incorrect because *I want to work in the garden* is an independent clause. Choice *B* is incorrect because *in the garden* has no subject and is a prepositional phrase. Choice *C* is incorrect because *are too tired* is not a clause because it has no subject.

4. C: A noun phrase is a noun and all of its modifiers; in this case, *long* and *black* are adjectives modifying the noun *limousine* and *the* is an article modifying *limousine*. Choice *A* is incorrect because it identifies the compound subject of the sentence. Choice *B* is incorrect because it includes the verb *rode*. Choice *D* is incorrect because it includes a subject and a verb, and phrases do not have both.

5. B: Choice *B* is correct because the idea of the original sentences is Armani getting lost while walking through Paris. Choice *A* is incorrect because it replaces third person with second person. Choice *C* is incorrect because the word *should* indicates an obligation to get lost. Choice *D* is incorrect because it is not specific to the original sentence but instead makes a generalization about getting lost.

6. C: There is no gerund phrase in the sentence. Choice *A* is incorrect because *swimming several laps* is a gerund phrase serving as the noun subject of the sentence. Choice *B* is incorrect because *using the flippers* is a gerund phrase serving as the noun object of the sentence. Choice *D* is incorrect because *learning to swim* is a gerund phrase serving as the noun subject of the sentence.

7. A: *My second cousin* is a nonessential appositive phrase renaming *Carrie Fisher*. Because it is nonessential, it is set off by commas in the sentence. Choice *B* is incorrect because *Harrison Ford* is an essential appositive explaining which actor is being discussed. Choice *C* is incorrect because there is no appositive phrase in the sentence. Choice *D* is incorrect because *Star Wars* is an essential appositive explaining which movie is being discussed.

8. B: *The fire crackling* is an absolute phrase that includes a participle following a noun and has nothing to do with the rest of the sentence but cannot stand alone as its own sentence. Choice *A* is incorrect because *going camping in the forest* is a gerund phrase serving as the noun object of the sentence. Choice *C* is incorrect because *hot cocoa and coffee* is a nonessential appositive phrase renaming *the best drinks*. Choice *D* is incorrect because *for school-age children* is a prepositional phrase.

9. C: Choice *C* is correct because it shows that Phoenix buried his cat with her favorite toys after she died, which is true of the original statement. Although Choices *A*, *B*, and *D* mention a backyard, the meanings of these choices are skewed. Choice *A* says that Phoenix buried his cat alive, which is incorrect. Choice *B* says his cat died in the backyard, which we do not know to be true. Choice *D* says Phoenix buried his cat after he buried her toys, which is also incorrect.

10. D: Choice *D* is correct because it expresses the sentiment of a moment of joy bringing tears to one's eyes as one sees a sunset while in a helicopter. Choice *A* is incorrect because it implies that the person was outside of the helicopter watching it from afar. Choice *B* is incorrect because the original sentence does not portray the sunset *flying up* into the sky. Choice *C* is incorrect because, while the helicopter may have been facing the sunset, this is not the reason that tears were in the speaker's eyes.

11. A: Answer Choice *A* uses the best, most concise word choice. Choice *B* uses the pronoun *that* to refer to people instead of *who*. *Choice C* incorrectly uses the preposition *with*. Choice *D* uses the preposition *for* and the additional word *any*, making the sentence wordy and less clear.

12. B: Choice *B* uses the best choice of words to create a subordinate and independent clause. In Choice *A, because* makes it seem like this is the reason they enjoy working from home, which is incorrect. In Choice *C,* the word *maybe* creates two independent clauses, which are not joined properly with a comma. Choice *D* uses *with*, which does not make grammatical sense.

13. B: The original sentence focuses on how politicians are using the student debt issue to their advantage, so Choice *B* is the best answer choice. Choice *A* says politicians want students' votes but suggests that it is the reason for student loan debt, which is incorrect. Choice *C* shifts the focus to voters, when the sentence is really about politicians. Choice *D* is vague and doesn't best restate the original meaning of the sentence.

14. A: This answer best matches the meaning of the original sentence, which states that seasoned runners offer advice to new runners because they have complaints of injuries. Choice *B* may be true, but it doesn't mention the complaints of injuries by new runners. Choice *C* may also be true, but it does not match the original meaning of the sentence. Choice *D* does not make sense in the context of the sentence.

15. D: A noun phrase consists of the noun and all of its modifiers. In this case, the subject of the sentence is the noun *puppy*, but it is preceded by several modifiers—adjectives that give more information about what kind of puppy, which are also part of the noun phrase. Thus, *A* is incorrect. Charlotte is the owner of the puppy and a modifier of the puppy, so *B* is false. *C* is incorrect because it contains some, but not all, of the modifiers pertaining to the puppy. *D* is correct because it contains all of them.

16. B: Both verb phrases are introduced with the word *who*, creating parallelism. Choice *A* is incorrect. The introductory words for the verb phrases do not match. Choice *C* is incorrect. The introductory words for the verb phrases do not match and the word *that* would modify an object, not a person. Use *who* for a person. Choice *D* is incorrect. The word *that* in the sentence should be used to modify an object not a person, and the clown is a person.

17. A: The linking verbs *have been* are the same in both verb phrases, creating parallelism. Choice *B* is incorrect. *Have been traveling* does not match with *were sightseeing*. Choice *C* is incorrect. Again, *were*

277

traveling does not match with *have been sightseeing.* Choice *D* is incorrect. The tenses of the verbs do not match. *Have been traveling* does not match with *they are sightseeing.*

18. D: To make *the building was sturdy and solid* subordinate to *the building crumbled in the earthquake,* create a dependent clause with the less important piece of information. Choice *A* is incorrect. It is two independent clauses joined with a semicolon and neither piece of information is subordinate to the other. Choice *B* is incorrect. This sentence implies that the building was still sturdy and solid after crumbling in the earthquake because the word *although* is misplaced. Choice *C* is incorrect because, even though it is a grammatically correct sentence, neither piece of information is subordinate to the other.

19. C: This sentence uses verbs in a parallel series, so each verb must follow the same pattern. In order to fit with the helping verb "would," each verb must be in the present tense. In Choices *A, B,* and *D,* one or more of the verbs switches to past tense. Only Choice *C* remains in the same tense, maintaining the pattern.

20. C: The second sentence tells of an unexpected outcome of the first sentence. Choice *A,* Choice *B,* and Choice *D* indicate a logical progression, which does not match this surprise. Only Choice *C* indicates this unexpected twist.

21. A: Only two of these suffixes, *–ize* and *–en,* can be used to form verbs, so *B* and *D* are incorrect. Those choices create adjectives. The suffix *–ize* means "to convert or turn into." The suffix *–en* means "to become." Because this sentence is about converting ideas into money, money+–ize or *monetize* is the most appropriate word to complete the sentence, so *C* is incorrect.

22. C: The suffix *-fy* means to make, cause, or cause to have. Choices *A,* B, and D are incorrect because they show meanings of other suffixes. Choice *A* shows the meaning of the suffix *-ous.* Choice *B* shows the meaning of the suffix *–ist,* and Choice *D* shows the meaning of the suffix *-age.*

23. A: *After* and *then* are transitional words that indicate time or position. Choice *B* is incorrect because the words *at, with,* and *to* are used as prepositions in this sentence, not transitions. Choice *C* is incorrect because the words *had* and *took* are used as verbs in this sentence. In Choice *D, a* and *the* are used as articles in the sentence.

24. A: Choice *A* includes all of the words functioning as nouns in the sentence. Choice *B* is incorrect because it includes the words *final* and *academic,* which are functioning as adjectives in this sentence. The word *he* makes Choice *C* incorrect because it is a pronoun. This example also includes the word *library,* which can function as a noun, but is functioning as an adjective modifying the word *databases* in this sentence. Choice *D* is incorrect because it leaves out the proper noun *Robert.*

25. C: The dependent adjective clause *cute and cuddly* does not modify *the children,* it modifies *teddy bears.* The modifier is misplaced. Choice *A* does not contain a misplaced modifier. It is a grammatically correct independent clause. Choice *B* does not have a misplaced modifier. It is a grammatically correct compound sentence with two independent clauses joined with a semicolon. Choice *D* does not have a misplaced modifier. The modifier *cute and cuddly* correctly modifies *teddy bears.* The sentence is grammatically correct.

26. B: *Dissatisfied* and *accommodations* are both spelled correctly in Choice *B*. These are both considered commonly misspelled words. One or both words are spelled incorrectly in Choices *A*, *C*, and *D*.

27. A: It is necessary to put a comma between the date and the year. It is also required to put a comma between the day of the week and the month. Choice *B* is incorrect because it is missing the comma between the day and year. Choice *C* is incorrect because it adds an unnecessary comma between the month and date. Choice *D* is missing the necessary comma between day of the week and the month.

28. D: To create parallelism, make both verbal gerunds. Choice *A* is incorrect. *Chewing* is a gerund and *to play* is an infinitive. Choice *B* is incorrect. *To chew* is an infinitive and *playing* is a gerund. Choice *C* is incorrect. *To chew* and *to play* are both infinitives, but they do not match with the verb *enjoy*.

29. D: In Choice *D*, the word function is a noun. While the word *function* can also act as a verb, in this particular sentence it is acting as a noun as the object of the preposition *at*. Choices *A* and *B* are incorrect because the word *function* cannot be used as an adjective or adverb.

30. C: Cacti is the correct plural form of the word *cactus*. Choice *A* (*tomatos*) includes an incorrect spelling of the plural of *tomato*. Both Choice *B* (*analysis*) and Choice *D* (*criterion*) are incorrect because they are in singular form. The correct plural form for these choices would be *criteria* and *analyses*.

31. B: Quotation marks are used to indicate something someone said. The example sentences feature a direct quotation that requires the use of double quotation marks. Also, the end punctuation, in this case a question mark, should always be contained within the quotation marks. Choice *A* is incorrect because there is an unnecessary period after the quotation mark. Choice *C* is incorrect because it uses single quotation marks, which are used for a quote within a quote. Choice *D* is incorrect because it places the punctuation outside of the quotation marks.

32. A: Choice *A* is correct because *has* is the same tense and number as the subject *Garth*, so the verb and subject agree. Choice *B* is incorrect because *had* is past tense while the sentence is clearly present tense, indicated by *that he cares for*. Choice *C* incorrectly uses *have*, which is plural and doesn't agree with the singular subject. Choice *D* is incorrect because *haves* is a plural noun indicating people with possessions, not a verb as is needed here.

33. D: In Choice *D,* the word *part* functions as an adjective that modifies the word *Irish*. Choices *A* and *C* are incorrect because the word *part* functions as a noun in these sentences. Choice *B* is incorrect because the word *part* functions as a verb.

34. C: *All of Shannon's family and friends* is the complete subject because it includes who or what is doing the action in the sentence as well as the modifiers that go with it. Choice *A* is incorrect because it only includes the simple subject of the sentence. Choices *B* and *D* are incorrect because they only include part of the complete subject.

35. D: Choice *D* directly addresses the reader, so it is in second person point of view. This is an imperative sentence since it issues a command; imperative sentences have an *understood you* as the subject. Choice *A* uses first person pronouns *I* and *my*. Choices *B* and *C* are incorrect because they use third person point of view.

36. A: The word *prodigious* is defined as very impressive, amazing, or large. In this sentence, the meaning can be drawn from the words *they became nervous about climbing its distant peak*, as this would be an appropriate reaction upon seeing a very large peak that's far in the distance. Choices *B, C,* and D do not accurately define the word *prodigious*, so they are incorrect.

37. D: Choice *D* correctly places a hyphen after the prefix *ex* to join it to the word *husband*. Words that begin with the prefixes *great, trans, ex, all,* and *self,* require a hyphen. Choices *A* and *C* place hyphens in words where they are not needed. *Beagle mix* would only require a hyphen if coming before the word *Henry*, since it would be serving as a compound adjective in that instance. Choice *B* contains hyphens that are in the correct place but are formatted incorrectly since they include spaces between the hyphens and the surrounding words.

38. C: Choice *C* is correct because quotation marks should be used for the title of a short work such as a poem. Choices *A,* B, and D are incorrect because the titles of novels, films, and newspapers should be placed in italics, not quotation marks.

39. C: This question focuses on the correct usage of the commonly confused word pairs of *it's/its* and *then/than*. *It's* is a contraction for *it is* or *it has*. *Its* is a possessive pronoun. The word *than* shows comparison between two things. *Then* is an adverb that conveys time. Choice *C* correctly uses *it's* and *than*. *It's* is a contraction for *it has* in this sentence, and *than* shows comparison between *work* and *rest*. None of the other answers choices use both of the correct words.

40. C: The original sentence states that firefighting is dangerous, making it necessary for firefighters to wear protective gear. The portion of the sentence that needs to be rewritten focuses on the gear, not the dangers, of firefighting. Choices *A, B*, and *D* all discuss the danger, not the gear, so *C* is the correct answer.

41. D: The original sentence states that though the sites are popular, they can be dangerous for teens, so *D* is the best choice. Choice *A* does state that there is danger, but it doesn't identify teens and limits it to just one site. Choice *B* repeats the statement from the beginning of the sentence, and Choice *C* says the sites are used too much, which is not the point made in the original sentence.

42. A: The affix *circum–* originates from Latin and means *around or surrounding*. It is also related to other round words, such as circle and circus. The rest of the choices do not relate to the affix *circum–* and are therefore incorrect.

43. C: The rules for "me" and "I" is that one should use "I" when it is the subject pronoun of a sentence, and "me" when it is the object pronoun of the sentence. Break the sentence up to see if "I" or "me" should be used. To say "Those are memories that I have now shared" is correct, rather than "Those are memories that me have now shared." Choice *A* is incorrect because "my siblings" should come before "I."

44. D: Choice *D* is correct because there should be a comma between the city and state. Choice *A* is incorrect because the order of the sentence designates that Chicago, Illinois is in Maywood, which is incorrect. Choice *B* is incorrect because the comma after "Maywood" interrupts the phrase "Maywood of Chicago." Choice *C* is incorrect because a comma after "Illinois" is unnecessary.

45. D: Choice *D* is correct because the Committee is one entity, therefore the possession should show the "Committee's approach" with the apostrophe between the "y" and the "s." Choice *A* is incorrect

280

because the word "Committies" is spelled wrong. Choice *B* is incorrect because the word "Committees" should not be plural and should have an apostrophe to show possession. Choice *C* is incorrect because the apostrophe indicates that the word "Committees" is plural.

46. A: Choice *A* is correct because the conjunction "and" is the best way to combine the two independent clauses. Choice *B* is incorrect because the conjunction "but" indicates a contrast, and there is no contrast between the two clauses. Choice *C* is incorrect because the introduction of the comma after "house" with no conjunction creates a comma splice. Choice *D* is incorrect because the word "he" becomes repetitive since the two clauses can be joined together.

47. B: Choice *B* is correct because it provides the correct verb tense and also makes sense within the context of the passage. Choice *A* is incorrect because the verb tense is inconsistent with the rest of the sentence. Choice *C* is incorrect because, with this use of the sentence, it would create a fragment because the verb "holding" has no helping verb in front of it. Choice *D* is incorrect because it changes the meaning of the sentence.

48. B: Choice *B* is correct. Choice *A* is incorrect because the sentence "In 2015." is a fragment. Choice *C* is incorrect because there should be a comma after introductory phrases in general, such as "In 2015," and Choice *C* omits a comma. Choice *D* is incorrect because there should be an independent clause on either side of a semicolon, and the phrase "In 2015" is not an independent clause.

49. B: Choice *B* is correct. Here, a colon is used to introduce an explanation. Colons either introduce explanations or lists. Additionally, the quote ends with the punctuation inside the quotes, unlike Choice *C*.

50. B: The word "raising" in Choice *A* makes the sentence grammatically incorrect. Choice *C* adds an apostrophe at the end of "its." While adding an apostrophe to most words would indicate possession, adding 's to the word "it" indicates a contraction. The possessive form of the word "it" is "its." The contraction "it's" denotes "it is." Thus, Choice *D* is incorrect.

51. B: *B* is correct because like the original sentence, it expresses their plan to go to the party if friends also go. Choice *A* is incorrect because it does not follow the meaning of the original sentence. Choice *C* is incorrect because it states that their friends are going, even though that is not known. Choice *D* is incorrect because it would make the new sentence mean the opposite of the original sentence.

52. C: Choice *C* is correct because the original sentence states that his recovery time was long because his leg was broken before the accident. Choice *A* is incorrect because there is no indication that the man had two broken legs. Choice *B* is incorrect because it indicates that he broke his leg during the car accident, not before. Choice *D* is incorrect because there is no indication that he broke his leg after the car accident.

53. A: Choice *A* is correct because it expresses the fact that the birthday and the party were both after Halloween. Choice *B* is incorrect because it says that the birthday was on Halloween, even though that was not stated in the original sentence. Choice *C* is incorrect because it says the party was specifically a Halloween party and not a birthday party. Choice *D* is incorrect because the party was after Halloween, not before.

54. D: The best answer is Choice *D* because it keeps the original meaning of the sentence with the transitional phrase *due to*. Choice *A* is incorrect; the sentence says that the animals thrive *with* these changing traits over time, but it does not say the animals thrive *because of* these traits. Choice *B* is incorrect because the sentence suggests it is the *environments* and not the *animals* that contain the traits. Choice *C* is incorrect; it says that animals thrive and that they have changing traits that develop, but it fails to show a connection between the two.

55. A: Choice *A* is correct because the meaning is the closest in similarity to the original; there is learning that occurs from the past lectures the speaker has sat through. Choice *B* is incorrect because it changes the tense of the act of sitting through lectures. Choice *C* is incorrect because it uses the conjunction *and* which fails to connect the two clauses. Choice *D* is incorrect because although it uses similar language, it changes the meaning to say that the speaker *goes away* to lectures.

Biology

1. A: It is the genetic code. Choice *B* is incorrect because DNA does not provide energy—that's the job of carbohydrates and glucose. Choice *C* is incorrect because DNA is double-stranded. Because Choices *B* and *C* are incorrect, Choice *D,* all of the above, is incorrect.

2. A: The Golgi apparatus is designed to tag, package, and ship out proteins destined for other cells or locations. The centrioles typically play a large role only in cell division when they ratchet the chromosomes from the mitotic plate to the poles of the cell. The mitochondria are involved in energy production and are the powerhouses of the cell. The cell structure responsible for cellular storage, digestion and waste removal is the lysosome. Lysosomes are like recycle bins. They are filled with digestive enzymes that facilitate catabolic reactions to regenerate monomers.

3. C: Cellulose and starch are both polysaccharides, which are long chains of glucose molecules, but they are connected by different types of bonds, which gives them different structures and different functions.

4. D: All of the above. Let's label *R* as the right-handed allele and *r* as the left-handed allele. Esther has to have the combination rr since she's left-handed. She had to get at least one recessive allele from each parent. So, mom could either be Rr or rr (right-handed or left-handed), and dad can also be Rr or rr. As long as each parent carries one recessive allele, it is possible that Esther is left-handed. Therefore, all answer choices are possible.

5. D: 1/16. The probability of each specified genotype can be determined by individual Punnett squares. Each probability should then be then multiplied (law of multiplication) to find the value, which in this case is ½ x ½ x ½ x ½=1/16.

	A	a
A	AA	Aa
A	AA	Aa

	B	b
b	Bb	bb
b	Bb	bb

	C	C
c	Cc	cc
c	Cc	cc

	D	d
D	DD	Dd
D	DD	Dd

Probabilities: AA=½   bb=½   cc=½   DD=½

6. D: *Choice A* is incorrect because meiosis produces haploid cells. *Choice B* is incorrect because there is no interphase II (otherwise gametes would be diploid instead of haploid). *Choice C* is incorrect because the resulting cells only have one set of chromosomes. *Choice D* is the only correct answer because each chromosome set goes through a process called crossing over, which jumbles up the genes on each chromatid, during meiosis I.

7. D: DNA serves as the hereditary material for prokaryotic and eukaryotic cells.

8. C: Oxygen. Water (*A*) is a reactant that gets sucked up by the roots. Carbon dioxide (*D*) is a reactant that goes into the stomata, and sunlight (*B*) inputs energy into the reaction in order to create the high-energy sugar.

9. C: Breaking down food to release energy. Breathing (*B*) is not cellular respiration; breathing is an action that takes place at the organism level with the respiratory system. Making high-energy sugars (*A*) is photosynthesis, not cellular respiration. Perspiration (*D*) is sweating, and has nothing to do with cellular respiration.

10. D: Algae can perform photosynthesis. One indicator that a plant is able to perform photosynthesis is the color green. Plants with the pigment chlorophyll are able to absorb the warmer colors of the light spectrum, but are unable to absorb green. That's why they appear green. Choices *A* and *C* are types of fungi, and are therefore not able to perform photosynthesis. Fungi obtain energy from food in their environment. Choice *B,* ant, is also unable to perform photosynthesis, since it is an animal.

11. B: The Linnaean system is the commonly used taxonomic system today. It classifies species based on their similarities and moves from comprehensive to more general similarities. The system is based on the following order: species, genus, family, order, class, phylum, and kingdom.

12. A: Homo is the human genus. Sapiens are the only remaining species in the homo genus.

13. A: The nucleus, chloroplast, and mitochondria are all bound by two layers of membrane. The Golgi apparatus, lysosome, and ER only have one membrane layer.

14. D: Human gametes each contain 23 chromosomes. This is referred to as haploid—half the number of the original germ cell (46). Germ cells are diploid precursors of the haploid egg and sperm. Meiosis has two major phases, each of which is characterized by sub-phases similar to mitosis. In Meiosis I, the DNA of the parent cell is duplicated in interphase, just like in mitosis. Starting with prophase I, things become a little different. Two homologous chromosomes form a tetrad, cross over, and exchange genetic content. Each shuffled chromosome of the tetrad migrates to the cell's poles, and two haploid daughter cells are formed. In Meiosis II, each daughter undergoes another division more similar to mitosis (with the exception of the fact that there is no interphase), resulting in four genetically-different cells, each with only ½ of the chromosomal material of the original germ cell.

15. B: Plants use chloroplasts to turn light energy into glucose. Animal cells do not have this ability. Chloroplasts can be found in the plant cell but not the animal cell.

16. D: Both steps of photosynthesis usually occur during daylight because even though the Calvin cycle is not dependent on light energy, it *is* dependent upon the ATP and NADPH produced by the light reactions. This is because that energy can be invested into bonds to create high-energy sugars. For each G3P molecule produced, the Calvin cycle requires the investment of 9 ATP molecules and 6 NADPH molecules.

17. A: The net products of anaerobic glycolysis from one 6-carbon glucose molecule are two 3-carbon pyruvate molecules; 2 reduced nicotinamide adenine dinucleotide (NADH) molecules, which are created when the electron carrier oxidized nicotinamide adenine dinucleotide (NAD+) peels off 2 electrons and a hydrogen atom; and 2 ATP molecules. Glycolysis requires 2 ATP molecules to drive the process forward, and since the gross end product is 4 ATP molecules, the net is 2 ATP molecules.

18. C: Glycolysis produces 2 pyruvate molecules per glucose molecule that gets broken down because glucose is a 6-carbon sugar and pyruvate is a 3-carbon sugar. Each pyruvate molecule oxidizes into a single acetyl-CoA molecule, which then enters the citric acid cycle. Therefore, 2 citric acid cycles can be completed per glucose molecule that initially entered glycolysis.

19. D: Oxidative phosphorylation includes two steps: the electron transport chain and chemiosmosis. These two processes help generate ATP molecules by transferring two electrons and a proton (H^+) from each NADH and $FADH_2$ to channel proteins, pumping the hydrogen ions to the inner-membrane space using energy from the high-energy electrons to create a concentration gradient. In chemiosmosis, ATP synthase uses facilitated diffusion to deliver protons across the concentration gradient from the inner mitochondrial membrane to the matrix.

20. C: The nucleolus is always located inside the nucleus. It contains important hereditary information about the cell that is critical for the reproductive process. Chloroplasts, Choice *A*, are only located in plant cells. It is not found in the mitochondria, Choice *B*, or attached to the cell membrane, Choice *D*.

21. C: The mitochondrion is often called the powerhouse of the cell and is one of the most important structures for maintaining regular cell function. It is where aerobic cellular respiration occurs and where most of the cell's ATP is generated. The number of mitochondria in a cell varies greatly from organism to organism and from cell to cell. Cells that require more energy, like muscle cells, have more mitochondria.

22. A: Photosynthesis is the process of converting light energy into chemical energy, which is then stored in sugar and other organic molecules. The photosynthetic process takes place in the thylakoids inside chloroplast in plants. Chlorophyll is a green pigment that lives in the thylakoid membranes and absorbs photons from light.

23. B: Carbohydrates consist of sugars. The simplest sugar molecule is called a monosaccharide and has the molecular formula of CH_2O, or a multiple of that formula. Monosaccharides are important molecules for cellular respiration. Their carbon skeleton can also be used to rebuild new small molecules. Lipids are fats, proteins are formed via amino acids, and nucleic acid is found in DNA and RNA.

24. A: The Calvin cycle is dependent upon the ATP and NADPH produced by the light reactions. Nine ATP molecules and six NADPH molecules are invested into the Calvin cycle for every one molecule of glyceraldehyde 3-phosphate (G3P) produced. In the endergonic reduction reaction, NADPH uses energy from ATP to add a hydrogen to each molecule of 3-phosphoglycerate. This converts the six molecules of 3-PGA into the 3-carbon sugar G3P. ATP supplies energy by donating a phosphate group (Pi) (becoming ADP), and NADPH loses a hydrogen to become $NADP^+$.

25. D: The cell membrane surrounds the cell and regulates which molecules can move in and out of the cell. Ribosomes build proteins, Choice *A*. Lysosomes, Choice *B*, break down large molecules. The nucleus, Choice *C*, contains the cell's DNA.

26. C: The lagging strand of DNA falls behind the leading strand because of its discontinuous synthesis. DNA helicase unzips the DNA helices so that synthesis can take place, and RNA primers are created by the RNA primase for the polymerases to attach to and build from. The lagging strand is synthesizing DNA in a direction that is hard for the polymerase to build, so multiple primers are laid down so that the entire length of DNA can be synthesized simultaneously, piecemeal. These short pieces of DNA being synthesized are known as Okazaki fragments and are joined together by DNA ligase.

27. B: Sunlight comes into the greenhouse as short-wavelength IR. As it is absorbed by surfaces in the greenhouse, it is converted to long-wavelength IR. The long-wavelength IR gets trapped inside the greenhouse and bounces off the surfaces and glass and remains inside the greenhouse. Since short-wavelength IR can enter the greenhouse, it also has the ability to leave the greenhouse, making Choice *A* incorrect. The greenhouse feels warmer, not cooler, than outside, so Choice *C* is incorrect. Water is not involved in the reaction noted in Figure 1, so Choice *D* is also incorrect.

28. D: Looking at the graph in Figure 2, the greenhouse plant grew taller than the outside plant. The bars representing the greenhouse plant are taller at 3 time points that Scientist A measured. Greenhouses trap sunlight, warm air, and gases, such as CO_2 inside the greenhouse, so plants have an increased rate of photosynthesis, allowing them to grow faster. The plants are also protected from pests inside the greenhouse.

29. B: Sunlight enters the greenhouse as short-wavelength IR and gets converted to long-wavelength IR. This process also gives off heat and makes the greenhouse feel warmer than the outside climate. Water and oxygen, Choices *A* and *D*, are not involved in this reaction. The plants remain the same and do not get converted into anything else, Choice *C*.

30. A: Short-wavelength IR enters the greenhouse in the form of sunlight. It can pass easily through the glass and can therefore pass easily back out to the outside environment. The long-wavelength IR, Choice *D*, gets trapped inside the greenhouse.

Chemistry

1. C: Conversion within the metric system is as simple as the movement of decimal points. The prefix *kilo-* means "one thousand," or three zeros, so the procedure to convert kilometers to the primary unit (meters) is to move the decimal point three units to the right. To get to centimeters, the decimal point must be moved an additional two places to the right: $0.78 \rightarrow 78,000$. Choice A is false because the decimal point has only been moved one place to right. Choice B is incorrect because the decimal point is moved two units in the wrong direction. Choice D is false because the decimal has only been moved three units to the right. The problem can also be solved by using the following conversion equation:

$$0.78 \text{ km} \times \frac{1,000 \text{ m}}{1 \text{ km}} \times \frac{100 \text{ cm}}{1 \text{ m}} = 78,000 \text{ cm}$$

The kilometer (km) units cancel each other out, as do the meter (m) units. The only units left are centimeters (cm).

2. A: Keratin is a structural protein and it is the primary constituent of things like hair and nails. Choice B is incorrect antigens are immune proteins that help fight disease. Hormonal proteins are responsible for initiating the signal transduction cascade to regulate gene expression. Choice C is incorrect because channel proteins are transport proteins that help move molecules into and out of a cell. Marker proteins help identify or distinguish a cell. Lastly, Choice D is incorrect because actin, like myosin, is a motor protein because it is involved in the process of muscle contraction.

3. B: Biological catalysts are termed *enzymes*, which are proteins with conformations that specifically manipulate reactants into positions which decrease the reaction's activation energy. Lipids do not usually affect reactions, and cofactors, while they can aid or be necessary to the proper functioning of enzymes, do not make up the majority of biological catalysts.

4. D: Protons have a positive charge. An atom is structured with a nucleus in the center that contains neutral neutrons and positive protons. Surrounding the nucleus are orbiting electrons that are negatively charged. Choice D is the only correct answer.

5. B: The set of results is close to the actual value of the acceleration due to gravity, making the results accurate. However, there is a different value recorded every time, so the results aren't precise, which makes Choice B the correct answer.

6. D: Sucrose, lactose, and maltose are disaccharides. Mannose is a monosaccharide.

7. D: Preparing a solution from a stock is simply a process of dilution by adding a certain amount of the stock to water. The amount of stock to use can be calculated using a formula and algebra with the given values for the stock molarity (15.0 M), the diluted volume (250 ml), and diluted molarity (1.50 M):

$$V_S = \frac{M_D V_D}{M_S}$$

$$V_S = \frac{(1.50 \text{ M})(250 \text{ ml})}{12.0 \text{ M}} = 31.3 \text{ ml}$$

Because the given values are written to three significant figures, the answer should also be written in three significant figures, making Choice *D* the correct answer. The other answer choices are either incorrect values or reported to an incorrect number of significant figures.

8. B: When a solution is on the verge of—or in the process of—crystallization, it is called a *supersaturated* solution. This can also occur in a solution that seems stable, but if it is disturbed, the change can begin the crystallization process. To display the relationship between the mass of a solute that a solvent holds and a given temperature, a *solubility curve* is used. If a reading is on the solubility curve, the solvent is *saturated*; it is full and cannot hold more solute. If a reading is above the curve, the solvent is *supersaturated* and unstable from holding more solute than it should. If a reading is below the curve, the solvent is *unsaturated* and could hold more solute. Choices *A*, *C*, and *D* are all stable, whereas Choice *B* is unstable.

9. D: Electrons orbit the nucleus of the atom in atomic shells or orbitals. The first atomic shell, closest to the nucleus, can accommodate two electrons. The second atomic shell can hold a maximum of eight electrons, and the third atomic shell can also house a maximum of eight electrons. The tendency to want to fill the outer orbital completely (called the valence shell), or get rid of a sole electron in the valence shell, influences the degree to which an atom will readily form chemical bonds.

10 A: The metallic substance in an ionic bond often has low ionization energy. Coupled with the fact that the nonmetal has a high electron affinity, the metallic substance readily transfers an electron to the nonmetal. Choice *B* is incorrect because it is the nonmetallic substance, not the metallic one, that has a high electron affinity. Choice *C* is incorrect because ionic bonds are very strong. As such, ionic compounds have high melting and boiling points and are brittle and crystalline. Lastly, Choice *D* is incorrect because the reactions that forms ionic bonds are exothermic.

11. B: Electronegativity, or the measure of an atom's tendency to attract a bonding pair of electrons, doesn't quite follow the general trend in the Periodic table, so the order should be memorized. Although it generally increases diagonal from the lower left corner to the upper right corner, some of the common elements do not fall along this diagonal. The most electronegative element is fluorine. The following order of decreasing electronegativity should be helpful:

$$F > O > Cl > N > Br > I > S > C > H > \text{metals}$$

12. B: Unlike in ionic bonds where electrons are transferred between the bonding atoms, covalent bonds are formed when two atoms share electrons. The atoms in covalent compounds are bonded together because of the balance of attraction and repulsion between their protons and electrons. Two atoms can be joined by single, double, or triple covalent bonds. As the number of electrons that are shared increases, the length of the bond decreases because the atoms are held together more closely.

13. A: The metric prefix for 10^{-3} is "milli." 10^{-3} is $\frac{1}{10^3}$ or $\frac{1}{1,000}$ or 0.001. If this were grams, 10^{-3} would represent 1 milligram or $\frac{1}{1,000}$ of a gram. For multiples of 10, the prefixes are as follows: deca $= 10^1$, hecta $= 10^2$, kilo $= 10^3$, mega $= 10^6$, giga $= 10^9$, tera $= 10^{12}$, peta $= 10^{15}$, and so on. For sub-units of 10, the prefixes are as follows: deci $= 10^{-1}$, centi $= 10^{-2}$, milli $= 10^{-3}$, micro $= 1^{-6}$, nano $= 10^{-9}$, pico $= 10^{-12}$, femto $= 10^{-15}$, and so on. Metric units are usually abbreviated by using the first letter of the prefix (except for micro, which is the Greek letter mu, or μ). Abbreviations for multiples greater than 10^3 are capitalized.

287

14. B: Metallic compounds can conduct electricity by creating a current, which is formed by passing energy through the freely moving electrons. The electrons are shared by many metal cations are more fluid than those in ionic structures. They float around the bonded metals and form a sea of electrons. Lewis structures are not usually depicted for metallic structures because of this free-roaming ability of the electrons.

15. C: The qualitative definition of a gas or element's ionization energy is the amount of energy needed to remove a valence electron, or the one most loosely bound, from that substance and form a cation. Choice *A,* refers to atomic radius, Choice *B* refers to electronegativity, and Choice *D* refers to electron affinity. All four of these properties follow trends on the Periodic table.

16. D: Recall that the rate of a reaction is the measure of the change in concentration of the reactants or products over a certain period of time. When the reactants are in the gaseous state, increases in pressure increase the frequency of collisions between molecules because they are compressed; therefore, the reaction rate increases because of these increased interactions and collisions. The reverse is true when pressure decreases; thus, the reaction rate decreases because there are fewer collisions between the gas molecules.

17. C: Equilibrium occurs when the rate of reactants forming products is equal to the rate of the products reverting back to the reactants. In equilibrium conditions, the concentration of reactants and products in the system doesn't change. The reaction shown is an example of heterogenous equilibrium because the substances are in different phases when equilibrium is reached. If, for example, the reactants and products were all gases, as in the conversion of sulfur dioxide to sulfur trioxide, and equilibrium is reached, it is considered homogenous equilibrium. There is not enough information provided in the equation to decide whether the system is in static or dynamic equilibrium because there is no indication about the whether the forward and reverse reactions are still occurring (dynamic equilibrium), or if all reactions have ceased (static equilibrium). Therefore, Choices *A* and *B* are incorrect.

18. C: Increasing temperature increases the rate of reactions due to increases in the kinetic energy of atoms and molecules. This increased movement results in increased collisions between reactants (with each other as well as with enzymes), which is the cause of the rate increase.

19. A: A chemical change alters the chemical makeup of the original object. When a piece of paper burns it cannot be returned to its original chemical makeup because it has formed new materials. Physical change refers to changing a substance's form, but not the composition of that substance. In physical science, "sedimentary change" and "potential change" are not terms used to describe any particular process.

20. C: An acid increases the concentration of H^+ ions when it is dissolved in water. It is a proton donor in a chemical equation, or acts an electron-pair acceptor. A base increases the concentration of OH^- ions when it is dissolved in water, accepts a proton in a chemical reaction, or is an electron-pair donor. Therefore, only Choice *C* is correct.

21. A: A synthesis reaction occurs when two or more elements or compounds are joined together to form a single product. Choice *A* shows the chemical equation for the synthesis of nitrogen dioxide (NO_2) from nitric oxide (NO) and oxygen (O_2). Choice *B* is a decomposition reaction because a single reactant (carbonic acid, which is in soft drinks) is broken down into two or more products (in this case, water and

288

carbon dioxide). Choices C and D are single displacement reactions, which occur when a single element or ion takes the place of another element in a compound.

22. B: The reaction between methane (CH_4) and oxygen is a combustion reaction, which is a special type of double displacement reaction. Double displacement reactions occur when two elements or ions exchange a single element to form two different compounds. This means that the final compounds have different combinations of cations and anions than the reactants did. Redox reactions and acid-base reactions are also special types of double replacement reactions. In combustion reactions, a hydrocarbon reacts with oxygen to form carbon dioxide and water.

23. B: The percent yield for a reaction is the actual yield is divided by the theoretical yield and then multiplied by 100. Since 65 grams of CaO were expected, this value is the theoretical yield. The actual yield is the 45 grams produced. Thus, the percent yield is:

$$\frac{45 \text{ g}}{65 \text{ g}} \times 100 = 69\%$$

24. B: An atom, ion, or molecule that loses electrons and becomes more positively charged has been oxidized. A substance is reduced when it gains electrons and becomes more negatively charged. Choices C and D are incorrect because when electrons, which carry a negative charge are lost, the amount of negative charge of the substance that lost them becomes less. Therefore, the charge of the substance that lost the electrons becomes less negative or more positive.

25. A: A conjugate base is the ion that is formed when an acid it is paired with loses a proton. HSO_4^- is the conjugate base of the acid H_2SO_4. Choice B is incorrect because it reverses the relationship. Remember that the acid donates a proton, so the conjugate base pair of an acid has the same molecular formula of the acid, except it has one fewer proton (H^+). Therefore, the conjugate base ion has lost a positive charge, so it should have a negative charge. Thus, Choice C is incorrect.

26. C: The correct answer is Choice C. Crystalline solids do not become soft before they melt. Amorphous solids become soft and pliable before melting because some of the bonds between the nonidentical units break before others. In crystalline solids, the bonds all break at the same time, Choice D, because the bonds between the identical repeating units are all equal in strength. This also gives the crystalline solid an exact melting point, Choice A. Crystalline solids also display cleavage and break across a plane, Choice B.

27. D: The correct answer is Choice D; the molecule is methanol. There are three hydrogen atoms attached to the carbon atom, giving CH_3, and one hydrogen atom attached to an oxygen atom, giving OH, which makes the formula CH_3OH. Choices A, B, and C do not have the correct number of carbon, hydrogen, or oxygen atoms as depicted in the Lewis diagram.

28. D: Semiconductors are covalent network solids that are in between being good insulators and good conductors but are neither in entirety. Choice D is the correct answer. Covalent network solids are formed between nonmetals with strong covalent bonds. Metallic solids, Choice A, are good conductors because of the delocalized electrons that transfer electricity. The electrons in ionic solids, Choice C, are held tightly in place, so they cannot conduct electricity at all.

29. A: When fossil fuels react with oxygen gas, they are burning, which causes a combustion reaction. Combustion reactions create carbon dioxide and water vapor. Combination reactions, Choice B, take

289

two smaller molecules and make one larger molecule. Choice *C*, vaporization, would indicate liquids becoming gases, and Choice *D*, solidification, would indicate liquids becoming solids, neither of which is occurring in this reaction.

30. B: For a chemical equation to be balanced, the same quantity of each element must be present on each side of the equation. On the left side of the equation, there is one Fe atom, and there are six oxygen atoms and three carbon atoms. On the right side of the equation, there is one iron atom and the rest of the oxygen and carbon atoms must be accounted for by the carbon dioxide molecules. Having three carbon dioxide molecules would give three carbon atoms and six oxygen atoms, which is equivalent to the reactants' side of the equation.

Anatomy and Physiology

1. C: Eosinophils, like neutrophils, basophils, and mast cells, are a type of leukocyte in a class called granulocytes. They are found underneath mucous membranes in the body and they primarily secrete destructive enzymes and defend against multicellular parasites like worms. Choice *A* describes basophils and mast cells, and Choices *B* and *D* describe neutrophils. Unlike neutrophils, which are aggressive phagocytic cells, eosinophils have low phagocytic activity.

2. B: The innermost epidermal tissue is a single layer of cells called the stratum basale. The melanocytes in the stratum basale produce melanin, an important pigment that absorbs UV rays to protect the skin from sun damage. The outermost epidermal layer, called the stratum corneum, helps repel water; therefore, Choice *A* is incorrect. The stratum granulosum produces keratin, so Choice *C* is incorrect. The dermis, which is underneath the epidermis, contains the oil glands that produce and secrete oil.

3. C: Tendons connect muscle to bone. Ligaments connect bone to bone. Both are made of dense, fibrous connective tissue (primary Type 1 collagen) to give strength. However, tendons are more organized, especially in the long axis direction like muscle fibers themselves, and they have more collagen. This arrangement makes more sense because muscles have specific orientations of their fibers, so they contract in somewhat predictable directions. Ligaments are less organized and more of a woven pattern because bone connections are not as organized as bundles of muscle fibers, so ligaments must have strength in multiple directions to protect against injury.

4. D: Cartilage is avascular, which is one reason why it is limited in its ability to repair itself following an injury. It receives materials such as nutrients via diffusion.

5. D: The smallest functional unit of the body is the cell. Groups of similar cells are arranged into *tissues,* such as nervous tissue, epithelial tissue, and adipose tissue. From there, different tissues are arranged into *organs,* and organs that work together form entire *organ systems.*

6. C: Oil glands, like sweat glands, are exocrine glands of the skin. Oil glands, which are attached to hair follicles, secrete sebum. Sebum is an oily substance that moisturizes the skin, protects it from water loss, helps keep the skin elastic, and provides a chemical defense against bacterial and fungal infections due to its slight acidity. Evaporative cooling, which is when the hottest water particles on the skin evaporate and leave behind the coolest ones to help cool the body, is not a function of sebum. In hot conditions, the hypothalamus will initiate a pathway that vasodilates blood vessels near the surface of the skin to increase heat loss and stimulate sweating.

7. A: Skeletal muscle fibers are made of myofibrils, which interact when a muscle contracts in a model called the sliding filament theory. The myofibrils are arranged in each muscle fibers in functional units called sarcomeres. The thicker filaments, called myosin, are in between the thinner actin filaments, which are anchored to Z lines. One sarcomere is defined as the region between two adjacent Z lines. Myosin filaments are attached to a central M line. When a muscle is at rest, there is a gap between the Z line and the myosin filaments; in fact, it is the arrangement of filaments that gives skeletal muscle its striated appearance. When the muscle contracts, the heads of the myosin filaments attach to the actin and form cross-bridges, which are used to pull the actin filaments closer to the M line.

8. D: Epithelial tissue covers the external surfaces of organs and lines many of the body's cavities. It can be arranged into four patterns. Transitional epithelium is noted for its ability to expand and contract. Choice *A* is incorrect because it describes simple epithelial tissue. Choice *B* is incorrect because it describes pseudostratified epithelial tissue. Choice *C* is incorrect because although transitional epithelial tissue does help protect the body from invading microbes, this ability is not unique to transitional epithelium. Instead, it is a shared characteristic of all epithelial tissue.

9. A: Antibodies. Antibiotics (*B*) fight bacteria, but the body does not make them naturally. White blood cells, not red blood cells (*D*) are the blood cells produced that fight the bacteria. Vaccines (*C*) are given to create antibodies and prevent future illness.

10. B: Red blood cells are the chief transport vehicle for oxygen. Red blood cells contain hemoglobin, a protein that helps transport oxygen throughout the circulatory system.

11. C: The axial skeleton includes the bones of the skull and face (so the mandible, or jaw bone is included), the ribs, the vertebral column (so the atlas, which is the name of the first cervical bone, is included), the sternum, and the hyoid. The bones of the shoulder girdle, clavicles, pelvis, and limbs are considered the bones the comprise the appendicular skeleton. Therefore, the illium, a bone of the pelvis, is not part of the axial skeleton.

12. C: The epididymis stores sperm and is a coiled tube located near the testes. The immature sperm that enters the epididymis from the testes migrates through the 20-foot long epididymis tube in about two weeks, where viable sperm are concentrated at the end. The vas deferens is a tube that transports mature sperm from the epididymis to the urethra. Seminal vesicles are pouches attached that add fructose to the ejaculate to provide energy for sperm. The prostate gland excretes fluid that makes up about a third of semen released during ejaculation. The fluid reduces semen viscosity and contains enzymes that aid in sperm functioning; both effects increase sperm motility and ultimate success.

13. C: The female reproductive system is a symphony of different hormones that work together in order to propagate the species. Below, find the function of each one:

Hormone	Source	Action
GnRH	Hypothalamus	Stimulates anterior pituitary to secrete FSH and LH
FSH	Anterior Pituitary	Stimulates ovaries to develop mature follicles (with ova); follicles produce increasingly high levels of estrogen
LH	Anterior Pituitary	Stimulates the release of the ovum by the follicle; follicle then converted into a corpus luteum that secretes progesterone
Estrogen	Ovary (follicle); placenta	Stimulates repair of endometrium of uterus; negative feedback effect inhibits hypothalamus production of GnRH
Progesterone	Ovary (corpus luteum); placenta	Stimulates thickening of and maintains endometrium; negative feedback inhibits pituitary production of LH
Prolactin	Anterior pituitary	Stimulates milk production after childbirth
Oxytocin	Posterior pituitary	Stimulates milk "letdown"
Androgens	Adrenal glands	Stimulates sexual drive
hCG	Embryo (if pregnancy)	Stimulates production of progesterone

14. A: Epithelial cells line cavities and surfaces of body organs and glands, and the three main shapes are squamous, columnar, and cuboidal. Epithelial cells contain no blood vessels, and their functions involve absorption, protection, transport, secretion, and sensing. Simple squamous epithelial are flat cells that are present in lungs and line the heart and vessels. Their flat shape aids in their function, which is diffusion of materials. The tunica intima, the inner layer of blood vessels, is lined with simple squamous epithelial tissue that sits on the basement membrane. Simple cuboidal epithelium is found in ducts, and simple columnar epithelium is found in tubes with projections (uterus, villi, bronchi). Any of these types of epithelial cells can be stacked, and then they are called stratified, not simple.

15. B: The position of the clavicle relative to the humerus is medial. Anatomical directions are referenced to the midline (medial, and lateral); to the center (proximal and distal); to the front and rear (anterior and posterior); toward the head and tail (cephalic and caudal); and to the head and feet (superior and inferior). In anatomical position, the body stands erect with palms facing forward. The clavicle would be clearly medial and superior to the humerus as it is closer to the midline and head.

16. A: The coronal, or frontal, plane is a vertical plane positioned so that it divides the body into front (ventral) and back (dorsal) regions. The plane is positioned so that the face, kneecap, and toes are on the ventral side, and the vertebrae and heel are on the dorsal side. The coronal plane is one of three body planes. The other two are the transverse and sagittal planes. The transverse plane divides the anatomy into upper (cranial or head) and lower (caudal or tail) regions. The sagittal plane runs front/back perpendicular to the frontal plane and divides the anatomy into right and left regions.

17. C: Cartilage adds mechanical support to joints. It provides a flexible cushion that aids in mobility while offering support. The first two choices are switched—it is ligaments that connect bones at joints and tendons that attach skeletal muscles to bones. *D* is incorrect because arteries, not veins, deliver oxygenated blood.

18. B: The dermis is the skin layer that contains nerves, blood vessels, hair follicles, and glands. These structures are called skin appendages. These appendages are scattered throughout the connective

292

tissue (elastin and collagen), and the connective tissue provides support to the outer layer, the epidermis. The epidermal surface is a thin layer (except feet and palms where it is thick) of continually-regenerating cells that don't have a blood supply of their own, which explains why superficial cuts don't bleed. The hypodermis is the subcutaneous layer underneath the dermis, and it is composed primarily of fat in order to provide insulation.

19. D: Receptors in the dermis help the body maintain homeostasis, for example, in terms of regulating body temperature. Signals travel to the hypothalamus, which then secretes hormones that activate effectors to keep internal temperature at a set point of 98.6°F (37°C). For example, if the environment is too cold, the hypothalamus will initiate a pathway that will cause the muscles to shiver because shivering helps heat the body.

20. B: The radius and ulna are the bones from the elbow to the wrist, and the humerus is the bone between the elbow and the shoulder. The tibia and fibula are the bones from the knee to the ankle, and the femur is the bone from the knee to the hip. The other choices are bones in the body as well, just not limb bones. The mandible is the jaw, the scapula is the shoulder blade, and the carpal bones are in the wrist.

21. B: In the Haversian system found in compact bone, concentric layers of bone cells are called lamellae. Between the lamellae are lacunae, which are gaps filled with osteocytes. The Haversian canals on the outer regions of the bone contain capillaries and nerve fibers. Spongy (cancellous) bone is on the extremities of long bones, which makes sense because the ends are softer due to the motion at joints (providing flexibility and cushion). The middle of the bone between the two spongy regions is called the diaphysis region. Spongy bone is highly vascular and is the site of red bone marrow (the marrow that makes red blood cells). Long bones, on the other hand, are long, weight-bearing bones like the tibia or femur that contain yellow marrow in adulthood. Trabeculae is a dense, collagenous, rod-shaped tissue that add mechanical support to the spongy regions of bone. Muscular trabeculae can be found in the heart and are similar in that they offer physical reinforcement.

22. A: Carbon dioxide-rich blood is delivered from systemic circulation to the right atrium. It is pumped into the right ventricle. The tricuspid valve prevents backflow between the two chambers. From there, the pulmonary artery takes blood to the lungs where diffusion causes gas exchange. Then, oxygenated blood returns to the left atrium before getting pumped into the left ventricle. The mitral valve prevents the backflow of blood from the left ventricle to the atrium. Finally, blood is ejected from the left ventricle through the aorta to enter systemic circulation.

23. B: Smooth, skeletal, and cardiac muscle have defining characteristics, due to their vastly different functions. All have actin and myosin microfilaments that slide past each other to contract.

Skeletal muscles have long fibers made of clearly defined sarcomeres, which make them appear striated. Sarcomeres consist of alternating dark A bands (thick myosin) and light I bands (thin actin). Upon muscle contraction, fibers slide past each. Skeletal muscles are attached to bone via tendons and are responsible for voluntary movement; their contraction brings bones together. They contain multiple nuclei, due to their bundling into fibers.

Cardiac muscles also contain sarcomeres and appear striated, but are branched cells with a single nucleus. Branching allows each cell to connect with several others, forming a huge network that has more strength (the whole is greater than the sum of its parts).

Smooth muscles are non-striated and are responsible for involuntary movement (such as digestion). They do not form cylindrical fibers like skeletal muscles. Their lack of striations is because they have no sarcomeres, and the filaments are randomly arranged.

24. B: The reflex arc is the simplest nerve pathway. The stimulus bypasses the brain, going from sensory receptors through an afferent (incoming) neuron to the spinal cord. It synapses with an efferent (outgoing) neuron in the spinal cord and is transmitted directly to muscle. There is no interneuron involved in a reflex arc. The classic example of a reflex arc is the knee jerk response. Tapping on the patellar tendon of the knee stretches the quadriceps muscle of the thigh, resulting in contraction of the muscle and extension of the knee.

25. A: The sternum is medial to the deltoid because it is much closer (typically right on) the midline of the body, while the deltoid is lateral at the shoulder cap. Superficial means that a structure is closer to the body surface and posterior means that it falls behind something else. For example, skin is superficial to bone and the kidneys are posterior to the rectus abdominis.

26. C: The relative density of eccrine sweat glands varies in different areas of the body. The palms and soles of the feet have the highest density, reaching values of approximately 400 sweat glands per square centimeter of epidermis. The head also has a high density of sweat glands, though significantly less than on the palms and soles. Areas such as the upper arms and thighs have only around 80 eccrine sweat glands per square inch of skin.

27. C: The cerebellum is important for balance and motor coordination. Aside from the brainstem and cerebellum, the outside portion of the brain is the cerebrum, which is the advanced operating system of the brain and is responsible for learning, emotion, memory, perception, and voluntary movement. The amygdala (emotions), language areas, and corpus collosum all exist within the cerebrum.

28. A: Choice *B* might be an attractive answer choice, but neutrophils are part of the innate immune system and are not considered part of the primary immune response. The first event that happens in a primary immune response is that macrophages ingest pathogens and display their antigens. Then, they secrete interleukin 1 to recruit helper T cells. Once helper T cells are activated, they secrete interleukin 2 to simulate plasma B cell and killer T cell production. Only then can plasma B cells make the pathogen specific antibodies.

29. D: Cartilage and synovial fluid are the primary sources of cushioning to joints during impact. The proprioceptive system is responsible for body awareness, coordinated reflexes for balance, and modifying movements based on neural feedback.

30. A: When a muscle is stretched, the embedded spindles are also stretched, activating sensory neurons in the spindles. This activation sends an impulse to the spinal cord, where the sensory neurons synapse with motor neurons. These motor neurons exit the spinal cord and travel back towards the limb, where they innervate the extrafusal fibers, which receive the message to relax.

Physics

1. D: Circular motion occurs around an invisible line around which an object can rotate. This invisible line is called an axis. Choice *A*, center of mass, is the average location of an object's mass. Choice *B*, the center of matter, is not a real term. Choice *C,* elliptical, describes an elongated circle and is not a viable selection.

2. D: An object at rest has forces acting upon it, including gravitational, normal, and frictional forces. All of these forces are in balance with each other and cause no movement in the object's position. This is equilibrium. An object in constant motion is also considered to be in equilibrium or a state of balanced forces.

3. B: For charges, *like charges repel* each other and *opposite charges attract* each other. Negatives and positives will attract, while two positive charges or two negative charges will repel each other. Charges have an effect on each other, so Choices *C* and *D* are incorrect.

4. D: Mass refers to the amount or quantity there is of an object. Light, sound, and heat are all forms of energy that can travel in waves.

5. C: Motion with one dimension or measurement is known as a *scalar quantity,* and includes things such as length, speed, or time. Motion with two dimensions is known as a *vector quantity*. This would be speed with a direction, or velocity. Choices *A, B,* and *C* (mass, length, speed) are all measurements of magnitudes—one-dimensional scalar quantities.

6. B: It appears to bend because of the refraction of light traveling from air to water. When light travels from one material to another it can reflect, refract, and go through different materials. Choice *A* is incorrect, as the pencil does not actually become warped but only *appears* to be warped. Choice *C* is incorrect; although the pencil appears to bend because of its immersion into separate mediums where speed is different, the pencil does not become temporarily warped—it only appears to be warped. Choice *D* is incorrect; it is the refraction of light, not reflection. The latter happens within the same medium, which makes the answer choice incorrect.

7. A: According to Ohm's Law: *V=IR*, so using the given variables: 3.0 V=I × 6.0 Ω

Solving for I: I=3.0 V/6.0 Ω=0.5 A

Choice *B* incorporates a miscalculation in the equation by multiplying 3.0 V by 6.0 Ω, rather than dividing these values. Choices *C* and *D* are labeled with the wrong units; Joules measure energy, not current.

8. C: This is a fundamental law of thermodynamics. Energy can only transfer, transform, or travel. The amount of energy in a system is always the same.

9. D: When electricity is run through a wire, it is carrying current and current has a charge. Therefore, there is a charge running down the wire, which creates a magnetic field that can attract and repel just like any magnet.

10. B: In broad terms, energy is divided into kinetic and potential energy. Kinetic energy refers to an object in motion. It is the product of mass and velocity ($KE = \frac{1}{2}mv^2$). Potential energy refers to the capacity for doing work. Its gravitational configuration is the product of mass, acceleration due to gravity, and height ($PE = mgh$). Examples of kinetic energy include heat (which is the thermal energy from atoms and molecules moving around), waves like light, and physical motion. Potential energy examples include gravitational energy and chemical energy stored in bonds.

11. C: The answer is 1800 seconds:

$$\left(45\ km \times \frac{1000\ m}{km}\right) \Big/ 25\frac{m}{s} = 1800\ seconds$$

12. D: The answer is 3.6 kilometers east of its point of departure. The ship is traveling faster than the current, so it will be east of the starting location. Its net forward velocity is 0.5 m/s which is 1.8 kilometers/hour, or 3.6 kilometers in two hours.

13. B: The answer is 2 m/s²:

$$a = \frac{\Delta v}{\Delta t} = \frac{132\frac{km}{h} - 60\frac{km}{h}}{10\ s}$$

$$\frac{72\frac{km}{h} \times 1000\frac{m}{km} \times \frac{h}{3600\ s}}{10\ s}$$

$$2\ m/s^2$$

14. C: The answer is 50,000 N. The equation $F = ma$ should be memorized. All of the values are given in the correct units (kilogram-meter-second) so plug them in to the equation:

$$F = 100,000\ kg \times 0.5\frac{m}{s^2} = 50,000\ N$$

15. B: The answer is 200 kilograms. This is actually a trick question. The mass of the astronaut is the same everywhere (it is the weight that varies from planet to planet). The astronaut's mass in kilograms is calculated by dividing his weight on Earth by the acceleration of gravity on Earth:

$$\frac{1962\ N}{9.81\ m/s^2} = 200\ kg$$

16. A: The answer is that the upward velocity is at a maximum when it leaves the punter's toe. The acceleration due to gravity reduces the upward velocity every moment thereafter. The speed is the same at points A and E, but the velocity is different. At point E, the velocity has a maximum *negative* value.

17. C: The answer is her angular velocity increases from (a) to (b) as she pulls her arms in close to her body and reduces her moment of inertia.

18. B: The answer is 14 m/s. Remember that the cannonball at rest, y meters off the ground, has a potential energy of $PE = mgy$. As it falls, the potential energy is converted to kinetic energy until (at ground level) the kinetic energy is equal to the total original potential energy:

$$\frac{1}{2}mv^2 = mgy$$

Rearranged to solve for velocity, the equation is:

$$v = \sqrt{2gy}$$

296

This makes sense because all objects fall at the same rate, so the velocity *must* be independent of the mass; thus, Choice *D* is incorrect. Plugging the values into the equation, the result is 14 m/s. Remember, the way to figure this quickly is to have *g* equal to 10 m/s² rather than 9.81 m/s².

19. B: The answer is at Point C, the bottom of the arc. The bottom of the arc must have the greatest kinetic energy because it is the point with the least potential energy, since the total energy is equivalent to the sum of both potential and kinetic energy.

20. C: This question isn't difficult, but it must be read carefully:

A is incorrect. Even though the total energy is at a maximum at Points A and E, it isn't equal at only those points. The total energy is the same at *all* points. *B* is incorrect. The kinetic energy is at a maximum at C, but not the *total* energy. The correct answer is *C*. The total energy is conserved, so it's the same at *all* points on the arc. *D* is incorrect. The motion of a pendulum is independent of the mass. Just like how all objects fall at the same rate, all pendulum bobs swing at the same rate, dependent on the length of the cord.

Mathematics

1. If a car can travel 300 miles in 4 hours, how far can it go in an hour and a half?
    a. 100 miles
    b. 112.5 miles
    c. 135.5 miles
    d. 150 miles

2. At the store, Jan spends $90 on apples and oranges. Apples cost $1 each and oranges cost $2 each. If Jan buys the same number of apples as oranges, how many oranges did she buy?
    a. 20
    b. 25
    c. 30
    d. 35

3. $\frac{11}{6} - \frac{3}{8} =$

    a. $\frac{5}{4}$

    b. $\frac{51}{36}$

    c. $\frac{35}{24}$

    d. $\frac{3}{2}$

4. A train traveling 50 miles per hour takes a trip lasting 3 hours. If a map has a scale of 1 inch per 10 miles, how many inches apart are the train's starting point and ending point on the map?
    a. 14
    b. 12
    c. 13
    d. 15

5. A traveler takes an hour to drive to a museum, spends 3 hours and 30 minutes there, and takes half an hour to drive home. What percentage of their time was spent driving?
    a. 15%
    b. 30%
    c. 40%
    d. 60%

6. Simplify the following fraction:

$$\frac{\frac{5}{7}}{\frac{9}{11}}$$

a. $\frac{55}{63}$

b. $\frac{7}{1000}$

c. $\frac{13}{15}$

d. $\frac{5}{11}$

7. Greg buys a $10 lunch with 5% sales tax. He leaves a $2 tip after his bill. How much money does he spend?
   a. $12.50
   b. $12
   c. $13
   d. $13.25

8. Marty wishes to save $150 over a 4-day period. How much must Marty save each day on average?
   a. $37.50
   b. $35
   c. $45.50
   d. $41

9. Bernard can make $80 per day. If he needs to make $300 and only works full days, how many days will this take?
   a. 6
   b. 3
   c. 5
   d. 4

10. A couple buys a house for $150,000. They sell it for $165,000. By what percentage did the house's value increase?
    a. 10%
    b. 13%
    c. 15%
    d. 17%

11. A school has 15 teachers and 20 teaching assistants. They have 200 students. What is the ratio of faculty to students?
    a. 3 : 20
    b. 4 : 17
    c. 5 : 54
    d. 7 : 40

299

12. A map has a scale of 1 inch per 5 miles. A car can travel 60 miles per hour. If the distance from the start to the destination is 3 inches on the map, how long will it take the car to make the trip?
    a. 12 minutes
    b. 15 minutes
    c. 17 minutes
    d. 20 minutes

13. Taylor works two jobs. The first pays $20,000 per year. The second pays $10,000 per year. She donates 15% of her income to charity. How much does she donate each year?
    a. $4500
    b. $5000
    c. $5500
    d. $6000

14. Keith's bakery had 252 customers go through its doors last week. This week, that number increased to 378. Express this increase as a percentage.
    a. 26%
    b. 50%
    c. 35%
    d. 12%

15. Kristen purchases $100 worth of CDs and DVDs. The CDs cost $10 each and the DVDs cost $15. If she bought four DVDs, how many CDs did she buy?
    a. 5
    b. 6
    c. 3
    d. 4

16. If Sarah reads at an average rate of 21 pages in four nights, how long will it take her to read 140 pages?
    a. 6 nights
    b. 26 nights
    c. 8 nights
    d. 27 nights

17. Mom's car drove 72 miles in 90 minutes. There are 5280 feet per mile. How fast did she drive in feet per second?
    a. 0.8 feet per second
    b. 48.9 feet per second
    c. 0.009 feet per second
    d. 70.4 feet per second

18. If $6t + 4 = 16$, what is t?
    a. 1
    b. 2
    c. 3
    d. 4

19. After a 30% sale discount, Frank purchased a new refrigerator for $660. How much did he save from the original price?
    a. $282.86
    b. $212.50
    c. $105.75
    d. $200

20. $3.4 + 2.35 + 4 =$
    a. 5.35
    b. 9.2
    c. 9.75
    d. 10.25

21. $5.88 \times 3.2 =$
    a. 18.816
    b. 16.44
    c. 20.352
    d. 17

22. $\frac{3}{25} =$
    a. 0.15
    b. 0.1
    c. 0.9
    d. 0.12

23. Which of the following is largest?
    a. 0.45
    b. 0.096
    c. 0.3
    d. 0.313

24. Which of the following is NOT a way to write 40 percent of N?
    a. $(0.4)N$

    b. $\frac{2}{5}N$

    c. $40N$

    d. $\frac{4N}{10}$

25. Which is closest to 17.8×9.9?
    a. 140
    b. 180
    c. 200
    d. 350

301

26. A student gets an 85% on a test with 20 questions. How many answers did the student solve correctly?
    a. 15
    b. 16
    c. 17
    d. 18

27. Four people split a bill. The first person pays for $\frac{1}{5}$, the second person pays for $\frac{1}{4}$, and the third person pays for $\frac{1}{3}$. What fraction of the bill does the fourth person pay?

    a. $\frac{13}{60}$

    b. $\frac{47}{60}$

    c. $\frac{1}{4}$

    d. $\frac{4}{15}$

28. 6 is 30% of what number?
    a. 18
    b. 20
    c. 24
    d. 26

29. $2\frac{1}{3} - 2\frac{1}{5} =$

    a. $\frac{2}{15}$

    b. $\frac{1}{15}$

    c. $\frac{1}{3}$

    d. $\frac{1}{5}$

30. What is $\frac{420}{98}$ rounded to the nearest integer?
    a. 4
    b. 3
    c. 5
    d. 6

31. $4\frac{1}{3} + 3\frac{3}{4} =$

    a. $6\frac{5}{12}$

    b. $8\frac{1}{12}$

    c. $8\frac{2}{3}$

    d. $7\frac{7}{12}$

32. There are $4x + 1$ treats in each party favor bag. If a total of $60x + 15$ treats are distributed, how many bags are given out?

    a. 15
    b. 16
    c. 20
    d. 22

33. Apples cost $2 each, while bananas cost $3 each. Maria purchased 10 fruits in total and spent $22. How many apples did she buy?

    a. 5
    b. 6
    c. 7
    d. 8

34. If $\frac{5}{2} \div \frac{1}{3} = n$, then n is between:

    a. 5 and 7
    b. 7 and 9
    c. 9 and 11
    d. 3 and 5

35. A closet is filled with red, blue, and green shirts. If $\frac{1}{3}$ of the shirts are green and $\frac{2}{5}$ are red, what fraction of the shirts are blue?

    a. $\frac{4}{15}$

    b. $\frac{1}{5}$

    c. $\frac{7}{15}$

    d. $\frac{1}{2}$

36. Shawna buys $2\frac{1}{2}$ gallons of paint. If she uses $\frac{1}{3}$ of it on the first day, how much does she have left?

    a. $1\frac{5}{6}$ gallons

    b. $1\frac{1}{2}$ gallons

    c. $1\frac{2}{3}$ gallons

    d. 2 gallons

37. A drug needs to be stored at room temperature (68 °F). What is the equivalent temperature in degrees Celsius?
    a. 36 °C
    b. 72 °C
    c. 68 °C
    d. 20 °C

38. Add 4.33 + 7.688.
    a. 12.018
    b. 3.358
    c. 8.121
    d. 33.289

39. Add and express in reduced form 7/12 + 2/9.
    a. 9/12
    b. 14/108
    c. 29/36
    d. 2/3

40. Subtract 37.517 − 18.664.
    a. 18.853
    b. 56.181
    c. 35.6506
    d. 18.032

41. Subtract 401.2 − 82.56.
    a. 118.66
    b. 318.64
    c. 315.94
    d. 483.76

42. Subtract and express in reduced form 39/45 − 8/15.
    a. 15/45
    b. 31/45
    c. 2/3
    d. 1/3

43. Multiply 13.7 × 0.3.
    a. 45.66
    b. 4.11
    c. 14.0
    d. 41.1

44. Multiply 1,413 × 0.07.
    a. 1414
    b. 98.91
    c. 989.1
    d. 9.891

45. Multiply and reduce 15/21 × 48/108.
    a. 20/63
    b. 33/87
    c. 60/189
    d. 720/2268

46. Divide, express with a fraction remainder 1,107 ÷ 34.
    a. 31 39/34
    b. 3 29/34
    c. 32/34
    d. 32 19/34

47. Divide and reduce 14/28 ÷ 23/9.
    a. 9/19
    b. 9/23
    c. 9/46
    d. 23/46

48. Express as a reduced mixed number 55/12.
    a. 4 7/12
    b. 4 7/55
    c. 4 3/12
    d. 4 12/55

49. Express as an improper fraction 9 5/6.
    a. 54/6
    b. 59/6
    c. 45/6
    d. 45/9

50. Round to the nearest thousandth 2,718.0354.
    a. 3,000
    b. 2,718.04
    c. 2,718.035
    d. 2,718.036

51. For the following similar triangles, what are the values of x and y (rounded to one decimal place)?

 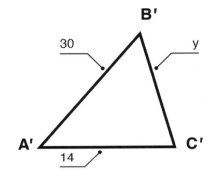

    a. $x = 16.5, y = 25.1$
    b. $x = 19.5, y = 24.1$
    c. $x = 17.1, y = 26.3$
    d. $x = 26.3, y = 17.1$

52. The square and circle have the same center. The circle has a radius of r. What is the area of the shaded region?

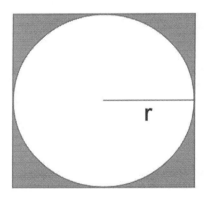

    a. $r^2 - \pi r^2$
    b. $4r^2 - 2\pi r$
    c. $(4 - \pi)r^2$
    d. $(\pi - 1)r^2$

53. Which equation is not a function?
    a. $y = |x|$
    b. $y = \sqrt{x}$
    c. $x = 3$
    d. $y = 4$

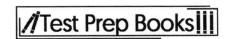

54. On Monday, Robert mopped the floor in 4 hours. On Tuesday, he did it in 3 hours. If on Monday, his average rate of mopping was p sq. ft. per hour, what was his average rate on Tuesday?

a. $\frac{4}{3}p$ sq. ft. per hour

b. $\frac{3}{4}p$ sq. ft. per hour

c. $\frac{5}{4}p$ sq. ft. per hour

d. $p + 1$ sq. ft. per hour

55. The table below displays the number of three-year-olds at Kids First Daycare who are potty-trained and those who still wear diapers.

	Potty-trained	Wear diapers	
Boys	26	22	48
Girls	34	18	52
	60	40	

What is the probability of a three-year-old girl from the school being potty-trained?
a. 52%
b. 34%
c. 65%
d. 57%

Reading Comprehension

Questions 1–10 are based on the following excerpt from a novel set in nineteenth-century France, where two friends, Albert de Morcerf and the Count of Monte Cristo, discuss Parisian social life.

"Mademoiselle Eugénie is pretty—I think I remember that to be her name."

"Very pretty, or rather, very beautiful," replied Albert, "but of that style of beauty which I don't appreciate; I am an ungrateful fellow."

"Really," said Monte Cristo, lowering his voice, "you don't appear to me to be very enthusiastic on the subject of this marriage."

"Mademoiselle Danglars is too rich for me," replied Morcerf, "and that frightens me."

"Bah," exclaimed Monte Cristo, "that's a fine reason to give. Are you not rich yourself?"

"My father's income is about 50,000 francs per annum; and he will give me, perhaps, ten or twelve thousand when I marry."

"That, perhaps, might not be considered a large sum, in Paris especially," said the count; "but everything doesn't depend on wealth, and it's a fine thing to have a good name, and to occupy a high station in society. Your name is celebrated, your position magnificent; and then the Comte de Morcerf is a soldier, and it's pleasing to see the integrity of a Bayard united to the poverty of a Duguesclin; disinterestedness is the brightest ray in which a noble sword can shine. As for me, I consider the union with Mademoiselle Danglars a most suitable one; she will enrich you, and you will ennoble her."

Albert shook his head, and looked thoughtful. "There is still something else," said he.

"I confess," observed Monte Cristo, "that I have some difficulty in comprehending your objection to a young lady who is both rich and beautiful."

"Oh," said Morcerf, "this repugnance, if repugnance it may be called, isn't all on my side."

"Whence can it arise, then? for you told me your father desired the marriage."

"It's my mother who dissents; she has a clear and penetrating judgment, and doesn't smile on the proposed union. I cannot account for it, but she seems to entertain some prejudice against the Danglars."

"Ah," said the count, in a somewhat forced tone, "that may be easily explained; the Comtesse de Morcerf, who is aristocracy and refinement itself, doesn't relish the idea of being allied by your marriage with one of ignoble birth; that is natural enough."

1. The meaning of the word "repugnance" is closest to:
   a. Strong resemblance
   b. Strong dislike
   c. Extreme shyness
   d. Extreme dissimilarity

2. What can be inferred about Albert's family?
   a. Their finances are uncertain.
   b. Albert is the only son in his family.
   c. Their name is more respected than the Danglars'.
   d. Albert's mother and father both agree on their decisions.

3. What is Albert's attitude towards his impending marriage?
   a. Pragmatic
   b. Romantic
   c. Indifferent
   d. Apprehensive

4. What is the best description of the Count's relationship with Albert?
   a. He's like a strict parent, criticizing Albert's choices.
   b. He's like a wise uncle, giving practical advice to Albert.
   c. He's like a close friend, supporting all of Albert's opinions.
   d. He's like a suspicious investigator, asking many probing questions.

5. Which sentence is true of Albert's mother?
    a. She belongs to a noble family.
    b. She often makes poor choices.
    c. She is primarily occupied with money.
    d. She is unconcerned about her son's future.

6. Based on this passage, what is probably NOT true about French society in the 1800s?
    a. Children often received money from their parents.
    b. Marriages were sometimes arranged between families.
    c. The richest people in society were also the most respected.
    d. People were often expected to marry within their same social class.

7. Why is the Count puzzled by Albert's attitude toward his marriage?
    a. He seems reluctant to marry Eugénie, despite her wealth and beauty.
    b. He is marrying against his father's wishes, despite usually following his advice.
    c. He appears excited to marry someone he doesn't love, despite being a hopeless romantic.
    d. He expresses reverence towards Eugénie, despite being from a higher social class than her.

8. The passage is made up mostly of what kind of text?
    a. Narration
    b. Dialogue
    c. Description
    d. Explanation

9. What does the word "ennoble" mean in the middle of the passage?
    a. to create beauty in another person
    b. to endow someone with wealth
    c. to make someone chaste again
    d. to give someone a noble rank or title

10. Why is the count said to have a "forced tone" in the last paragraph?
    a. Because he is in love with Mademoiselle Eugénie and is trying to keep it a secret.
    b. Because he finally agrees with Albert's point of view but still doesn't understand it.
    c. Because he finally understands Albert's point of view but still doesn't agree with it.
    d. Because he is only pretending that Albert is his friend to get information out of him.

Questions 11–12 are based on the following passage:

Four hundred years ago, in 1612, the north-west of England was the scene of England's biggest peacetime witch trial: the trial of the Lancashire witches. Twenty people, mostly from the Pendle area of Lancashire, were imprisoned in the castle as witches. Ten were hanged, one died in gaol, one was sentenced to stand in the pillory, and eight were acquitted. The 2012 anniversary sees a small flood of commemorative events, including works of fiction by Blake Morrison, Carol Ann Duffy, and Jeanette Winterson. How did this witch trial come about, and what accounts for its enduring fame?

We know so much about the Lancashire Witches because the trial was recorded in unique detail by the clerk of the court, Thomas Potts, who published his account soon afterwards as *The Wonderful Discovery of Witches in the County of Lancaster*. I have recently published a modern-

309

English edition of this book, together with an essay piecing together what we know of the events of 1612. It has been a fascinating exercise, revealing how Potts carefully edited the evidence, and also how the case against the "witches" was constructed and manipulated to bring about a spectacular show trial. It all began in mid-March when a pedlar from Halifax named John Law had a frightening encounter with a poor young woman, Alizon Device, in a field near Colne. He refused her request for pins and there was a brief argument during which he was seized by a fit that left him with "his head ... drawn awry, his eyes and face deformed, his speech not well to be understood; his thighs and legs stark lame." We can now recognize this as a stroke, perhaps triggered by the stressful encounter. Alizon Device was sent for and surprised all by confessing to the bewitching of John Law and then begged for forgiveness.

When Alizon Device was unable to cure the pedlar, the local magistrate, Roger Nowell was called in. Characterized by Thomas Potts as "God's justice" he was alert to instances of witchcraft, which were regarded by the Lancashire's puritan-inclined authorities as part of the cultural rubble of "popery"—Roman Catholicism—long overdue to be swept away at the end of the country's very slow protestant reformation. "With weeping tears" Alizon explained that she had been led astray by her grandmother, "old Demdike," well-known in the district for her knowledge of old Catholic prayers, charms, cures, magic, and curses. Nowell quickly interviewed Alizon's grandmother and mother, as well as Demdike's supposed rival, "old Chattox" and her daughter Anne. Their panicky attempts to explain themselves and shift the blame to others eventually only ended up incriminating them, and the four were sent to Lancaster gaol in early April to await trial at the summer assizes. The initial picture revealed was of a couple of poor, marginal local families in the forest of Pendle with a longstanding reputation for magical powers, which they had occasionally used at the request of their wealthier neighbours. There had been disputes but none of these were part of ordinary village life. Not until 1612 did any of this come to the attention of the authorities.

The net was widened still further at the end of April when Alizon's younger brother James and younger sister Jennet, only nine years old, came up between them with a story about a "great meeting of witches" at their grandmother's house, known as Malkin Tower. This meeting was presumably to discuss the plight of those arrested and the threat of further arrests, but according to the evidence extracted from the children by the magistrates, a plot was hatched to blow up Lancaster castle with gunpowder, kill the gaoler, and rescue the imprisoned witches. It was, in short, a conspiracy against royal authority to rival the gunpowder plot of 1605—something to be expected in a county known for its particularly strong underground Roman Catholic presence.

Those present at the meeting were mostly family members and neighbours, but they also included Alice Nutter, described by Potts as "a rich woman [who] had a great estate, and children of good hope: in the common opinion of the world, of good temper, free from envy or malice." Her part in the affair remains mysterious, but she seems to have had Catholic family connections, and may have been one herself, providing an added motive for her to be prosecuted.

"The Lancashire Witches 1612–2012" by Robert Poole.

11. According to the passage, how many people were arrested as witches in the Lancashire trials?
    a. 10
    b. 20
    c. 30
    d. 40

12. As it is used in the first paragraph, the word *commemorative* most nearly means:
    a. Associated with being acquitted
    b. An act of disloyalty
    c. A circumstance to be disliked
    d. In honor of something

Questions 13–14 refer to the following paragraph:

> The Brookside area is an older part of Kansas City, developed mainly in the 1920s and 30s, and is considered one of the nation's first "planned" communities with shops, restaurants, parks, and churches all within a quick walk. A stroll down any street reveals charming two-story Tudor and Colonial homes with smaller bungalows sprinkled throughout the beautiful tree-lined streets. It is common to see lemonade stands on the corners and baseball games in the numerous "pocket" parks tucked neatly behind rows of well-manicured houses. The Brookside shops on 63rd street between Wornall Road and Oak Street are a hub of commerce and entertainment where residents freely shop and dine with their pets (and children) in tow. This is also a common "hangout" spot for younger teenagers because it is easily accessible by bike for most. In short, it is an idyllic neighborhood just minutes from downtown Kansas City.

13. Which of the following states the main idea of this paragraph?
    a. The Brookside shops are a popular hangout for teenagers.
    b. There are a number of pocket parks in the Brookside neighborhood.
    c. Brookside is a great place to live.
    d. Brookside has a high crime rate.

14. According to this paragraph, which of the following is unique to this neighborhood?
    a. It is old.
    b. It is in Kansas City.
    c. It has shopping.
    d. It is one of the nation's first planned communities.

Questions 15–18 refer to the following passage, titled "Education is Essential to Civilization."

> Early in my career, a master teacher shared this thought with me: "Education is the last bastion of civility." While I did not completely understand the scope of those words at the time, I have since come to realize the depth, breadth, truth, and significance of what he said. Education provides society with a vehicle for raising its children to be civil, decent, human beings with something valuable to contribute to the world. It is really what makes us human and what distinguishes us as civilized creatures.
>
> Being "civilized" humans means being "whole" humans. Education must address the mind, body, and soul of students. It would be detrimental to society if our schools were myopic in their focus, only meeting the needs of the mind. As humans, we are multi-dimensional, multi-faceted

311

beings who need more than head knowledge to survive. The human heart and psyche have to be fed in order for the mind to develop properly, and the body must be maintained and exercised to help fuel the working of the brain.

Education is a basic human right, and it allows us to sustain a democratic society in which participation is fundamental to its success. It should inspire students to seek better solutions to world problems and to dream of a more equitable society. Education should never discriminate on any basis, and it should create individuals who are self-sufficient, patriotic, and tolerant of other's ideas.

All children can learn, although not all children learn in the same manner. All children learn best, however, when their basic physical needs are met, and they feel safe, secure, and loved. Students are much more responsive to a teacher who values them and shows them respect as individual people. Teachers must model at all times the way they expect students to treat them and their peers. If teachers set high expectations for their students, the students will rise to that high level. Teachers must make the well-being of their students their primary focus and must not be afraid to let their students learn from their own mistakes.

In the modern age of technology, a teacher's focus is no longer the "what" of the content, but more importantly, the "why." Students are bombarded with information and have access to ANY information they need right at their fingertips. Teachers have to work harder than ever before to help students identify salient information and to think critically about the information they encounter. Students have to read between the lines, identify bias, and determine who they can trust in the milieu of ads, data, and texts presented to them.

Schools must work in consort with families in this important mission. While children spend most of their time in school, they are dramatically and indelibly shaped by the influences of their family and culture. Teachers must not only respect this fact but must strive to include parents in the education of their children and must work to keep parents informed of progress and problems. Communication between classroom and home is essential for a child's success.

Humans have always aspired to be more, do more, and to better ourselves and our communities. This is where education lies, right at the heart of humanity's desire to be all that we can be. Education helps us strive for higher goals and better treatment of ourselves and others. I shudder to think what would become of us if education ceased to be the "last bastion of civility." We must be unapologetic about expecting excellence from our students—our very existence depends upon it.

15. Which of the following best summarizes the author's main point?
    a. Education as we know it is over-valued in modern society, and we should find alternative solutions.
    b. The survival of the human race depends on the educational system, and it is worth fighting for to make it better.
    c. The government should do away with all public schools and require parents to home school their children instead.
    d. While education is important, some children simply are not capable of succeeding in a traditional classroom.

16. Based on this passage, which of the following can be inferred about the author?
    a. The author feels passionately about education.
    b. The author does not feel strongly about his point.
    c. The author is angry at the educational system.
    d. The author is unsure about the importance of education.

17. Based on this passage, which of the following conclusions could be drawn about the author?
    a. The author would not support raising taxes to help fund much needed reforms in education.
    b. The author would support raising taxes to help fund much needed reforms in education, as long as those reforms were implemented in higher socio-economic areas first.
    c. The author would support raising taxes to help fund much needed reforms in education for all children in all schools.
    d. The author would support raising taxes only in certain states to help fund much needed reforms in education.

18. According to the passage, which of the following is not mentioned as an important factor in education today?
    a. Parent involvement
    b. Communication between parents and teachers
    c. Impact of technology
    d. Cost of textbooks

Questions 19–27 are based upon the following passage:

This excerpt is an adaptation from Charles Dickens' speech in Birmingham in England on December 30, 1853 on behalf of the Birmingham and Midland Institute.

> My Good Friends,—When I first imparted to the committee of the projected Institute my particular wish that on one of the evenings of my readings here the main body of my audience should be composed of working men and their families, I was animated by two desires; first, by the wish to have the great pleasure of meeting you face to face at this Christmas time, and accompany you myself through one of my little Christmas books; and second, by the wish to have an opportunity of stating publicly in your presence, and in the presence of the committee, my earnest hope that the Institute will, from the beginning, recognise one great principle—strong in reason and justice—which I believe to be essential to the very life of such an Institution. It is, that the working man shall, from the first unto the last, have a share in the management of an Institution which is designed for his benefit, and which calls itself by his name.
>
> I have no fear here of being misunderstood—of being supposed to mean too much in this. If there ever was a time when any one class could of itself do much for its own good, and for the welfare of society—which I greatly doubt—that time is unquestionably past. It is in the fusion of different classes, without confusion; in the bringing together of employers and employed; in the creating of a better common understanding among those whose interests are identical, who depend upon each other, who are vitally essential to each other, and who never can be in unnatural antagonism without deplorable results, that one of the chief principles of a Mechanics' Institution should consist. In this world a great deal of the bitterness among us arises

313

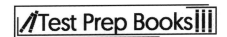

from an imperfect understanding of one another. Erect in Birmingham a great Educational Institution, properly educational; educational of the feelings as well as of the reason; to which all orders of Birmingham men contribute; in which all orders of Birmingham men meet; wherein all orders of Birmingham men are faithfully represented—and you will erect a Temple of Concord here which will be a model edifice to the whole of England.

Contemplating as I do the existence of the Artisans' Committee, which not long ago considered the establishment of the Institute so sensibly, and supported it so heartily, I earnestly entreat the gentlemen—earnest I know in the good work, and who are now among us,—by all means to avoid the great shortcoming of similar institutions; and in asking the working man for his confidence, to set him the great example and give him theirs in return. You will judge for yourselves if I promise too much for the working man, when I say that he will stand by such an enterprise with the utmost of his patience, his perseverance, sense, and support; that I am sure he will need no charitable aid or condescending patronage; but will readily and cheerfully pay for the advantages which it confers; that he will prepare himself in individual cases where he feels that the adverse circumstances around him have rendered it necessary; in a word, that he will feel his responsibility like an honest man, and will most honestly and manfully discharge it. I now proceed to the pleasant task to which I assure you I have looked forward for a long time.

19. Which word is most closely synonymous with the word *patronage* as it appears in the following statement?

...that I am sure he will need no charitable aid or condescending patronage

a. Auspices
b. Aberration
c. Acerbic
d. Adulation

20. Which term is most closely aligned with the definition of the term *working man* as it is defined in the following passage?

You will judge for yourselves if I promise too much for the working man, when I say that he will stand by such an enterprise with the utmost of his patience, his perseverance, sense, and support...

a. Plebeian
b. Viscount
c. Entrepreneur
d. Bourgeois

314

21. Based upon the contextual evidence provided in the passage above, what is the meaning of the term *enterprise* in the third paragraph?
    a. Company
    b. Courage
    c. Game
    d. Cause

22. The speaker addresses his audience as *My Good Friends*—what kind of credibility does this salutation give to the speaker?
    a. The speaker is an employer addressing his employees, so the salutation is a way for the boss to bridge the gap between himself and his employees.
    b. The speaker's salutation is one from an entertainer to his audience and uses the friendly language to connect to his audience before a serious speech.
    c. The salutation gives the serious speech that follows a somber tone, as it is used ironically.
    d. The speech is one from a politician to the public, so the salutation is used to grab the audience's attention.

23. According to the aforementioned passage, what is the speaker's second desire for his time in front of the audience?
    a. To read a Christmas story
    b. For the working man to have a say in his institution which is designed for his benefit
    c. To have an opportunity to stand in their presence
    d. For the life of the institution to be essential to the audience as a whole

24. The speaker's tone in the passage can be described as:
    a. Happy and gullible
    b. Lazy and entitled
    c. Confident and informed
    d. Angry and frustrated

25. One of the main purposes of the last paragraph is:
    a. To persuade the audience to support the Institute no matter what since it provided so much support to the working class.
    b. To market the speaker's new book while at the same time supporting the activities of the Institute.
    c. To inform the audience that the Institute is corrupt and will not help them out when the time comes to give them compensation.
    d. To provide credibility to the working man and share confidence in their ability to take on responsibilities if they are compensated appropriately.

26. According to the passage, what does the speaker wish to erect in Birmingham?
    a. An Educational Institution
    b. The Temple of Concord
    c. A Writing Workshop
    d. A VA Hospital

315

27. As it is used in the second paragraph, the word *antagonism* most nearly means:
    a. Conformity
    b. Opposition
    c. Affluence
    d. Scarcity

Questions 28–31 refer to the following passage:

> Although many Missourians know that Harry S. Truman and Walt Disney hailed from their great state, probably far fewer know that it was also home to the remarkable George Washington Carver. At the end of the Civil War, Moses Carver, the slave owner who owned George's parents, decided to keep George and his brother and raise them on his farm. As a child, George was driven to learn and he loved painting. He even went on to study art while in college but was encouraged to pursue botany instead. He spent much of his life helping others by showing them better ways to farm; his ideas improved agricultural productivity in many countries. One of his most notable contributions to the newly emerging class of Black farmers was to teach them the negative effects of agricultural monoculture, i.e. growing the same crops in the same fields year after year, depleting the soil of much needed nutrients and resulting in a lesser yielding crop. Carver was an innovator, always thinking of new and better ways to do things, and is most famous for his over three hundred uses for the peanut. Toward the end of his career, Carver returned to his first love of art. Through his artwork, he hoped to inspire people to see the beauty around them and to do great things themselves. When Carver died, he left his money to help fund ongoing agricultural research. Today, people still visit and study at the George Washington Carver Foundation at Tuskegee Institute.

28. Which of the following describes the kind of writing used in the above passage?
    a. Narrative
    b. Persuasive
    c. Technical
    d. Expository

29. According to the passage, what was George Washington Carver's first love?
    a. Plants
    b. Art
    c. Animals
    d. Soil

30. According to the passage, what is the best definition for agricultural monoculture?
    a. The practice of producing or growing a single crop or plant species over a wide area and for a large number of consecutive years
    b. The practice of growing a diversity of crops and rotating them from year to year
    c. The practice of growing crops organically to avoid the use of pesticides
    d. The practice of charging an inflated price for cheap crops to obtain a greater profit margin

31. Which of the following is the best summary of this passage?
    a. George Washington Carver was born at a time when scientific discovery was at a virtual standstill.
    b. Because he was African American, there were not many opportunities for George Washington Carver.
    c. George Washington Carver was an intelligent man whose research and discoveries had an impact worldwide.
    d. George Washington Carver was far more successful as an artist than he was as a scientist.

Questions 32–36 are based upon the following passage:

This excerpt is an adaptation from *The Life-Story of Insects,* by Geo H. Carpenter.

> Insects as a whole are preeminently creatures of the land and the air. This is shown not only by the possession of wings by a vast majority of the class, but by the mode of breathing to which reference has already been made, a system of branching air-tubes carrying atmospheric air with its combustion-supporting oxygen to all the insect's tissues. The air gains access to these tubes through a number of paired air-holes or spiracles, arranged segmentally in series.
>
> It is of great interest to find that, nevertheless, a number of insects spend much of their time under water. This is true of not a few in the perfect winged state, as for example aquatic beetles and water-bugs ('boatmen' and 'scorpions') which have some way of protecting their spiracles when submerged, and, possessing usually the power of flight, can pass on occasion from pond or stream to upper air. But it is advisable in connection with our present subject to dwell especially on some insects that remain continually under water till they are ready to undergo their final moult and attain the winged state, which they pass entirely in the air. The preparatory instars of such insects are aquatic; the adult instar is aerial. All may-flies, dragon-flies, and caddis-flies, many beetles and two-winged flies, and a few moths thus divide their life-story between the water and the air. For the present we confine attention to the Stone-flies, the May-flies, and the Dragon-flies, three well-known orders of insects respectively called by systematists the Plecoptera, the Ephemeroptera and the Odonata.
>
> In the case of many insects that have aquatic larvae, the latter are provided with some arrangement for enabling them to reach atmospheric air through the surface-film of the water. But the larva of a stone-fly, a dragon-fly, or a may-fly is adapted more completely than these for aquatic life; it can, by means of gills of some kind, breathe the air dissolved in water.

32. Which statement best details the central idea in this passage?
    a. It introduces certain insects that transition from water to air.
    b. It delves into entomology, especially where gills are concerned.
    c. It defines what constitutes as insects' breathing.
    d. It invites readers to have a hand in the preservation of insects.

33. Which definition most closely relates to the usage of the word *moult* in the passage?
    a. An adventure of sorts, especially underwater
    b. Mating act between two insects
    c. The act of shedding part or all of the outer shell
    d. Death of an organism that ends in a revival of life

34. What is the purpose of the first paragraph in relation to the second paragraph?
    a. The first paragraph serves as a cause, and the second paragraph serves as an effect.
    b. The first paragraph serves as a contrast to the second.
    c. The first paragraph is a description for the argument in the second paragraph.
    d. The first and second paragraphs are merely presented in a sequence.

35. What does the following sentence most nearly mean:

    The preparatory instars of such insects are aquatic; the adult instar is aerial.

    a. The volume of water is necessary to prep the insect for transition rather than the volume of the air.
    b. The abdomen of the insect is designed like a star in the water as well as the air.
    c. The stage of preparation in between molting is acted out in the water, while the last stage is in the air.
    d. These insects breathe first in the water through gills yet continue to use the same organs to breathe in the air.

36. Which of the statements reflect information that one could reasonably infer based on the author's tone?
    a. The author's tone is persuasive and attempts to call the audience to action.
    b. The author's tone is passionate due to excitement over the subject and personal narrative.
    c. The author's tone is informative and exhibits interest in the subject of the study.
    d. The author's tone is somber, depicting some anger at the state of insect larvae.

Questions 37–39 are based on the following passage:

Random Lake Advertisement

> Who needs the hassle of traveling far away? This summer, why not rent a house on Random Lake? Located conveniently ten miles away from Random City, Random Lake has everything a family needs. Swimming, kayaking, boating, fishing, volleyball, mini-golf, go-cart track, eagle watching, nature trails—there are enough activities here to keep a family busy for a month, much less a week.

> Random Lake hotels are available for every lifestyle and budget. Prefer a pool or free breakfast? Prefer quiet? Historical? Modern? No problem. The Random Lake area has got you covered. House rentals are affordable too. During the summer months, rentals can go as cheaply as 600 dollars a week. Even better deals can be found during the off season. Most homes come fully furnished, and pontoon boats, kayaks, and paddle boats are available for rental. With the Legends and the Broadmoor developments slated for grand openings in March, the choices are endless!

37. The main purpose of this passage is to do what?
    a. Describe
    b. Inform
    c. Persuade
    d. Entertain

38. Which of the following sentences is out of place and should be removed?
    a. "This summer, why not rent a house on Random Lake?"
    b. "There are enough activities here to keep a family busy for a month."
    c. "Pontoon boats, kayaks, and paddle boats are available for rental."
    d. "With several new housing developments slated for grand opening in March, the choices are endless!"

39. Which of the following can be deduced from Passages 1 and 2?
    a. Random City is more populated than Random Lake.
    b. The Random Lake area is newer than Random City.
    c. The Random Lake area is growing.
    d. Random Lake prefers families to couples.

Questions 40–42 are based upon the following passage:

This excerpt is an adaptation from "What to the Slave is the Fourth of July?" Rochester, New York, July 5, 1852.

Fellow citizens—Pardon me, and allow me to ask, why am I called upon to speak here today? What have I, or those I represent, to do with your national independence? Are the great principles of political freedom and of natural justice, embodied in that Declaration of Independence, extended to us? And am I therefore called upon to bring our humble offering to the national altar, and to confess the benefits, and express devout gratitude for the blessings, resulting from your independence to us?

Would to God, both for your sakes and ours, ours that an affirmative answer could be truthfully returned to these questions! Then would my task be light, and my burden easy and delightful. For who is there so cold that a nation's sympathy could not warm him? Who so obdurate and dead to the claims of gratitude that would not thankfully acknowledge such priceless benefits? Who so stolid and selfish, that would not give his voice to swell the hallelujahs of a nation's jubilee, when the chains of servitude had been torn from his limbs? I am not that man. In a case like that, the dumb may eloquently speak, and the lame man leap as an hart.

But, such is not the state of the case. I say it with a sad sense of the disparity between us. I am not included within the pale of this glorious anniversary. Oh pity! Your high independence only reveals the immeasurable distance between us. The blessings in which you this day rejoice, I do not enjoy in common. The rich inheritance of justice, liberty, prosperity, and independence, bequeathed by your fathers, is shared by *you*, not by *me*. This Fourth of July is *yours,* not *mine.* You may rejoice, *I* must mourn. To drag a man in fetters into the grand illuminated temple of liberty, and call upon him to join you in joyous anthems, were inhuman mockery and sacrilegious irony. Do you mean,

319

citizens, to mock me, by asking me to speak today? If so there is a parallel to your conduct. And let me warn you that it is dangerous to copy the example of a nation whose crimes, towering up to heaven, were thrown down by the breath of the Almighty, burying that nation and irrecoverable ruin! I can today take up the plaintive lament of a peeled and woe-smitten people.

By the rivers of Babylon, there we sat down. Yea! We wept when we remembered Zion. We hanged our harps upon the willows in the midst thereof. For there, they that carried us away captive, required of us a song; and they who wasted us required of us mirth, saying, "Sing us one of the songs of Zion." How can we sing the Lord's song in a strange land? If I forget thee, O Jerusalem, let my right hand forget her cunning. If I do not remember thee, let my tongue cleave to the roof of my mouth.

40. What is the tone of the first paragraph of this passage?
   a. Exasperated
   b. Inclusive
   c. Contemplative
   d. Nonchalant

41. Which word CANNOT be used synonymously with the term *obdurate* as it is conveyed in the text below?

Who so obdurate and dead to the claims of gratitude, that would not thankfully acknowledge such priceless benefits?

   a. Steadfast
   b. Stubborn
   c. Contented
   d. Unwavering

42. What is the central purpose of this text?
   a. To demonstrate the author's extensive knowledge of the Bible
   b. To address the hypocrisy of the Fourth of July holiday
   c. To convince wealthy landowners to adopt new holiday rituals
   d. To explain why minorities often relished the notion of segregation in government institutions

Questions 43–46 are based on the following passage:

The more immediately after the commission of a crime a punishment is inflicted, the more just and useful it will be. It will be more just, because it spares the criminal the cruel and superfluous torment of uncertainty, which increases in proportion to the strength of his imagination and the sense of his weakness; and because the privation of liberty, being a punishment, ought to be inflicted before condemnation, but for as short a time as possible. Imprisonments, I say, being only the means of securing the person of the accused, until he be tried, condemned, or acquitted, ought not only to be of as short duration, but attended with as little severity as possible. The time should be determined by the necessary preparation for the trial, and the right of priority in the oldest prisoners. The confinement ought not to be closer than is requisite to prevent his flight, or his concealing the proofs of the crime; and the trial should be conducted

320

with all possible expedition. Can there be a more cruel contrast than that between the indolence of a judge, and the painful anxiety of the accused; the comforts and pleasures of an insensible magistrate, and the filth and misery of the prisoner? In general, as I have before observed, *the degree of the punishment, and the consequences of a crime, ought to be so contrived, as to have the greatest possible effect on others, with the least possible pain to the delinquent*. If there be any society in which this is not a fundamental principle, it is an unlawful society; for mankind, by their union, originally intended to subject themselves to the least evils possible.

An immediate punishment is more useful; because the smaller the interval of time between the punishment and the crime, the stronger and more lasting will be the association of the two ideas of *Crime* and *Punishment;* so that they may be considered, one as the cause, and the other as the unavoidable and necessary effect. It is demonstrated, that the association of ideas is the cement which unites the fabric of the human intellect; without which, pleasure and pain would be simple and ineffectual sensations. The vulgar, that is, all men who have no general ideas or universal principles, act in consequence of the most immediate and familiar associations; but the more remote and complex only present themselves to the minds of those who are passionately attached to a single object, or to those of greater understanding, who have acquired an habit of rapidly comparing together a number of objects, and of forming a conclusion; and the result, that is, the action in consequence, by these means, becomes less dangerous and uncertain.

It is, then, of the greatest importance, that the punishment should succeed the crime as immediately as possible, if we intend, that, in the rude minds of the multitude, the seducing picture of the advantage arising from the crime, should instantly awake the attendant idea of punishment. Delaying the punishment serves only to separate these two ideas; and thus affects the minds of the spectators rather as being a terrible sight than the necessary consequence of a crime; the horror of which should contribute to heighten the idea of the punishment.

There is another excellent method of strengthening this important connexion between the ideas of crime and punishment; that is, to make the punishment as analogous as possible to the nature of the crime; in order that the punishment may lead the mind to consider the crime in a different point of view, from that in which it was placed by the flattering idea of promised advantages.

Crimes of less importance are commonly punished, either in the obscurity of a prison, or the criminal is *transported*, to give, by his slavery, an example to societies which he never offended; an example absolutely useless, because distant from the place where the crime was committed. Men do not, in general, commit great crimes deliberately, but rather in a sudden gust of passion; and they commonly look on the punishment due to a great crime as remote and improbable. The public punishment, therefore, of small crimes will make a greater impression, and, by deterring men from the smaller, will effectually prevent the greater.

(Cesare Beccaria, "Punishments, Advantages of Immediate," *The Criminal Recorder,* 1810).

43. What is the main purpose of this passage?
    a. To describe
    b. To inform
    c. To persuade
    d. To entertain

44. Which of the following excerpts best exemplifies the main idea of this passage?
    a. "The vulgar, that is, all men who have no general ideas or universal principles, act in consequence of the most immediate and familiar associations."
    b. "Crimes of less importance are commonly punished, either in the obscurity of a prison, or the criminal is *transported*, to give, by his slavery, an example to societies which he never offended."
    c. "Men do not, in general, commit great crimes deliberately, but rather in a sudden gust of passion; and they commonly look on the punishment due to a great crime as remote and improbable."
    d. "The more immediately after the commission of a crime a punishment is inflicted, the more just and useful it will be."

45. With which of the following statements would the author most likely disagree?
    a. Criminals are incapable of connecting crime and punishment.
    b. A punishment should quickly follow the crime.
    c. Most criminals do not think about the consequences of their actions.
    d. Where a criminal is punished is just as important as when.

46. Walking through the heavily wooded park by the river in October, I was amazed at the beautiful colors of the foliage, the bright blue sky, and the crystal-clear water.

    Using the context clues in the preceding sentence, which of the following words is the correct meaning of the word foliage?

    a. Leaves of the trees
    b. Feathers of the birds
    c. Tree bark
    d. Rocks on the path

Questions 47–55 are based on the following passage:

I heartily accept the motto, "that government is best which governs least," and I should like to see it acted up to more rapidly and systematically. Carried out, it finally amounts to this, which also I believe—"that government is best which governs not at all," and when men are prepared for it, that will be the kind of government which they will have. Government is at best but an expedient; but most governments are usually, and all governments are sometimes, inexpedient. The objections which have been brought against a standing army, and they are many and weighty, and deserve to prevail, may also at last be brought against a standing government. The standing army is only an arm of the standing government. The government itself, which is only the mode which the people have chosen to execute their will, is equally liable to be abused and perverted before the people can act through it. Witness the present Mexican war, the work of comparatively a few individuals using the standing government as their tool; for, in the outset, the people would not have consented to this measure.

322

This American government—what is it but a tradition, though a recent one, endeavoring to transmit itself unimpaired to posterity, but each instant losing some of its integrity? It has not the vitality and force of a single living man; for a single man can bend it to his will. It is a sort of wooden gun to the people themselves. But it is not the less necessary for this; for the people must have some complicated machinery or other, and hear its din, to satisfy that idea of government which they have. Governments show thus how successfully men can be imposed on, even impose on themselves, for their own advantage. It is excellent, we must all allow. Yet this government never of itself furthered any enterprise, but by the alacrity with which it got out of its way. It does not keep the country free. It does not settle the West. It does not educate. The character inherent in the American people has done all that has been accomplished; and it would have done somewhat more, if the government had not sometimes got in its way. For government is an expedient by which men would fain succeed in letting one another alone; and, as has been said, when it is most expedient, the governed are most let alone by it. Trade and commerce, if they were not made of India-rubber, would never manage to bounce over the obstacles which legislators are continually putting in their way; and, if one were to judge these men wholly by the effects of their actions and not partly by their intentions, they would deserve to be classed and punished with those mischievous persons who put obstructions on the railroads.

But, to speak practically and as a citizen, unlike those who call themselves no-government men, I ask for, not at once no government, but at once a better government. Let every man make known what kind of government would command his respect, and that will be one step toward obtaining it.

Excerpt from *Civil Disobedience* by Henry David Thoreau

47. Which phrase best encapsulates Thoreau's use of the term *expedient* in the first paragraph?
    a. A dead end
    b. A state of order
    c. A means to an end
    d. Rushed construction

48. Which best describes Thoreau's view on the Mexican War?
    a. Government is inherently corrupt because it must wage war.
    b. Government can easily be manipulated by a few individuals for their own agenda.
    c. Government is a tool for the people, but it can also act against their interest.
    d. The Mexican War was a necessary action, but not all the people believed this.

49. What is Thoreau's purpose for writing?
    a. His goal is to illustrate how government can function if ideals are maintained.
    b. He wants to prove that true democracy is the best government, but it can be corrupted easily.
    c. Thoreau reflects on the stages of government abuses.
    d. He is seeking to prove that government is easily corruptible and inherently restrictive of individual freedoms that can simultaneously affect the whole state.

323

50. Which example best supports Thoreau's argument?
    a. A vote carries in the Senate to create a new road tax.
    b. The president vetoes the new FARM bill.
    c. Prohibition is passed to outlaw alcohol.
    d. Trade is opened between the United States and Iceland.

51. Which best summarizes this section from the following passage?

    "This American government—what is it but a tradition, though a recent one, endeavoring to transmit itself unimpaired to posterity, but each instant losing some of its integrity? It has not the vitality and force of a single living man; for a single man can bend it to his will. It is a sort of wooden gun to the people themselves."

    a. The government may be instituted to ensure the protections of freedoms, but this is weakened by the fact that it is easily manipulated by individuals.
    b. Unlike an individual, government is uncaring.
    c. Unlike an individual, government has no will, making it more prone to be used as a weapon against the people.
    d. American government is modeled after other traditions but actually has greater potential to be used to control people.

52. According to Thoreau, what's the main reason why government eventually fails to achieve progress?
    a. There are too many rules.
    b. Legislation eventually becomes a hindrance to the lives and work of everyday people.
    c. Trade and wealth eventually become the driving factor of those in government.
    d. Government doesn't separate religion and state.

53. As it is used in the first paragraph, the word *liable* most nearly means:
    a. Paramount
    b. Inconceivable
    c. Susceptible
    d. Detrimental

54. According to the passage, which government is Thoreau talking about?
    a. Mexican
    b. American
    c. Chinese
    d. British

55. As it is used in the second paragraph, the word *posterity* most nearly means:
    a. Persons of royal lineage.
    b. All future generations of people.
    c. A person involved in directing education.
    d. A person who offers views on important life questions

324

Vocabulary

1. What word meaning "harshly criticizing" best fits in the following sentence:

The charge nurse was fired for frequently _____ the staff.

a. Macerating
b. Extoling
c. Lauding
d. Denigrating

2. Select the correct meaning of the underlined word in the following sentence:

The patient's cheeks appeared <u>ruddy</u>.

a. Swollen or puffy
b. Edematous
c. Flushed
d. Discolored or blotchy

3. What word meaning "to infer" best fits in the following sentence:

The nurse was able to _____ that the patient was allergic to the ointment.

a. Deduce
b. Induce
c. Conjecture
d. Construct

4. What word meaning "unexpected and unfortunate" best fits in the following sentence:

It was _____ circumstances that landed the patient in the ER.

a. Adversary
b. Untoward
c. Undulated
d. Unobstructed

5. What is the best definition of the word *chorea*?
a. A digestive condition common in infants
b. An abnormal discharge from any body orifice, particularly the ears or eyes
c. Any disorder of the nervous system that includes involuntary, jerky movements
d. Weakness of the peripheral muscles

6. Select the correct meaning of the underlined word in the following sentence:

The nurse informed the toddler's mother that the boy should start to sleep better once the cause of his <u>pruritis</u> was identified and treated.

a. Vomiting
b. Ringing in the ears
c. Insomnia
d. Itchiness

7. What word meaning "on the same side" best fits in the following sentence:

The patient complained of _____ shoulder and wrist pain.

a. Bilateral
b. Ipsilateral
c. Contralateral
d. Alateral

8. Select the correct meaning of the underlined word in the following sentence:

The medication side effects that the patient experienced were <u>diaphoresis</u> and dizziness.

a. Excessive sweating
b. Dyspnea
c. Wheezing
d. Frequent urination

9. Select the correct meaning of the underlined word in the following sentence:

The nurse explained the risk factors for contracting a <u>venereal</u> disease.

a. Vector-borne
b. Sexually-transmitted
c. Relating to the gums
d. Parasitic

10. What word meaning "to renounce" best fits in the following sentence:

After witnessing the consequences of smoking on his dental health, the patient decided to _____ his beliefs that smoking was harmless.

a. Abstain
b. Inculcate
c. Abjure
d. Interrogate

11. What is the best definition of the word *deleterious*?
    a. Removable
    b. Excision
    c. Harmful
    d. Deferable

12. What word meaning "inability to feel pleasure" best fits in the following sentence:

    The nurse referred the patient to a psychologist on account of his insomnia and _____.

    a. Athetosis
    b. Depression
    c. Contentment
    d. Anhedonia

13. Select the correct meaning of the underlined word in the following sentence:

    The doctor studied the newborn's face for <u>nuances</u> in expression.

    a. Apparent disparities
    b. Subtle differences
    c. Drastic changes
    d. Visual cues

14. What word meaning "further from the trunk" best fits in the following sentence:

    The ankle is _____ to the knee.

    a. Dorsal
    b. Distal
    c. Proximal
    d. Ventral

15. What word meaning "apathetic" or "composed" best fits in the following sentence:

    The _____ demeanor of the patient made it difficult to read his true level of pain.

    a. Egregious
    b. Insolent
    c. Impervious
    d. Phlegmatic

16. What word meaning "caused or produced by an agent outside the body" best fits in the following sentence:

Use of _____ testosterone had reduced his body's ability to produce the hormone.

    a. Steroid
    b. Organic
    c. Exogenous
    d. Endogenous

17. Fortify most nearly means which of the following?
    a. Foster
    b. Barricade
    c. Strengthen
    d. Undermine

18. What word meaning "body wasting usually due to chronic illness" best fits in the following sentence:

Over time, it became clear that her uncontrolled AIDS had caused _____.

    a. Catatonia
    b. Anorexia
    c. Ataxia
    d. Cachexia

19. What is the best definition of the word *palpate*?
    a. Fluttering
    b. An abnormal heartbeat
    c. To physically examine using touch
    d. To splint or support a body part

20. Select the correct meaning of the underlined word in the following sentence:

The patient with the transtibial amputation used crutches as an <u>auxiliary</u> aid.

    a. Relating to the armpit
    b. Prosthetic
    c. Ambulatory
    d. Ancillary

21. What word meaning "innocent" best fits in the following sentence:

The young child's _____ expression was sweet and endearing.

    a. Guileless
    b. Cunning
    c. Begrudging
    d. Vapid

22. What is the best definition of the word *vacuous*?
    a. Inane
    b. A cellular organelle
    c. Suction
    d. Ingenious

23. Select the correct meaning of the underlined word in the following sentence:

    The charge nurse was a good leader because she had <u>gravitas</u> and commanded respect.

    a. Intelligence
    b. Dignity
    c. Gratitude
    d. Somberness

24. What word meaning "sticking together of membranous surfaces" best fits in the following sentence:

    The biker had _____ along his scar tissue.

    a. Adhesions
    b. Abrasions
    c. Contusions
    d. Avulsions

25. Select the correct meaning of the underlined word in the following sentence:

    An ultrasound was ordered to image the patient's <u>hepatic</u> portal system.

    a. Relating to the pancreas
    b. Relating to the liver
    c. Relating to the kidney
    d. Relating to gallbladder

26. What is the best definition of the word *peritoneum*?
    a. The smooth muscular contractions that propel food along the digestive tract
    b. The region between the anus and scrotum
    c. The outer connective tissue layer covering bones
    d. The serous membrane lining the abdominal cavity

27. Select the correct meaning of the underlined word in the following sentence:

    The <u>vehement</u> speeches from former patients motivated many donors to increase their pledges.

    a. Ardent
    b. Motivational
    c. Novel
    d. Virulent

329

28. What word meaning "the space inside a hollow or tubular structure" best fits in the following sentence:

The atherosclerotic plaques decreased the volume of the arterial _____.

   a. Lumen
   b. Constriction
   c. Angioplasty
   d. Vessel

29. What word meaning "confused" best fits in the following sentence:

Upon waking from the procedure, the patient was _____.

   a. Lucid
   b. Anesthetized
   c. Befuddled
   d. Diffident

30. Select the medical term for a "bed sore."
   a. Decubitus ulcer
   b. Duodenal ulcer
   c. Neurotropic ulcer
   d. Ischemic ulcer

31. What word meaning to "conduct towards something" best fits in the following sentence:

The _____ nerve carried the signal from the receptor to the spinal cord.

   a. Stimuli
   b. Interneuron
   c. Efferent
   d. Afferent

32. What is the best definition of the word *eschar*?
   a. Scar tissue
   b. Skin ulcer
   c. Dark scab
   d. Fistula

33. What is the best definition of the word *pallor*?
   a. Turgor
   b. Flushed skin
   c. Wan
   d. Febrile

34. What is the best definition of the word *rhinorrhea*?
    a. Nasal discharge
    b. Sinus pressure
    c. Sneezing
    d. Nosebleed

35. Select the correct meaning of the underlined word in the following sentence:

    The medication had an <u>intrathecal</u> route of administration.

    a. Under tongue
    b. Around the spinal cord
    c. In the ear
    d. Inside the cheek

36. What is the best definition of the word *lament*?
    a. Verbally express grief
    b. Reconcile
    c. Encourage
    d. Verbally extol

37. What is the best definition of the word *noxious*?
    a. Relating to oxygen
    b. Innocuous
    c. Irritating
    d. Harmful

38. What is the best definition of the word *kyphosis*?
    a. An abnormal lateral curvature of the spine
    b. An inward curvature of the cervical spine
    c. An outward curvature of the thoracic spine
    d. Swayback or the commonly seen excessive curvature of the lumbar spine

39. Select the correct meaning of the underlined word in the following sentence:

    The graduate student's thesis was focused on <u>gerontology</u>.

    a. The study of diseases
    b. The study of growth
    c. The study of genes
    d. The study of aging

40. For which suspected condition might an endoscopy be ordered?
    a. Ulcerative colitis
    b. Peptic ulcer
    c. Angina
    d. Pulmonary embolism

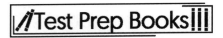

41. What word meaning "uncompromising" best fits in the following sentence:

    The patient remained _____ in his refusal to take medications.

    a. Intransigent
    b. Complacent
    c. Inexplicable
    d. Confound

42. Blood pressure would be recorded as which of the following?
    a. Subjective data
    b. Objective data
    c. Assessment
    d. Plan

43. What is a terminal illness?
    a. One from which a patient will likely not recover
    b. The most recent illness a patient had
    c. One that is not infectious
    d. One that the patient is born with

44. Where is the popliteal fossa located?
    a. The knee
    b. The skull
    c. The hip
    d. The scapula

45. What word meaning "a model of perfection" best fits in the following sentence:

    Her chart notes were a _____ of medical records.

    a. Parable
    b. Paradox
    c. Paragon
    d. Paraphrase

46. Select the correct meaning of the underlined word in the following sentence:

    The hospital room looked <u>pristine</u>.

    a. Unorganized and dingy
    b. Unfriendly
    c. Sterile
    d. Clean and new

47. What is tinnitus?
   a. Ringing in the ear
   b. Temporary deafness
   c. Grinding the teeth
   d. Clicking jaw

48. What does the suffix -itis mean?
   a. Pain
   b. Disease
   c. Inflammation
   d. Tumor

49. What is dysphagia?
   a. Difficulty breathing
   b. Difficulty recognizing faces
   c. Difficulty swallowing
   d. Difficulty speaking

50. What is urticaria?
   a. Burning urine
   b. Kidney stones
   c. Bladder infection
   d. Hives

51. What is the best definition of the word *elucidate*?
   a. Learn
   b. Enlighten
   c. Plan
   d. Corroborate

52. What is the best definition of the word *verify*?
   a. Criticize
   b. Change
   c. Teach
   d. Substantiate

53. What is the best definition of the word *inspire*?
   a. Motivate
   b. Impale
   c. Exercise
   d. Patronize

54. What is the best definition of the word *mendacious*?
   a. Earnest
   b. Bold
   c. Criminal
   d. Liar

333

55. What is the best definition of the word *mitigate*?
    a. alleviate
    b. focus
    c. fiery
    d. conspire

Grammar

1. Which sentence is grammatically correct?
    a. The baseball that is autographed belongs to whom?
    b. The baseball which is autographed belongs to who?
    c. Whom does the baseball which is autographed belong to?
    d. Whom does the baseball that is autographed belong to?

2. Which of the following words is spelled incorrectly?
    a. Caffiene
    b. Counterfeit
    c. Sleigh
    d. Receipt

3. Which sentence is grammatically incorrect?
    a. Will you please bring me the water before you take her the pizza?
    b. Can I put the box on the shelf where you can reach?
    c. Will you lend me your pen so I can sign for my loan?
    d. What if the two of us were to gather too many flowers?

4. Which word combination properly completes the following sentence:

    I hurt my ankle_____ but now it feels _____.

    a. badly/good
    b. bad/good
    c. bad/well
    d. badly/well

5. Which of the following sentences is a fragment?
    a. We went to the zoo to see the tigers and lions.
    b. Instead we saw elephants, zebras and giraffes.
    c. Because the lion and tiger habitat was closed.
    d. What sound does a giraffe make anyway?

6. Which of the following is a run-on sentence?
    a. I love to go water-skiing, I love alpine skiing, I also love Nordic skiing.
    b. The best way to learn to ski is to take lessons.
    c. All three types of skiing require different skills and different equipment.
    d. It takes a long time to learn how to ski; waterskiing takes the longest time.

334

7. Which sentence has a dangling modifier?
    a. Eating a large meal, I had to chew my food slowly.
    b. Eating a large meal, my food had to be chewed slowly.
    c. Eating a large meal, I was too full afterward.
    d. Eating a large meal, I was more full than I have ever been.

8. Which sentence is an example of a double negative?
    a. She couldn't find anything to say.
    b. He did like something she said.
    c. They didn't like nothing I said.
    d. I cannot say I don't disapprove of that.

9. What is the subject complement in the following sentence:

Pulling heavy rope helps strengthen muscles.

    a. Heavy rope
    b. Muscles
    c. Strengthen
    d. Pulling heavy rope

10. Which version of the following sentence has correct capitalization?

"i told mother about my favorite book: *all the light we cannot see,*" said martha. "she liked it."

    a. "i Told mother about my Favorite Book: *all the light we cannot see,*" Said martha. "she Liked it.
    b. "I told mother about my favorite Book: *All The Light We Cannot See,*" Said Martha. "she liked it."
    c. "I told Mother about my favorite book: *All the Light We Cannot See,*" said Martha. "She liked it."
    d. I told Mother about my favorite book: ALL THE LIGHT WE CANNOT SEE," said Martha. "She liked it."

11. Which sentence below is punctuated correctly with periods?
    a. It's 2 pm and I've forgotten my appointment with Dr Samson
    b. It's 2PM and I've forgotten my appointment with Dr. Samson
    c. It's 2 P.M. and I've forgotten my appointment with Dr. Samson.
    d. It's 2 P.M. and I've forgotten. my appointment with Dr Samson.

12. Which sentence below is punctuated correctly with a question mark?
    a. Can you please take the garbage out?
    b. I wonder if anyone has taken the garbage out?
    c. Miles asked Lisa if she'd taken out the garbage?
    d. Didn't anybody take the garbage out?

13. Which sentence below is punctuated correctly with an exclamation mark?
    a. Can you eat more than one slice of pizza!
    b. Yikes! That startled me!
    c. The cow jumped over the moon?!
    d. That's impossible!!!!!

335

14. Which sentence below is punctuated correctly with commas?
    a. The sample consisted of several cheeses, two, meats, and three, crackers.
    b. Mother Teresa, a humanitarian, said, "Be kind to one another."
    c. Hello friend, how have you been, lately?
    d. He ate too much food, consequently, he had a stomachache and heartburn.

15. Which sentence is punctuated correctly with colons and semicolons?
    a. There are four people who are most important to me; my husband Harold; my daughter Sarah; my friend Debbie; and my sister Jenna.
    b. There are four people; who are most important to me: my husband Harold, my daughter Sarah, my friend Debbie, and my sister Jenna.
    c. There are four people who are most important to me; my husband: Harold, my daughter: Sarah, my friend: Debbie, and my sister: Jenna
    d. There are four people who are most important to me: my husband, Harold; my daughter, Sarah; my friend, Debbie; and my sister, Jenna.

16. Which quotation is punctuated correctly?
    a. Daniel said, "I want to travel to Mars."
    b. Daniel said "I want to travel to Mars".
    c. Daniel said, I want to "travel to Mars".
    d. "Daniel said I want to travel to Mars."

17. Which subject/verb agreement makes the following sentence grammatically correct?

    The _____ _____ at the championship on March 7ᵗʰ.

    a. teams/competes
    b. teams/wins
    c. team/competes
    d. team/win

18. Which sentence shows grammatically correct subject/verb agreement?
    a. The professor of physics compliments the student.
    b. The professor of physics compliment the student.
    c. The professors of physics compliments the student.
    d. The professors of physics will compliments the student.

19. Which sentence below does not contain an error in comma usage for dates?
    a. My niece arrives from Australia on Monday, February 4, 2016.
    b. My cousin's wedding this Saturday June 9, conflicts with my best friend's birthday party.
    c. The project is due on Tuesday, May, 17, 2016.
    d. I can't get a flight home until Thursday September 21.

20. Which of the following sentences uses correct spelling?
    a. Although he believed himself to be a consciensious judge of character, his judgment in this particular situation was grossly erroneous.
    b. Although he believed himself to be a conscientious judge of character, his judgment in this particular situation was grossly erroneous.
    c. Although he believed himself to be a conscientious judge of character, his judgement in this particular situation was grossly erroneous.
    d. Although he believed himself to be a conciencious judge of character, his judgemant in this particular situation was grossly erroneous.

21. The stress of preparing for the exam was starting to take its toll on me.

    In the preceding sentence, what part of speech is the word *stress*?

    a. Verb
    b. Noun
    c. Adjective
    d. Adverb

22. Select the example that uses the correct plural form.
    a. Rooves
    b. Octopi
    c. Potatos
    d. Fishes

23. Which of these examples uses correct punctuation?
    a. The presenter said, "The award goes to," and my heart skipped a beat.
    b. The presenter said, "The award goes to" and my heart skipped a beat.
    c. The presenter said "The award goes to" and my heart skipped a beat.
    d. The presenter said, "The award goes to", and my heart skipped a beat.

24. Select the sentence in which the word *counter* functions as an adjective.
    a. The kitchen counter was marred and scratched from years of use.
    b. He countered my offer for the car, but it was still much higher than I was prepared to pay.
    c. Her counter argument was very well presented and logically thought out.
    d. Some of the board's proposals ran counter to the administration's policies.

25. In which of the following sentences does the pronoun correctly agree with its antecedent?
    a. Human beings on the planet have the right to his share of clean water, food, and shelter.
    b. Human beings on the planet have the right to their share of clean water, food, and shelter.
    c. Human beings on the planet have the right to its share of clean water, food, and shelter.
    d. Human beings on the planet have the right to her share of clean water, food, and shelter.

26. Every single one of my mother's siblings, their spouses, and their children met in Colorado for a week-long family vacation last summer.

   Which of the following is the complete subject of the preceding sentence?

   a. Every single one
   b. Siblings, spouses, children
   c. One
   d. Every single one of my mother's siblings, their spouses, and their children

27. Which of the following sentences incorrectly uses italics?
   a. *Old Yeller* is a classic in children's literature, yet very few young people today have read it or even seen the movie.
   b. My favorite musical of all time has to be *The Sound of Music* followed closely by *Les Miserables*.
   c. Langston Hughes's famous poem *Dreams* is the most anthologized of all his works.
   d. When I went to the Louvre, I was surprised at how small Leonardo de Vinci's *Mona Lisa* is compared to other paintings.

28. Which of the following sentences employs correct usage?
   a. It's always a better idea to ask permission first rather than ask for forgiveness later.
   b. Its always a better idea to ask permission first rather than ask for forgiveness later.
   c. It's always a better idea to ask permission first rather then ask for forgiveness later.
   d. Its always a better idea to ask permission first rather then ask for forgiveness later.

29. Which of the following is an imperative sentence?
   a. The state flower of Texas is the blue bonnet.
   b. Do you know if the team is playing in the finals or not?
   c. Take the first right turn, and then go one block west.
   d. We won in overtime!

30. Identify the compound sentence from the following examples:
   a. John and Adam met for coffee before going to class.
   b. As I was leaving, my dad called and needed to talk.
   c. I ran before work and went to the gym afterward for an hour or so.
   d. Felix plays the guitar in my roommate's band, and Alicia is the lead vocalist.

31. Jose had three exams on Monday, so he spent several hours in the library the day before and more time in his dorm room that night studying.

   Identify all the words that function as nouns in the preceding sentence:

   a. Jose, exams, hours, library, day, time, room, night
   b. Jose, exams, Monday, hours, library, day, time, room, night
   c. Jose, exams, Monday, he, hours, library, day, time, dorm, night
   d. Exams, Monday, hours, library, day, time, room, night

338

32. Identify the sentence that uses correct subject-verb agreement.
    a. Each of the students have completed the final project and presentation.
    b. Many players on the basketball team was injured in last night's game.
    c. My friends from school has been trying to talk me in to dance classes.
    d. Everyone in my family has broken a bone except for me.

33. Which of the following sentences has an error in capitalization?
    a. My Mom used to live on the East Coast.
    b. I registered for one semester of Famous Women in Film, but there is not enough room in my schedule.
    c. I prefer traveling on Southwest Airlines because they do not charge baggage fees.
    d. I have never been to Martha's Vineyard or to any other part of New England for that matter.

34. The exhilarating morning air, combined with the beautiful mountain scenery, inspired me to want to jump right out of bed every morning for a lengthy run.

    From the following words, select one that is used as an adjective in the preceding sentence.

    a. Air
    b. Inspired
    c. Exhilarating
    d. Morning

35. My favorite teacher gave _____ and _____ extra credit on our project.
    a. me, him
    b. he, I
    c. him, I
    d. him, me

36. Which of these sentences uses correct punctuation?
    a. We traveled through six states on our road trip; Texas, New Mexico, Colorado, Wyoming, Utah, and Montana.
    b. We traveled through six states on our road trip: Texas, New Mexico, Colorado, Wyoming, Utah, and Montana.
    c. We traveled through six states on our road trip -- Texas, New Mexico, Colorado, Wyoming, Utah, and Montana.
    d. We traveled through six states on our road trip, Texas, New Mexico, Colorado, Wyoming, Utah, and Montana.

37. Which of the following sentences employs correct usage?
    a. You're going to need to go there to get your backpack from their house.
    b. Your going to need to go there to get you're backpack from their house.
    c. You're going to need to go their to get your backpack from there house.
    d. Your going to need to go their to get you're backpack from there house.

339

38. Which of the following sentences correctly uses an apostrophe?
    a. The childrens' choir performed at the Music Hall on Tuesday.
    b. The Smith's went to Colorado with us last summer.
    c. The Joneses' house is currently unoccupied while they are out of the country.
    d. Peoples' attitudes about politics are sometimes apathetic.

39. Which of the following sentences uses incorrect parallel structure?
    a. We worked out every day by swimming, biking, and a run.
    b. The list of craft supplies included scissors, glue, tissue paper, and glitter.
    c. Before I can come over, I need to run to the bank, go to the grocery store, and stop by the dry cleaners.
    d. I love to eat good food, take long walks, and read great books.

Directions for questions 40–43: Rewrite the sentence in your head following the directions given below. Keep in mind that your new sentence should be well written and should have essentially the same meaning as the original sentence.

40. Although she was nervous speaking in front of a crowd, the author read her narrative with poise and confidence.

    Rewrite, beginning with <u>The author had poise and confidence while reading...</u> the next words will be:

    a. because she was nervous speaking in front of a crowd.
    b. but she was nervous speaking in front of a crowd.
    c. even though she was nervous speaking in front of a crowd.
    d. before she was nervous speaking in front of a crowd.

41. There was a storm surge and loss of electricity during the hurricane.

    Rewrite, beginning with <u>While the hurricane occurred,</u> the next words will be:

    a. there was a storm surge after the electricity went out.
    b. the storm surge caused the electricity to go out.
    c. the electricity surged into the storm.
    d. the electricity went out, and there was a storm surge.

42. When one elephant in a herd is sick, the rest of the herd will help it walk and bring it food.

    Rewrite, beginning with <u>An elephant herd will</u> the next words will be:

    a. be too sick and tired to walk
    b. help and support
    c. gather food when they're sick
    d. be unable to walk without food

340

43. They went out to eat after the soccer game.

    Rewrite, beginning with <u>They finished the soccer game</u> the next words will be:

    a. then went out to eat.
    b. after they went out to eat.
    c. so they could go out to eat.
    d. because they went out to eat.

Directions for questions 44 – 50: Select the best version of the underlined part of the sentence. If there is no mistake, choose Correct as is.

44. If teachers set high expectations for <u>there students</u>, the students will rise to that high level.
    a. thare students
    b. they're students
    c. their students
    d. *Correct as is*

45. What I like about Biology class is that we focus not on the "what" of the content, <u>but more importantly, the 'why.'</u>
    a. but more importantly, the "why".
    b. but more importantly, the "why."
    c. but more importantly, the 'why'.
    d. *Correct as is*

46. While kids spend most of their time in school, they are dramatically shaped <u>with the influences</u> of their family.
    a. by the influences
    b. for the influences
    c. to the influences
    d. *Correct as is*

47. Because Kevin broke his leg last year, <u>he must spend</u> time in physical therapy to get ready for football season.
    a. he was spent
    b. he must to spend
    c. he must spending
    d. *Correct as is*

48. Lisa is constantly worried about being late to <u>work. This</u> is her worst nightmare.
    a. Lisa is constantly worried about being late to work: this is her worst nightmare.
    b. Lisa is constantly worried about being late to work this is her worst nightmare.
    c. Lisa is constantly worried about being late to work, this is her worst nightmare.
    d. *Correct as is*

49. When Ariana <u>goes off to college</u>, she knew she would miss her high school friends.
    a. going off to college
    b. go off to college
    c. went off to college
    d. *Correct as is*

50. <u>Although, they were closed down, they are open again after remodeling.</u>
    a. Although they were closed down, they are open again after remodeling.
    b. Although they were closed down they are open again after remodeling.
    c. Although they were closed down. They are open again after remodeling.
    d. *Correct as is*

Directions for questions 51–55

Select the best version of the underlined part of the sentence. The first choice is the same as the original sentence. If you think the original sentence is best, choose the first answer.

51. While all dogs <u>descend through gray wolves</u>, it's easy to notice that dog breeds come in a variety of shapes and sizes.
    a. descend through gray wolves
    b. descend by gray wolves
    c. descend from gray wolves
    d. descended through gray wolves

52. With such a <u>drastic range of traits, appearances and body types</u> dogs are one of the most variable and adaptable species on the planet.
    a. drastic range of traits, appearances and body types
    b. drastic range of traits, appearances, and body types
    c. drastic range of traits and appearances and body types
    d. drastic range of traits, appearances, as well as body types

53. Since the first discovery of dinosaur bones, <u>scientists has made strides in technological development and methodologies used to investigate</u> these extinct animals.
    a. scientists has made strides in technological development and methodologies used to investigate
    b. scientists has made strides in technological development, and methodologies, used to investigate
    c. scientists have made strides in technological development and methodologies used to investigate
    d. scientists, have made strides in technological development and methodologies used, to investigate

54. Paleontologists know this sail exists and have ideas for the function of <u>the sail however they are uncertain of which idea is the true function.</u>
    a. the sail however they are uncertain of which idea is the true function.
    b. the sail however, they are uncertain of which idea is the true function.
    c. the sail however they are, uncertain, of which idea is the true function.
    d. the sail; however, they are uncertain of which idea is the true function.

342

55. Usually, all news <u>outlets have some sort of bias, it's just a question of how much</u> bias clouds the reporting.
    a. outlets have some sort of bias, it's just a question of how much
    b. outlets have some sort of bias. Just a question of how much
    c. outlets have some sort of bias it can just be a question of how much
    d. outlets have some sort of bias, its just a question of how much

Biology

1. What types of molecules can move through a cell membrane by passive transport?
    a. Complex sugars
    b. Non-lipid-soluble molecules
    c. Oxygen
    d. Molecules moving from areas of low concentration to areas of high concentration

2. What is ONE feature that both prokaryotes and eukaryotes have in common?
    a. A plasma membrane
    b. A nucleus enclosed by a membrane
    c. Organelles
    d. A nucleoid

3. Diffusion and osmosis are examples of what type of transport mechanism?
    a. Active
    b. Passive
    c. Extracellular
    d. Intracellular

4. How many daughter cells are formed from one parent cell during meiosis?
    a. One
    b. Two
    c. Three
    d. Four

5. The process of breaking large molecules into smaller molecules to provide energy is known as which of the following?
    a. Metabolism
    b. Bioenergetics
    c. Anabolism
    d. Catabolism

6. With which genotype would the recessive phenotype appear, if the dominant allele is marked with "A" and the recessive allele is marked with "a"?
    a. AA
    b. aa
    c. Aa
    d. aA

7. Which organelle is responsible for generating energy for the cell and is referred to as the powerhouse of the cell?
   a. Mitochondria
   b. Nucleus
   c. Ribosomes
   d. Cell wall

8. A color-blind male and a carrier female have three children. What is the probability that they are all color blind?
   a. 1/4
   b. 1/8
   c. 1/16
   d. 1/32

9. How are fungi similar to plants?
   a. They have a cell wall.
   b. They contain chloroplasts.
   c. They perform photosynthesis.
   d. They use carbon dioxide as a source of energy.

10. What important function are the roots of plants responsible for?
    a. Absorbing water from the surrounding environment
    b. Performing photosynthesis
    c. Conducting sugars downward through the leaves
    d. Supporting the plant body

11. Which subdiscipline of biology would a botanist study?
    a. Growth of an aloe plant
    b. Evolution of monkeys
    c. Genetic changes in human brain cancer
    d. Interaction between worker bees and a queen bee

12. What shape does a water molecule form?
    a. C-shape
    b. S-shape
    c. V-shape
    d. T-shape

13. Which type of biological molecule stores information?
    a. Carbohydrates
    b. Nucleic acids
    c. Proteins
    d. Lipids

14. What are chloroplasts responsible for in plant cells?
    a. Maintaining the cell's shape
    b. Containing the cell's DNA
    c. Converting energy from sunlight to glucose
    d. Building proteins

15. What changes in a reaction when an enzyme is added?
    a. The amount of free energy stored in the reactants
    b. The number of products that result from the reaction
    c. The amount of free energy stored in the products
    d. The amount of time needed for the reaction to occur

16. If a molecule were trying to enter an animal cell, which organelle would it have to pass through first?
    a. Cell wall
    b. Cell membrane
    c. Nucleus
    d. Endoplasmic reticulum

17. Which of the following represents a possible number of ATP molecules for oxidative phosphorylation to generate?
    a. 26
    b. 30
    c. 4
    d. 36

18. Which is a product of the photosynthetic reaction?
    a. CO_2
    b. H_2O
    c. O_2
    d. Solar energy

19. Which of the following is identical in both mitosis and meiosis?
    a. The number of divisions
    b. The number of daughter cells produced
    c. The synapsis of homologous chromosomes
    d. When DNA replication occurs

20. Which of the following is directly transcribed from DNA and represents the first step in protein building?
    a. siRNA
    b. rRNA
    c. mRNA
    d. tRNA

21. What information does a genotype give that a phenotype does not?
    a. The genotype necessarily includes the proteins coded for by its alleles.
    b. The genotype will always show an organism's recessive alleles.
    c. The genotype must include the organism's physical characteristics.
    d. The genotype shows what an organism's parents looked like.

	T	t
T		
t		

22. Which statement is supported by the Punnett square above, if "T"=Tall and "t"=short?
    a. Both parents are homozygous tall.
    b. 100% of the offspring will be tall because both parents are tall.
    c. There is a 25% chance that an offspring will be short.
    d. The short allele will soon die out.

23. Which of the following CANNOT be found in a human cell's genes?
    a. Sequences of amino acids to be transcribed into mRNA
    b. Lethal recessive traits like sickle cell anemia
    c. Mutated DNA
    d. DNA that codes for proteins the cell doesn't use

24. Which of Mendel's laws of inheritance states that a dominant phenotype will always be seen over a recessive phenotype?
    a. The law of dominance
    b. The law of similarity
    c. The law of segregation
    d. The law of independent assortment

25. Which base pairs up with adenine in DNA?
    a. Uracil
    b. Thymine
    c. Guanine
    d. Cytosine

Questions 26–30 pertain to the passage:

Scientist A wants to grow white flowered plants and is doing a series of crossbreeding experiments. She had each plant genetically tested so she knows which alleles comprise each plant. The dominant flowers are red (A) and the recessive allele (a) produces white flowers.

Figure 1 below represents the different flowers that underwent crossbreeding during Round #1A

Round #1A

Crossbreeding #1A			Crossbreeding #2A			Crossbreeding #3A		
	A	**a**		**a**	**a**		**a**	**a**
A	AA	Aa	**A**	Aa	Aa	**A**	Aa	Aa
A	AA	Aa	**A**	Aa	Aa	**a**	aa	aa

Figure 2 below represents the number of flowers that were red and white after the first round of crossbreeding experiments.

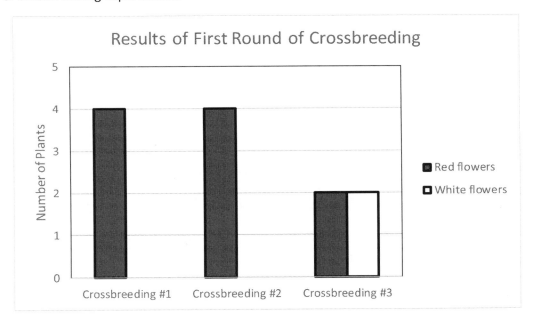

During her second round of crossbreeding, she adds in a plant of unknown genetic makeup with red flowers. She crosses it with a white-flowering plant. The results of her experiment are represented in the next figure.

347

Figure 3 represents the genetic results from the second round of crossbreeding.

Round #2

	a	a
?	Aa	Aa
?	aa	aa

Scientist A takes offspring plants from Round #1A and crossbreeds them with each other and calls this Round #1B.

Figure 4 below represents the results of crossbreeding from Round #1B.

Round #1B

Crossbreeding #1B			Crossbreeding #2B			Crossbreeding #3B		
	A	**a**		**A**	**a**		**a**	**a**
A	AA	Aa	**A**	AA	Aa	**a**	aa	aa
A	AA	Aa	**a**	Aa	aa	**a**	aa	aa

26. Crossbreeding which two plants will give her the highest likelihood of obtaining some white plants right away in Round #1A?
    a. AA × Aa
    b. Aa × aa
    c. AA × aa
    d. AA × AA

27. What percentage of plants are white after the first crossbreeding reactions?
    a. 12
    b. 50
    c. 16.7
    d. 25

28. What is the genetic makeup of the unknown plant from the second round of crossbreeding?
   a. aa
   b. Aa
   c. AA
   d. Cannot be determined

29. From which group of crossbreeding in Round #1B can she obtain 100% white flowers by the second generation?
   a. They are all equal.
   b. 1B
   c. 2B
   d. 3B

30. Which of her five senses did she use for the observation step of the scientific method here?
   a. Sight
   b. Smell
   c. Touch
   d. Hearing

Chemistry

1. Which of following about nuclear reactions is NOT true?
   a. They involve the release of energy
   b. The structure of the nucleus changes.
   c. They take place in the atom's nucleus.
   d. The reactants and products have equal mass.

2. What does the Lewis Dot structure of an element represent?
   a. The outer electron valence shell population
   b. The inner electron valence shell population
   c. The positioning of the element's protons
   d. The positioning of the element's neutrons

3. What is the chemical reaction when a compound is broken down into its basic components called?
   a. A synthesis reaction
   b. A decomposition reaction
   c. An organic reaction
   d. An oxidation reaction

4. Which of the following is a balanced chemical equation?
   a. $Na + Cl_2 \rightarrow NaCl$
   b. $2\,Na + Cl_2 \rightarrow NaCl$
   c. $2\,Na + Cl_2 \rightarrow 2\,NaCl$
   d. $2\,Na + 2\,Cl_2 \rightarrow 2\,NaCl$

349

5. What is the name of this compound: CO?
    a. Carbonite oxide
    b. Carbonic dioxide
    c. Carbonic monoxide
    d. Carbon monoxide

6. What is the molarity of a solution made by dissolving 4.0 grams of NaCl into enough water to make 120 mL of solution? The atomic mass of Na is 23.0 g/mol and Cl is 35.5 g/mol.
    a. 0.34 M
    b. 0.57 M
    c. 0.034 M
    d. 0.057 M

7. Considering a gas in a closed system, at a constant volume, what will happen to the temperature if the pressure is increased?
    a. The temperature will stay the same.
    b. The temperature will decrease.
    c. The temperature will increase.
    d. It cannot be determined with the information given.

8. Which of the following statements regarding proteins is FALSE?
    a. Two amino acids combine through a condensation reaction.
    b. The twenty amino acids differ by their side chains, but all include a central carbon atom.
    c. Two amino acids bond together at their amine groups.
    d. Protein chains may either be hydrophilic or hydrophobic.

9. What coefficients are needed to balance the following combustion equation?

$$\_\,C_2H_{10} + \_\,O_2 \rightarrow \_\,H_2O + \_\,CO_2$$

    a. 1:5:5:2
    b. 1:9:5:2
    c. 2:9:10:4
    d. 2:5:10:4

10. What is the purpose of a catalyst?

    a. To increase a reaction's rate by increasing the activation energy
    b. To increase a reaction's rate by increasing the temperature
    c. To increase a reaction's rate by decreasing the activation energy
    d. To increase a reaction's rate by decreasing the temperature

11. What is a change in state from a solid to a gas called?
    a. Evaporation
    b. Melting
    c. Condensation
    d. Sublimation

12. Salts like sodium iodide (NaI) and potassium chloride (KCl) use what type of bond?
    a. Ionic bonds
    b. Disulfide bridges
    c. Covalent bonds
    d. London dispersion forces

13. Which of the following is unique to covalent bonds?
    a. Most covalent bonds are formed between the elements H, F, N, and O.
    b. Covalent bonds are dependent on forming dipoles.
    c. Bonding electrons are shared between two or more atoms.
    d. Molecules with covalent bonds tend to have a crystalline solid structure.

14. Which of the following describes a typical gas?
    a. Indefinite shape and indefinite volume
    b. Indefinite shape and definite volume
    c. Definite shape and definite volume
    d. Definite shape and indefinite volume

15. Which of the following is a chief difference between evaporation and boiling?
    a. Liquids boil only at the surface while they evaporate equally throughout the liquid.
    b. Evaporating substances change from gas to liquid while boiling substances change from liquid to gas.
    c. Evaporation happens in nature while boiling is a manmade phenomenon.
    d. Evaporation can happen below a liquid's boiling point.

16. Which of the following is a special property of water?
    a. Water easily flows through phospholipid bilayers.
    b. A water molecule's oxygen atom allows fish to breathe.
    c. Water is highly cohesive which explains its high melting point.
    d. Water can self-hydrolyze and decompose into hydrogen and oxygen.

17. For any given element, an isotope is an atom with which of the following?
    a. A different atomic number.
    b. A different number of protons.
    c. A different number of electrons.
    d. A different mass number.

18. Which of the following regarding alpha particles is true?
    a. Their mass is greater than that of protons and neutrons
    b. Their mass is less than that of beta particles
    c. They have the greatest tissue penetration power
    d. They are high-energy electrons

19. According to the periodic table, which of the following elements is the least reactive?
    a. Fluorine
    b. Silicon
    c. Neon
    d. Gallium

20. Explain the Law of Conservation of Mass as it applies to this reaction: $2\,H_2 + O_2 \rightarrow 2\,H_2O$.
    a. Electrons are lost.
    b. The hydrogen loses mass.
    c. New oxygen atoms are formed.
    d. There is no decrease or increase of matter.

21. What type of chemical reaction produces a salt?
    a. An oxidation reaction
    b. A neutralization reaction
    c. A synthesis reaction
    d. A decomposition reaction

22. Which of the following correctly displays 8,600,000,000,000 in scientific notation?
    a. 8.6×10^{12}
    b. 8.6×10^{-12}
    c. 8.6×10^{11}
    d. 86×10^{11}

23. In the following reaction, which element is oxidized and which is reduced?

$$Fe(s) + CuSO_4(aq) \rightarrow FeSO_4(aq) + Cu(s)$$

    a. Fe is reduced and loses electrons, Cu is oxidized and gains electrons.
    b. Fe is reduced and gains electrons, Cu is oxidized and loses electrons.
    c. Fe is oxidized and loses electrons, Cu is reduced and gains electrons.
    d. Fe is oxidized and gains electrons, Cu is reduced and loses electrons.

24. In the reaction below, if 500 grams of hydrogen reacted with excess nitrogen, what is the mass of produced ammonia gas in the reaction? Use the following molar masses, if needed: N_2=28.0 g/mol, H_2=2.02 g/mol, and NH_3=17.0 g/mol.

$$3\,H_2(g) + N_2(g) \rightarrow 2\,NH_3(g)$$

    a. 230 grams of NH_3
    b. 280 grams of NH_3
    c. 2300 grams of NH_3
    d. 2800 grams of NH_3

25. A smooth sweet tea recipe calls for 150 grams of glucose ($C_6H_{12}O_6$) and 1400 grams of water. What is the molarity of this mixture? (Use the following molar masses for C, H, O: C=12.01 g/mol, H=1.008 g/mol, and O=16.0 g/mol. The density of water is 1 g/mL.)
    a. $M = 0.695\ mol/L$
    b. $M = 0.595\ mol/L$
    c. $M = 0.505\ mol/L$
    d. $M = 0.650\ mol/L$

26. Which characteristic is NOT a property of water?
    a. If it acts as an acid, it donates a proton.
    b. If it acts as a base, it donates a proton.
    c. If it donates a proton, it becomes a conjugate base in the form of hydroxide ions.
    d. If it accepts a proton, it becomes a conjugate acid in the form of hydronium ions.

27. In the following reaction, which elements experience changes in oxidation numbers, indicating an oxidation-reduction reaction?

Reaction	$I_2O_5 + 5CO_2 \rightarrow I_2 + 5CO$							
Elements	I_2	O_5	+ 5C	O_2	$\rightarrow$	I_2	+5C	O
Oxidation #s	+5	-2	-2	+2		0	+4	-2

    a. Iodine and carbon
    b. Carbon and oxygen
    c. Oxygen and Iodine
    d. Carbon monoxide

28. Scientist A is observing an unknown substance in the lab. Which observation describes a chemical property of the substance?
    a. She sees that it is green in color.
    b. She weighs it and measures the volume and finds the density to be 10 g/L.
    c. She applies pressure to it and finds that it breaks apart easily.
    d. She passes it through a flame and finds that it burns.

29. Which of the following processes can be SOLELY categorized as a chemical reaction process?
    a. The condensation of water vapor around the container of an ice-cold beverage
    b. Baking brownies with chocolate chips
    c. The shattering of a glass mason jar after falling on the floor
    d. The combination of sand (SiO_2) in water

30. What is the base-conjugate acid pair in the following chemical reaction: $H_2O + NH_3 \rightarrow NH_4^+ + OH^-$?
    a. H_2O and NH_4^+
    b. H_2O and NH_3
    c. NH_3 and NH_4^+
    d. NH_3 and OH^-

Anatomy and Physiology

1. What is the order of filtration in the nephron?
    a. Collecting Duct $\rightarrow$ Proximal tubule $\rightarrow$ Loop of Henle
    b. Proximal tubule $\rightarrow$ Loop of Henle $\rightarrow$ Collecting duct
    c. Loop of Henle $\rightarrow$ Collecting duct $\rightarrow$ Proximal tubule
    d. Loop of Henle $\rightarrow$ Proximal tubule $\rightarrow$ Collecting duct

2. Which are neurons that transmit signals from the CNS to effector tissues and organs?
   a. Motor
   b. Sensory
   c. Interneuron
   d. Reflex

3. Which statement about white blood cells is true?
   a. B cells are responsible for antibody production.
   b. White blood cells are made in the white/yellow cartilage before they enter the bloodstream.
   c. Platelets, a special class of white blood cell, function to clot blood and stop bleeding.
   d. The majority of white blood cells only activate during the age of puberty, which explains why children and the elderly are particularly susceptible to disease.

4. Which is NOT a function of the pancreas?
   a. Secretes the hormone insulin in response to growth hormone stimulation
   b. Secretes bicarbonate into the small intestine to raise the pH from stomach secretions
   c. Secretes enzymes used by the small intestine to digest fats, sugars, and proteins
   d. Secretes hormones from its endocrine portion in order to regulate blood sugar levels

5. Which organ is not a component of the lymphatic system?
   a. Thymus
   b. Spleen
   c. Tonsil
   d. Gall bladder

6. Which action is unrelated to blood pH?
   a. Exhalation of carbon dioxide
   b. Kidney reabsorption of bicarbonate
   c. ADH secretion
   d. Nephron secretion of ammonia

7. Which gland regulates calcium levels?
   a. Thyroid
   b. Pineal
   c. Adrenal
   d. Parathyroid

8. What are the functions of the hypothalamus?

   I. Regulate body temperature
   II. Send stimulatory and inhibitory instructions to the pituitary gland
   III. Receives sensory information from the brain

   a. I and II
   b. I and III
   c. II and III
   d. I, II, and III

9. Which muscle system is unlike the others?
   a. Bicep: Tricep
   b. Quadricep: Hamstring
   c. Gluteus maximus: Gluteus minimus
   d. Trapezius/Rhomboids: Pectoralis Major

10. How do muscle fibers shorten during contraction?
   a. The actin filaments attach to the myosin, forming cross-bridges, and pull the fibers closer together.
   b. Calcium enters the sarcoplasmic reticulum, initiating an action potential.
   c. Myosin cross-bridges attach, rotate, and detach from actin filaments causing the ends of the sarcomere to be pulled closer together.
   d. The t-tubule system allows the fibers to physically shorten during contraction.

11. In what way does the skeletal system support the immune system?
   a. Bones support and protect the spleen
   b. Calcium is stored in the bones
   c. The bone marrow is the site of WBC production
   d. The osteoclasts make new bone cells when necessary

12. The human anatomy is divided into geographical planes for the purpose of identifying structures. Which of the following definitions is correct?
   a. The sagittal plane is a horizontal line that divides the core of the body into the right and left sides.
   b. The caudal plane is a vertical line that divides the body into the right and left sides.
   c. The transverse plane is a horizontal line that divides the body into upper and lower sections.
   d. The coronal plane is a horizontal line that divides the body into upper or superior and lower or inferior sections.

13. After assessing a patient's passive range of motion in the knee, the therapist determines there is limitation in flexion. Which of the following list of structures may be responsible for the restricted range of motion?
   a. Quadriceps, ligaments, knee joint capsule, fascia
   b. Hamstrings, ligaments, knee joint capsule, fascia
   c. Gastrocnemius, ligaments, knee joint capsule, fascia
   d. Ligaments, knee joint capsule, fascia

14. Which of the following structures acts like a funnel by delivering the urine from the millions of collecting tubules to the ureters?
   a. The renal pelvis
   b. The renal cortex
   c. The renal medulla
   d. Bowman's capsule

15. Which of the following is NOT a component of a sarcomere?
   a. Actin
   b. D-line
   c. A-Band
   d. I-Band

355

16. Which of the following about the autonomic nervous system (ANS) is true?
    a. It controls the reflex arc
    b. It contains motor (efferent) neurons
    c. It contains sensory (afferent) neurons
    d. It contains both parasympathetic nerves and sympathetic nerves

17. Which of the following about epithelial tissue is NOT true?
    a. It does not contain blood vessels.
    b. The cells are more loosely packed than in connective tissue.
    c. It regenerates quickly.
    d. It covers exposed surfaces and lines internal cavities and passageways in the body.

18. Which of the following systems does not include a transportation system throughout the body?
    a. Cardiovascular system
    b. Endocrine system
    c. Immune system
    d. Nervous system

19. Which of the following upper body movements take place in the sagittal plane?

    I. Elbow extension
    II. Wrist flexion
    III. Shoulder abduction
    IV. Neck left tilt

    a. I and IV
    b. I, III, IV
    c. I and II
    d. II and III

20. What muscle is the primary antagonist in knee flexion?
    a. Hamstrings
    b. Quadriceps
    c. Gastrocnemius
    d. Tibialis anterior

21. What is the MAIN function of the respiratory system?
    a. To eliminate waste through the kidneys and bladder
    b. To exchange gas between the air and circulating blood
    c. To transform food and liquids into energy
    d. To excrete waste from the body

22. Which system comprises the 206 bones of the body?
    a. Skeletal
    b. Muscular
    c. Endocrine
    d. Reproductive

23. If a patient is having lower back pain, which term could they use to describe the area of their pain?
    a. Pedal
    b. Lumbar
    c. Axillary
    d. Cephalic

24. If a person falls and hits their head, which part of the skeleton protects their brain from injury?
    a. Pelvic girdle
    b. Ribs
    c. Vertebrae
    d. Cranium

25. The epidermis is composed of what type of cells?
    a. Osteoclasts
    b. Connective
    c. Dendritic
    d. Epithelial

26. Which of the following lists of joint types is in the correct order for increasing amounts of permitted motion (least mobile to most mobile)?
    a. Hinge, condyloid, saddle
    b. Saddle, hinge, condyloid
    c. Saddle, condyloid, hinge
    d. Hinge, saddle, condyloid

27. Which of the following correctly lists the structures of a muscle from largest to smallest?
    a. Fasciculus, muscle fiber, actin, myofibril
    b. Muscle fiber, fasciculus, myofibril, actin
    c. Sarcomere, fasciculus, myofibril, myosin
    d. Muscle fiber, myofibril, sarcomere, actin

28. Myosin cross-bridges attach to the actin filament when the sarcoplasmic reticulum is stimulated to release which of the following?
    a. Calcium ions
    b. Acetylcholine
    c. Troponin
    d. Adenosine triphosphate (ATP)

29. Which of the following types of joints are correctly matched with the anatomic joint example given?
    I. Cartilaginous: pubic symphysis
    II. Saddle: thumb carpal-metacarpal
    III. Plane: sutures in skull
    IV. Pivot: radial head on ulna

    a. Choices I, II, and III
    b. Choices I, II, and IV
    c. Choices I, III, and IV
    d. All are correct

357

30. A child complains of heavy breathing even when relaxing. They are an otherwise healthy child with no history of respiratory problems. What might be the issue?
    a. Asthma
    b. Blood clot
    c. Hyperventilation
    d. Exercising too hard

Physics

1. At what point in its swing does a pendulum have the most potential energy?
    a. At the top of its swing, just before going into motion
    b. At the bottom of its swing, in full motion
    c. Halfway between the top of its swing and the bottom of its swing
    d. It has the same amount of potential energy throughout its path

2. Which of the following is considered a force?
    a. Weight
    b. Mass
    c. Acceleration
    d. Gravity

3. What is the force that opposes motion?
    a. Reactive force
    b. Responsive force
    c. Friction
    d. Momentum

4. Which of the following is true regarding magnets?
    a. Opposite charges attract
    b. Like charges attract
    c. Opposite charges repel
    d. Like charges do not repel or attract

5. Who is credited for simplifying the laws of motion?
    a. Einstein
    b. Hawking
    c. Copernicus
    d. Newton

6. According to Newton's Three Laws of Motion, which of the following is true?
    a. Two objects cannot exert a force on each other without touching.
    b. An object at rest has no inertia.
    c. The weight of an object is the same as the mass of the object.
    d. The weight of an object is equal to the mass of an object multiplied by gravity.

7. Which of the following statements about parallel circuits is FALSE?
    a. If the resistance is different in each load, more current passes through the load with the lower resistance.
    b. If the resistance is different in each load, more current passes through the one with higher resistance.
    c. If the resistance is the same in both loads, then the same amount of current passes through each one.
    d. The voltage is the same across each resistor.

8. A spinning ice skater who extends their arms horizontally to slow down is demonstrating which of the following?
    a. Conservation of angular momentum
    b. Conservation of mechanical energy
    c. Conservation of matter
    d. Conservation of mass

9. When an ice skater spins on one skate in a circle, what happens if they extend their arms out like the letter "T"?
    a. They spin faster.
    b. They spin slower.
    c. They stop spinning.
    d. Nothing changes.

10. What is the acceleration of a vehicle starting from rest and reaching a velocity of 15 m/s in 5.0 s?
    a. 3.0 m/s
    b. 75 m/s
    c. 3.0 m/s^2
    d. 75 m/s^2

11. How do you calculate the useful work performed in lifting a 10-kilogram weight from the ground to the top of a 2-meter ladder?
    a. $10 \text{ kg} \times 2 \text{ m} \times 32 \text{ m/s}^2$
    b. $10 \text{ kg} \times 2 \text{ m}^2 \times 9.81 \text{ m/s}$
    c. $10 \text{ kg} \times 2 \text{ m} \times 9.81 \text{ m/s}^2$
    d. It can't be determined without knowing the ground elevation

359

12. A steel spring is loaded with a 10-newton weight and is stretched by 0.5 centimeters. What is the deflection if it's loaded with two 10-newton weights?

a. 0.5 centimeter
b. 1 centimeter
c. 2 centimeters
d. It can't be determined without knowing the Modulus of Elasticity of the steel.

13. A 1000-kilogram concrete block is resting on a wooden surface. Between these two materials, the coefficient of sliding friction is 0.4 and the coefficient of static friction is 0.5. How much more force is needed to get the block moving than to keep it moving?

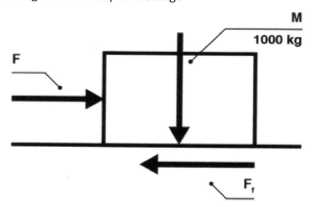

a. 981 N
b. 1962 N
c. 3924 N
d. 9810 N

14. The master cylinder (F1) of a hydraulic jack has a cross-sectional area of 0.1 m², and a force of 50 N is applied. What must the area of the drive cylinder (F2) be to support a weight of 800 N?

a. 0.4 m²
b. 0.8 m²
c. 1.6 m²
d. 3.2 m²

15. A gas with a volume V_1 is held down by a piston with a force of F newtons. The piston has an area of A. After heating the gas, it expands against the weight to a volume V_2. What was the work done?

(a)   (b)

a. $\frac{F}{A}$

b. $\frac{F}{A} \times V_1$

c. $\frac{F}{A} \times V_2$

d. $\frac{F}{A} \times (V_2 - V_1)$

361

16. A 1000-kilogram weight is raised 30 meters in 10 minutes. What is the approximate power expended in the period?

    a. 1000 Kg × m/s^2

    b. 500 N·m

    c. 500 J/s

    d. 100 watts

17. A 2-meter high, concrete block is submerged in a body of water 12 meters deep (as shown). Assuming that the water has a unit weight of 1000 N/m^3, what is the pressure acting on the upper surface of the block?

    a. 10,000 Pa

    b. 12,000 Pa

    c. 14,000 Pa

    d. It can't be calculated without knowing the top area of the block.

![Test Prep Books]

18. Closed Basins A and B each contain a 10,000-ton block of ice. The ice block in Basin A is floating in sea water. The ice block in Basin B is aground on a rock ledge (as shown). When all the ice melts, what happens to the water level in Basin A and Basin B?

Basin A   **Basin B**

    a. Water level rises in A but not in B
    b. Water level rises in B but not in A
    c. Water level rises in neither A nor B
    d. Water level rises in both A and B

19. An official 10-lane Olympic pool is 50 meters wide by 25 meters long. How long does it take to fill the pool to the recommended depth of 3 meters using a pump with a 750 liter per second capacity?
    a. 2500 seconds
    b. 5000 seconds
    c. 10,000 seconds
    d. 100,000 seconds

20. Water is flowing in a rectangular canal 10 meters wide by 2 meters deep at a velocity of 3 m/s. The canal is half full. What is the flow rate?
    a. 30 m³/s
    b. 60 m³/s
    c. 90 m³/s
    d. 120 m³/s

Answer Explanations #2

Mathematics

1. B: 300 miles in 4 hours is $\frac{300}{4} = 75$ miles per hour. In 1.5 hours, the car will go 1.5×75 miles, or 112.5 miles.

2. C: The best way to solve this problem is by using a system of equations. We know that Jan bought $90 worth of apples ($a$) and oranges ($o$) at $1 and $2 respectively. That means our first equation is:

$$1(a) + 2(o) = 90$$

We also know that she bought an equal number of apples and oranges, which gives us our second equation $a = o$. We can then replace a with o in the first equation to give:

$$1(o) + 2(o) = 90 \text{ or } 3(o) = 90$$

Which yields:

$$o = 30$$

Thus, Jan bought 30 oranges (and 30 apples).

3. C: To subtract fractions, they must have a common denominator. In this case, 24 can be used because it is the least common multiple of 6 and 8:

$$\frac{11}{6} - \frac{3}{8} = \frac{44}{24} - \frac{9}{24} = \frac{44 - 9}{24} = \frac{35}{24}$$

In the last step, 15 is factored out from the numerator and denominator, yielding $\frac{3}{2}$.

4. D: First, the train's journey in the real world is $3 \times 50 = 150$ miles. On the map, 1 inch corresponds to 10 miles, so that is equivalent to $\frac{150}{10} = 15$ inches on the map.

5. B: The total trip time is $1 + 3.5 + 0.5 = 5$ hours. The total time driving is $1 + 0.5 = 1.5$ hours. So, the fraction of time spent driving is $\frac{1.5}{5}$ or $\frac{3}{10}$. To get the percentage, convert this to a fraction out of 100. The numerator and denominator are multiplied by 10, with a result of $\frac{30}{100}$. The percentage is the numerator in a fraction out of 100, so 30%.

6. A: First simplify the larger fraction by separating it into two. When dividing one fraction by another, remember to *invert* the second fraction and multiply the two as follows:

$$\frac{5}{7} \times \frac{11}{9}$$

The resulting fraction $\frac{55}{63}$ cannot be simplified further, so this is the answer to the problem.

7. A: The tip is not taxed, so he pays 5% tax only on the $10. 5% of $10 is $0.05 \times 10 = \$0.50$. Add up $10 + \$2 + \$0.50$ to get $12.50.

8. A: In order to determine the savings needed per day, $\frac{150}{4} = 37.5$, so she needs to save an average of $37.50 per day.

9. D: The number of days can be found by taking the total amount Bernard needs to make and dividing it by the amount he earns per day:

$$\frac{300}{80} = \frac{30}{8} = \frac{15}{4} = 3.75$$

But Bernard is only working full days, so he will need to work 4 days, since 3 days is not a sufficient amount of time.

10. A: The value went up by $165,000 - \$150,000 = \$15,000$. Out of $150,000, this is $\frac{15,000}{150,000} = \frac{1}{10}$. Convert this to having a denominator of 100, the result is $\frac{10}{100}$ or 10%.

11. D: The total faculty is:

$$15 + 20 = 35$$

So, the ratio is $35 : 200$. Then, divide both of these numbers by 5, since 5 is a common factor to both, with a result of $7 : 40$.

12. B: The journey will be $5 \times 3 = 15$ miles. A car traveling at 60 miles per hour is traveling at 1 mile per minute. The resulting equation would be:

$$\frac{15 \text{ mi}}{1 \frac{\text{mi}}{\text{min}}} = 15 \text{ min}$$

Therefore, it will take 15 minutes to make the journey.

13. A: Taylor's total income is $20,000 + \$10,000 = \$30,000$. Fifteen percent as a fraction is $\frac{15}{100} = \frac{3}{20}$. So:

$$\frac{3}{20} \times \$30,000 = \frac{\$90,000}{20}$$

$$\frac{\$9,000}{2} = \$4,500$$

14. B: First, calculate the difference between the larger value and the smaller value.

$$378 - 252 = 126$$

To calculate this difference as a percentage of the original value, and thus calculate the percentage *increase*, divide 126 by 252, then multiply by 100 to reach the percentage 50%, Choice *B*.

15. D: Kristen bought four DVDs, which would cost a total of $4 \times 15 = \$60$. She spent a total of $100, so she spent $100 - \$60 = \$40$ on CDs. Since they cost $10 each, she must have purchased $\frac{40}{10} =$ four CDs.

16. D: This problem can be solved by setting up a proportion involving the given information and the unknown value. The proportion is:

$$\frac{21 \text{ pages}}{4 \text{ nights}} = \frac{140 \text{ pages}}{x \text{ nights}}$$

Solving the proportion by cross-multiplying, the equation becomes $21x = 4 \times 140$, where $x = 26.67$. Since it is not an exact number of nights, the answer is rounded up to 27 nights. Twenty-six nights would not give Sarah enough time.

17. D: This problem can be solved by using unit conversion. The initial units are miles per minute. The final units need to be feet per second. Converting miles to feet uses the equivalence statement 1 mile equals 5,280 feet. Converting minutes to seconds uses the equivalence statement, 1 minute equals 60 seconds. Setting up the ratios to convert the units is shown in the following equation:

$$\frac{72 \text{ mi}}{90 \text{ min}} \times \frac{1 \text{ min}}{60 \text{ s}} \times \frac{5,280 \text{ ft}}{1 \text{ mi}} = 70.4 \frac{\text{ft}}{\text{s}}$$

The initial units cancel out, and the new units are left.

18. B: First, subtract 4 from each side. This yields $6t = 12$. Now, divide both sides by 6 to obtain $t = 2$.

19. A: Since $660 is the price *after* a 30% discount, $660 represents 70% of the original price. To determine the original price, set up a proportion with the ratio of the sale price (660) to original price (unknown) equal to the ratio of sale percentage (where x represents the unknown original price):

$$\frac{660}{x} = \frac{70}{100}$$

To solve a proportion, cross multiply and set the products equal to each other:

$$(660)(100) = (70)(x)$$

Multiplying each side results in the equation:

$$66,000 = 70x$$

To solve for x, divide both sides by 70:

$$\frac{66,000}{70} = \frac{70x}{70}$$

$$x = 942.86$$

Remember that x represents the original price. Subtracting the sale price from the original price ($942.86 - \$660$) indicates that Frank saved $282.86.

366

20. C: The decimal points are lined up, with zeroes put in as needed. Then, the numbers are added just like integers:

$$
\begin{array}{r}
3.40 \\
2.35 \\
+\underline{4.00} \\
9.75
\end{array}
$$

21. A: This problem can be multiplied as 588×32, except at the end, the decimal point needs to be moved three places to the left. Performing the multiplication will give 18,816, and moving the decimal place over three places results in 18.816.

22. D: The fraction is converted so that the denominator is 100 by multiplying the numerator and denominator by 4, to get $\frac{3}{25} = \frac{12}{100}$. Dividing a number by 100 just moves the decimal point two places to the left, with a result of 0.12.

23. A: Figure out which is largest by looking at the first non-zero digits. Choice *B*'s first non-zero digit is in the hundredths place. The other three all have non-zero digits in the tenths place, so it must be *A*, *C*, or *D*. Of these, *A* has the largest first non-zero digit.

24. C: $40N$ would be 4,000% of N. All of the other coefficients are equivalent to $\frac{40}{100}$ or 40%.

25. B: Instead of multiplying these out, the product can be estimated by using $18 \times 10 = 180$. The error here should be lower than 15, since it is rounded to the nearest integer, and the numbers add to something less than 30.

26. C: 85% of a number means multiplying that number by 0.85. So, $0.85 \times 20 = \frac{85}{100} \times \frac{20}{1}$, which can be simplified to $\frac{17}{20} \times \frac{20}{1} = 17$.

27. A: To find the fraction of the bill that the first three people pay, the fractions need to be added, which means finding the common denominator. The common denominator will be 60.

$$
\frac{1}{5} + \frac{1}{4} + \frac{1}{3} = \frac{12}{60} + \frac{15}{60} + \frac{20}{60} = \frac{47}{60}
$$

The remainder of the bill is:

$$
1 - \frac{47}{60} = \frac{60}{60} - \frac{47}{60} = \frac{13}{60}
$$

28. B: 30% is 3/10. The number itself must be 10/3 of 6, or $\frac{10}{3} \times 6 = 10 \times 2 = 20$.

29. A: First, these numbers should be converted to improper fractions: $\frac{7}{3} - \frac{11}{5}$. Take 15 as a common denominator:

$$
\frac{7}{3} - \frac{11}{5} = \frac{35}{15} - \frac{33}{15} = \frac{2}{15}
$$

30. A: Dividing by 98 can be approximated by dividing by 100, which would mean shifting the decimal point of the numerator to the left by 2. The result is 4.2 and rounds to 4.

31. B:

$$4\frac{1}{3} + 3\frac{3}{4}$$

$$4 + 3 + \frac{1}{3} + \frac{3}{4}$$

$$7 + \frac{1}{3} + \frac{3}{4}$$

Adding the fractions gives:

$$\frac{1}{3} + \frac{3}{4} = \frac{4}{12} + \frac{9}{12} = \frac{13}{12} = 1 + \frac{1}{12}$$

Thus:

$$7 + \frac{1}{3} + \frac{3}{4} = 7 + 1 + \frac{1}{12} = 8\frac{1}{12}$$

32. A: Each bag contributes $4x + 1$ treats. The total treats will be in the form $4nx + n$ where n is the total number of bags. The total is in the form $60x + 15$, from which it is known $n = 15$.

33. D: Let a be the number of apples and b the number of bananas. Then, the total cost is $2a + 3b = 22$, while it also known that $a + b = 10$. Using the knowledge of systems of equations, cancel the b variables by multiplying the second equation by -3. This makes the equation $-3a - 3b = -30$. Adding this to the first equation, the b values cancel to get $-a = -8$, which simplifies to $a=8$.

34. B: $\frac{5}{2} \div \frac{1}{3} = \frac{5}{2} \times \frac{3}{1} = \frac{15}{2} = 7.5$

35. A: The total fraction taken up by green and red shirts will be:

$$\frac{1}{3} + \frac{2}{5} = \frac{5}{15} + \frac{6}{15} = \frac{11}{15}$$

The remaining fraction is:

$$1 - \frac{11}{15}$$

$$\frac{15}{15} - \frac{11}{15} = \frac{4}{15}$$

36. C: If she has used $\frac{1}{3}$ of the paint, she has 2/3 remaining. $2\frac{1}{2}$ gallons are the same as $\frac{5}{2}$ gallons. The calculation is:

$$\frac{2}{3} \times \frac{5}{2} = \frac{5}{3} = 1\frac{2}{3} \text{ gallons}$$

37. D: The correct answer of 20 °C can be found using the appropriate temperature conversion formula:

$$°C = (°F - 32) \times \frac{5}{9}$$

38. A: 12.018

Set up the problem, with the larger number on top and numbers lined up at the decimal. Place a zero at the end of the number with fewer digits to the right of the decimal (4.33 → 4.330), which does not change its value but makes for easier addition. Add, carrying anything over 9 into the next column to the left. Solve from right to left.

39. C: $\frac{29}{36}$

Set up the problem and find a common denominator for both fractions.

$$\frac{7}{12} + \frac{2}{9}$$

Multiply each fraction across by the equivalent of 1 to convert to a common denominator.

$$\frac{7}{12} \times \frac{3}{3} + \frac{2}{9} \times \frac{4}{4}$$

Once over the same denominator, add across the top. The total is over the common denominator.

$$\frac{21 + 8}{36} = \frac{29}{36}$$

40. A: 18.853

Set up the problem, larger number on top and numbers lined up at the decimal. Begin subtracting with the far-right column. Borrow 10 from the column to the left, when necessary.

41. B: 318.64

Set up the problem, with the larger number on top and numbers lined up at the decimal. Insert 0 in any blank spots to the right of the decimal as placeholders. Begin subtracting with the far-right column. Borrow 10 from the column to the left, when necessary.

42. D: $\frac{1}{3}$

Set up the problem and find a common denominator for both fractions.

$$\frac{39}{45} - \frac{8}{15}$$

Multiply each fraction across by 1 to convert to a common denominator.

$$\frac{39}{45} \times \frac{1}{1} - \frac{8}{15} \times \frac{3}{3}$$

369

Once over the same denominator, subtract across the top.

$$\frac{39 - 24}{45} = \frac{15}{45}$$

Reduce:

$$\frac{15 \div 15}{45 \div 15} = \frac{1}{3}$$

43. B: 4.11

Set up the problem, with the larger number on top. Multiply as if there are no decimal places. Add the answer rows together. Count the number of decimal places that were in the original numbers ($1 + 1 = 2$).

Place the decimal 2 places to the right for the final solution.

44. B: 98.91

Set up the problem, with the larger number on top. Multiply as if there are no decimal places. Add the answer rows together. Count the number of decimal places that were in the original numbers (2).

Place the decimal in that many spots from the right for the final solution.

45. A: $\frac{20}{63}$

Line up the fractions:

$$\frac{15}{21} \times \frac{48}{108}$$

Reduce the fractions prior to multiplying:

$$\frac{15 \div 3}{21 \div 3} = \frac{5}{7}$$

$$\frac{48 \div 4}{108 \div 4} = \frac{12}{27}$$

Multiply across the top and across the bottom:

$$\frac{5 \times 12}{7 \times 27} = \frac{60}{189}$$

Reduce:

$$\frac{60 \div 3}{189 \div 3} = \frac{20}{63}$$

46. D: $32\frac{19}{34}$

Set up the division problem.

$$34\overline{)1107}$$

34 does not go into 1 or 11 but will go into 110 so start there.

$$
\begin{array}{r}
32 \\
34\overline{)1107} \\
-102 \\
\hline
87 \\
-68 \\
\hline
19
\end{array}
$$

The answer is $32\frac{19}{34}$.

47. C: $\frac{9}{46}$

Set up the division problem.

$$\frac{14}{28} \div \frac{23}{9}$$

Flip the second fraction and multiply.

$$\frac{14}{28} \times \frac{9}{23}$$

Simplify and reduce with cross multiplication.

$$\frac{1}{2} \times \frac{9}{23}$$

Multiply across the top and across the bottom.

$$\frac{1 \times 9}{2 \times 23} = \frac{9}{46}$$

48. A: $4\frac{7}{12}$

Divide:

$$
\begin{array}{r}
4 \\
12\overline{)55} \\
-48 \\
\hline
7
\end{array}
$$

The result is $4\frac{7}{12}$.

This cannot be reduced.

49. B: $\frac{59}{6}$

The original number was $9\frac{5}{9}$. Multiply the denominator by the whole number portion. Add the numerator and put the total over the original denominator.

$$\frac{(6 \times 9) + 5}{6} = \frac{59}{6}$$

50. C: 2,718.035

To round 2,718.0354 to the nearest thousandths, use the digit in the ten-thousandths.

4 is less than 5, so round down in the thousandths.

2,718.035

51. C: Because the triangles are similar, the lengths of the corresponding sides are proportional. Therefore:

$$\frac{30 + x}{30} = \frac{22}{14} = \frac{y + 15}{y}$$

This results in the equation:

$$14(30 + x) = 22 \times 30$$

When solved, this gives:

$$x = 17.1$$

The proportion also results in the equation:

$$14(y + 15) = 22y$$

When solved, this gives:

$$y = 26.3$$

372

52. C: The area of the shaded region is the area of the square minus the area of the circle. The area of the circle is πr^2. The side of the square will be $2r$, so the area of the square will be $4r^2$. Therefore, the difference is:

$$4r^2 - \pi r^2 = (4 - \pi)r^2$$

53. C: The equation $x = 3$ is not a function because it does not pass the vertical line test. This test is made from the definition of a function, where each x-value must be mapped to one and only one y-value. This equation is a vertical line, so the x-value of 3 is mapped with an infinite number of y-values.

54. A: Robert accomplished his task on Tuesday in $\frac{3}{4}$ the time compared to Monday. He must have worked $\frac{4}{3}$ as fast.

55. C: There are 34 girls who are potty-trained out of a total of 52 girls:

$$34 \div 52 = 0.65 = 65\%$$

Reading Comprehension

1. B: Strong dislike. This vocabulary question can be answered using context clues. Based on the rest of the conversation, the reader can gather that Albert isn't looking forward to his marriage. As the Count notes that "you don't appear to me to be very enthusiastic on the subject of this marriage," and also remarks on Albert's "objection to a young lady who is both rich and beautiful," readers can guess Albert's feelings. The answer choice that most closely matches "objection" and "not . . . very enthusiastic" is *B*, "strong dislike."

2. C: Their name is more respected than the Danglars'. This inference question can be answered by eliminating incorrect answers. Choice *A* is tempting, considering that Albert mentions money as a concern in his marriage. However, although he may not be as rich as his fiancée, his father still has a stable income of 50,000 francs a year. Choice *B* isn't mentioned at all in the passage, so it's impossible to make an inference. Finally, Choice *D* is false because Albert's father arranged his marriage, but his mother doesn't approve of it. Evidence for Choice *C* can be found in the Count's comparison of Albert and Eugénie: "she will enrich you, and you will ennoble her." In other words, the Danglars are wealthier but the Morcerf family has a more noble background.

3. D: Apprehensive. There are many clues in the passage that indicate Albert's attitude towards his marriage—far from enthusiastic, he has many reservations. This question requires test takers to understand the vocabulary in the answer choices. "Pragmatic" is closest in meaning to "realistic," and "indifferent" means "uninterested." The only word related to feeling worried, uncertain, or unfavorable about the future is "apprehensive."

4. B: He is like a wise uncle, giving practical advice to Albert. Choice *A* is incorrect because the Count's tone is friendly and conversational. Choice *C* is also incorrect because the Count questions why Albert doesn't want to marry a young, beautiful, and rich girl. While the Count asks many questions, he isn't particularly "probing" or "suspicious"—instead, he's asking to find out more about Albert's situation and then give him advice about marriage.

373

5. A: She belongs to a noble family. Though Albert's mother doesn't appear in the scene, there's more than enough information to answer this question. More than once is his family's noble background mentioned (not to mention that Albert's mother is the Comtesse de Morcerf, a noble title). The other answer choices can be eliminated—she is deeply concerned about her son's future; money isn't her highest priority because otherwise she would favor a marriage with the wealthy Danglars; and Albert describes her "clear and penetrating judgment," meaning she makes good decisions.

6. C: The richest people in society were also the most respected. The Danglars family is wealthier but the Morcerf family has a more aristocratic name, which gives them a higher social standing. Evidence for the other answer choices can be found throughout the passage: Albert mentioned receiving money from his father's fortune after his marriage; Albert's father has arranged this marriage for him; and the Count speculates that Albert's mother disapproves of this marriage because Eugénie isn't from a noble background like the Morcerf family, implying that she would prefer a match with a girl from aristocratic society.

7. A: He seems reluctant to marry Eugénie, despite her wealth and beauty. This is a reading comprehension question, and the answer can be found in the following lines: "'I confess,' observed Monte Cristo, "that I have some difficulty in comprehending your objection to a young lady who is both rich and beautiful."' Choice *B* is the opposite (Albert's father is the one who insists on the marriage), Choice *C* incorrectly represents Albert's eagerness to marry, and Choice *D* describes a more positive attitude than Albert actually feels ("repugnance").

8. B: The passage is mostly made up of dialogue. We can see this in the way the two characters communicate with each other, in this case through the use of quotations marks, or dialogue. Narration is when the narrator (not the characters) is explaining things that are happening in the story. Description is when the narrator describes a specific setting and its images. Explanation is when the author is analyzing or defining something for the reader's benefit.

9. D: The meaning of the word "ennoble" in the middle of the paragraph means to give someone a noble rank or title. In the passage, we can infer that Albert is noble but not rich, and Mademoiselle Eugénie is rich but not noble.

10. C: Because he finally understands Albert's point of view but still doesn't agree with it. The other choices aren't mentioned anywhere in the passage. Remember, although this passage is part of a larger text, the test taker should only pay attention to what's in the passage itself in order to find the correct answer.

11. B: According to the passage, 20 people were arrested as witches in the Lancashire trials. The essay tells us that "ten were hanged, one died in goal (jail), one was sentenced to death in the pillory, and eight were acquitted."

12. D: The word *commemorative* means in honor of something. The context clue here includes the "works of fiction" by the authors Blake Morrison, Ann Duffy, and Jeanette Winterson, no doubt to celebrate the preserved history of the famous trial.

13. C: All the details in this paragraph suggest that Brookside is a great place to live, plus the last sentence states that it is an *idyllic neighborhood*, meaning it is perfect, happy, and blissful. Choices *A* and *B* are incorrect, because although they do contain specific details from the paragraph that support the main idea, they are not the main idea. Choice *D* is incorrect because there is no reference in the paragraph to the crime rate in Brookside.

14. D: In the first sentence, it states very clearly that the Brookside neighborhood is *one of the nation's first planned communities*. This makes it unique, as many other neighborhoods are old, many other neighborhoods exist in Kansas City, and many other neighborhoods have shopping areas. For these reasons, all the other answer choices are incorrect.

15. B: The author clearly states that education is crucial to the survival of the human race, and it can be easily inferred that if this is true, then improvements to our educational system are certainly worth fighting for. Choices *A* and *C* are incorrect because there is nothing in the passage that relates to these statements. Choice *D* is incorrect because it directly contradicts what the author states about all children's ability to learn.

16. A: Clearly, this author feels passionately about the importance of education. This is evident especially in the word choices. For this reason, all the other answer choices are incorrect.

17. C: Based on the author's passionate stance about the importance of education for all children, this answer choice makes the most sense. For this reason, all the other answer choices are incorrect.

18. D: The author mentions the importance of parent involvement and communication between school and home. He also devotes one full paragraph to the impact of technology on education. Nowhere in the passage does the author mention the cost of textbooks, so Choice *D* is correct.

19. A: The word *patronage* most nearly means *auspices*, which means *protection* or *support*. Choice *B*, *aberration*, means *deformity* and does not make sense within the context of the sentence. Choice *C*, *acerbic*, means *bitter* and also does not make sense in the sentence. Choice *D*, *adulation*, is a positive word meaning *praise*, and thus does not fit with the word *condescending* in the sentence.

20. D: *Working man* is most closely aligned with Choice *D*, *bourgeois*. In the context of the speech, the word *bourgeois* means *working* or *middle class*. Choice *A*, *Plebeian*, does suggest *common people*; however, this is a term that is specific to ancient Rome. Choice *B*, *viscount*, is a European title used to describe a specific degree of nobility. Choice *C*, *entrepreneur*, is a person who operates their own business.

21. D: *Enterprise* most closely means *cause*. Choices *A*, *B*, and *C* are all related to the term *enterprise*. However, Dickens speaks of a *cause* here, not a company, courage, or a game. *He will stand by such an enterprise* is a call to stand by a cause to enable the working man to have a certain autonomy over his own economic standing. The very first paragraph ends with the statement that the working man *shall . . . have a share in the management of an institution which is designed for his benefit.*

22. B: The speaker's salutation is one from an entertainer to his audience and uses the friendly language to connect to his audience before a serious speech. Recall in the first paragraph that the speaker is there to "accompany [the audience] . . . through one of my little Christmas books," making him an author there to entertain the crowd with his own writing. The speech preceding the reading is the passage itself, and, as the tone indicates, a serious speech addressing the "working man." Although the passage speaks of employers and employees, the speaker himself is not an employer of the audience, so Choice *A* is incorrect. Choice *C* is also incorrect, as the salutation is not used ironically, but sincerely, as the

375

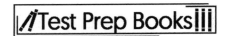

speech addresses the wellbeing of the crowd. Choice *D* is incorrect because the speech is not given by a politician, but by a writer.

23. B: For the working man to have a say in his institution which is designed for his benefit. Choice *A* is incorrect because that is the speaker's *first* desire, not his second. Choices *C* and *D* are tricky because the language of both of these is mentioned after the word *second*. However, the speaker doesn't get to the second wish until the next sentence. Choices *C* and *D* are merely prepositions preparing for the statement of the main clause, Choice *B*.

24. C: The speaker's tone can best be described as *confident and informed.* The speaker addresses the audience as "My good friends," and says, "I have no fear of being misunderstood," which implies confidence. Additionally, the speaker's knowledge of the proposal and topic can be seen in the text as well, especially in the second paragraph.

25. D: To provide credibility to the working man and share confidence in their ability to take on responsibilities if they are compensated appropriately. The speaker provides credibility by saying "he will stand by such an enterprise with the utmost of his patience," and displays their responsibilities by saying "he will feel his responsibility like an honest man."

26. A: The speaker says to "Erect in Birmingham a great Education Institution, properly educational." Choice *B* is close, but the speaker uses the name "Temple of Concord" in the passage as a metaphor, so this is incorrect. The other two choices aren't mentioned in the passage.

27. B: The word *antagonism* most nearly means opposition. Choice *A, conformity*, is the opposite of antagonism. Choice *C, affluence*, means abundance. Choice *D, scarcity*, means being deficient in something.

28. D: This is the correct answer choice because expository writing involves straightforward, factual information and analysis. It is unbiased and does not rely on the writer's personal feelings or opinions. Choice *A* is incorrect because narrative writing tells a story. Choice *B* is incorrect because persuasive writing is intended to change the reader's mind or position on a topic. Choice *C* is incorrect because technical writing attempts to outline a complex object or process.

29. B: This is the correct answer choice because the passage begins by describing Carver's childhood fascination with painting and later returns to this point when it states that at the end of his career "Carver returned to his first love of art." For this reason, all the other answer choices are incorrect.

30. A: This is the correct answer choice because the passage contains a definition of the term, *agricultural monoculture*, which is very similar to this answer.

31. C: This is the correct answer choice because there is ample evidence in the passage that refers to Carver's brilliance and the fact that his discoveries had a far-reaching impact both then and now. There is no evidence in the passage to support any of the other answer choices.

32. A: It introduces certain insects that transition from water to air. Choice *B* is incorrect because although the passage talks about gills, it is not the central idea of the passage. Choices *C* and *D* are incorrect because the passage does not "define" or "invite," but only serves as an introduction to stoneflies, dragonflies, and mayflies and their transition from water to air.

33. C: The act of shedding part or all of the outer shell. Choices *A*, *B*, and *D* are incorrect.

34. B: The first paragraph serves as a contrast to the second. Notice how the first paragraph goes into detail describing how insects are able to breathe air. The second paragraph acts as a contrast to the first by stating "[i]t is of great interest to find that, nevertheless, a number of insects spend much of their time under water." Watch for transition words such as "nevertheless" to help find what type of passage you're dealing with.

35: C: The stage of preparation in between molting is acted out in the water, while the last stage is in the air. Choices *A*, *B*, and *D* are all incorrect. *Instars* is the phase between two periods of molting, and the text explains when these transitions occur.

36. C: The author's tone is informative and exhibits interest in the subject of the study. Overall, the author presents us with information on the subject. One moment where personal interest is depicted is when the author states, "It is of great interest to find that, nevertheless, a number of insects spend much of their time under water."

37. C: This passage is designed to *persuade*. The whole purpose of the passage is to convince vacationers to come to Random Lake. There are some informative aspects of the passage, such as what's available – boating, house rentals, pontoon boats, but an extremely positive spin is put on the area, a spin that's designed to attract visitors. To prove it's persuasive, the argument can be reversed: Random Lake is *not* a good place to vacation. With a lack of adjectives and adverbs, there's a lack of *descriptive* detail, and this passage doesn't delight or *entertain* like a witty narrative might.

38. C: "Pontoon boats, kayaks, and paddle boats are available for rental" is out of place. The sentence before refers to fully furnished homes, and the sentence after refers to new developments. This sentence would have fit much better near, "Swimming, kayaking, boating, fishing, volleyball, mini-golf, go-cart track, eagle watching, nature trails," because the activities of the area are described. "This summer, why not rent a house on Random Lake?" is followed, logically, by a description of where Random Lake is. "There are enough activities there to keep a family busy for a month," is preceded by a listing of all those activities. "With several new housing developments slated for grand opening in March, the choices are endless!" links to "furnished houses," because this is an opportunity to find even more houses.

39. C: *The Random Lake area is growing.* This can be deduced with the passage, "With the Legends and The Broadmoor developments slated for grand openings in March, the choices are endless!" Considering buildings are being added, not razed, the Random Lake area would have to be growing. *Random City is more populated than Random Lake.* The word *city* is not necessarily indicative of size. There's simply not enough information to determine the size of either Random City or Random Lake. *The Random Lake area is newer than Random City.* Though this might seem logical with the addition of new buildings at Random Lake, there's no way to confirm this. The reader simply doesn't know enough about Random City to draw a comparison. *Random Lake prefers families to couples.* The ad definitely appeals to families but, "There are hotels available for every lifestyle and budget," proves that Random Lake is trying to appeal to everyone. Furthermore, "Prefer quiet? Historical? Modern?" proves that there are accommodations for every lifestyle.

40. A: The tone is exasperated. While contemplative is an option because of the inquisitive nature of the text, Choice *A* is correct because the speaker is frustrated by the thought of being included when he felt that the fellow members of his race were being excluded. The speaker is not nonchalant, nor accepting of the circumstances which he describes.

41. C: Choice *C, contented*, is the only word that has a different meaning. Furthermore, the speaker expresses objection and disdain throughout the entire text.

42. B: To address the hypocrisy of the Fourth of July holiday. While the speaker makes biblical references, it is not the main focus of the passage, thus eliminating Choice *A* as an answer. The passage also makes no mention of wealthy landowners and doesn't speak of any positive response to the historical events, so Choices *C* and *D* are not correct.

43. C: Throughout the entire text, the author maintains a persuasive tone. He argues that punishment should quickly follow the crime and gives a host of reasons why: it's more humane; it helps the prisoner to understand the nature of their crimes; it makes a better example for society. To confirm it's a persuasive stance, try reversing the argument. If the position cannot be reversed, then it's not persuasive. In this instance, the reader could argue in rebuttal that the punishment does not have to quickly follow the crime. Regardless of the veracity of this argument, simply creating it proves that the passage is persuasive.

44. D: "The more immediately after the commission of a crime a punishment is inflicted, the more just and useful it will be," best exemplifies the main idea of this passage. All subsequent discussion links back to this main idea and plays the role of supporting details. "The vulgar, that is, all men who have no general ideas or universal principles, act in consequence of the most immediate and familiar associations," supports this idea because the "vulgar," criminals, in other words, are used to making quick associations and are not used to delaying gratification or ignoring their impulses. "Crimes of less importance are commonly punished, either in the obscurity of a prison, or the criminal is transported, to give, by his slavery, an example to societies which he never offended," supports the main idea because the author argues that this is the wrong way to punish because if the punishment occurs in the same area the crime was committed, then the punishment will have more effect, since criminals will associate the areas with their crimes.

Furthermore, transferring a prisoner takes time and delays punishment. Lastly, the author states, "Men do not, in general, commit great crimes deliberately, but rather in a sudden gust of passion; and they commonly look on the punishment due to a great crime as remote and improbable." To reduce the sense of punishments being remote and improbable, criminals must, according to the author, receive an immediate punishment. Therefore, by removing a lengthy gap between crime and punishment, a criminal's punishment will be close and probable, which the author argues is the most humane way to punish and the mark of a civilized society.

45. A: The author would disagree most strongly with the statement *criminals are incapable of connecting crime and punishment*. Though the author states that criminals are often passionate and consider punishment unlikely in the heat of the crime, the entire premise of the passage is that reducing the time between crime and punishment increases the likelihood of an association. He also argues that if a society does this consistently, the probability that individuals will consider the consequences of their actions increases. *A punishment should quickly follow the crime* is a restatement of the main idea, supported by evidence throughout the passage. *Most criminals do not think about the consequences of*

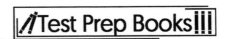

their actions. Though the author makes this clear, he goes on to say that, in general, reducing the time between crime and punishment will have the most positive effect on the prisoner and on society. *Where a criminal is being punished is just as important as when.* The author argues in the passage that a punishment should be immediate and near where the crime originally occurred.

46. A: The word *foliage* is defined as leaves on plants or trees. In this sentence, the meaning can be drawn from the fact that a heavily wooded area in October would be characterized by the beautiful changing colors of the leaves. The other answer choices do not accurately define the word *foliage*, so they are incorrect.

47. C: This is a tricky question, but it can be solved through careful context analysis and vocabulary knowledge. One can infer that the use of "expedient," while not necessarily very positive, isn't inherently bad in this context either. Note how in the next line, he says, "but most governments are usually, and all governments are sometimes, inexpedient." This use of "inexpedient" indicates that a government becomes a hindrance rather than a solution; it slows progress rather than helps facilitate progress. Thus, Choice *A* and Choice *D* can be ruled out because these are more of the result of government, not the intention or initial design. Choice *B* makes no logical sense. Therefore, Choice *C* is the best description of *expedient.* Essentially, Thoreau is saying that government is constructed as a way of developing order and people's rights, but the rigidity of government soon inhibits justice and human rights.

48. B: While Choice *D* is the only answer that mentions the Mexican War directly, Thoreau clearly thinks the war is unnecessary because the people generally didn't consent to the war. Choices *A*, *B*, and *C* are all correct to a degree, but the answer asks for the best description. Therefore, Choice *B* is the most accurate representation of Thoreau's views. Essentially, Thoreau brings to light the fact that the few people in power can twist government and policy for their own needs.

49. D: Choices *A* and *B* are completely incorrect. Thoreau is not defending government in any way. His views are set against government. As mentioned in the text, he appreciates little government but favors having no government structure at all. The text is reflective by nature but not reflective on the stages of government abuses as Choice *C* suggests. Choice *D* is the more appropriate answer because of the presence of evidence in the text. Thoreau cites current events and uses them to illustrate the point he's trying to make.

50. C: One of Thoreau's biggest criticisms of government is its capacity to impose on the people's freedoms and liberties, enacting rules that the people don't want and removing power from the individual. None of the scenarios directly impose specific regulations or restrictions on the people, except Prohibition. Prohibition removed the choice to consume alcohol in favor of abstinence, which was favored by the religious conservatives of the time. Thus, Thoreau would point out that this is a clear violation of free choice and an example of government meddling.

51. A: Choice *B* is totally irrelevant. Choice *C* is also incorrect; Thoreau never personifies government. Also, this doesn't coincide with his wooden gun analogy. Choice *D* is compelling because of its language but doesn't define the statement. Choice *A* is the most accurate summary of the main point of Thoreau's statement.

52. B: Thoreau specifically cites that legislators "are continually putting in their way." This reflects his suspicion and concern of government intervention. Recall that Thoreau continually mentions that

379

government, while meant as a way to establish freedom, is easily used to suppress freedom, piling on regulations and rules that inhibit progress. Choice *B* is the answer that most directly states how Thoreau sees government getting in the way of freedom.

53. C: The word *liable* most nearly means susceptible. The text says, "The government itself, which is only the mode which the people have chosen to execute their will, is equally liable to be abused and perverted before the people can act through it." Thoreau is saying here that the government is vulnerable enough to be abused. Choice *A, paramount,* means having importance. Choice *B, inconceivable,* means unbelievable. Choice *D, detrimental,* means damaging.

54. B: Thoreau is talking about the American government. We see this information in the beginning of the second paragraph. The passage mentions the Mexican War, but the passage itself does not relay the vulnerabilities of the Mexican government. The other two countries are not mentioned in the passage.

55. B: Posterity means all future generations of people. The sentence would say, "The American government—what is it but a tradition, though a recent one, endeavoring to transmit itself unimpaired to all future generations of people . . ." Choice *A* would be the definition of *royalty.* Choice *C* would be the definition of an *educator.* Choice *D* would be the definition of a *philosopher.*

Vocabulary

1. D: Denigrating. To *denigrate* is to disparage or belittle.

2. C: Flushed. *Ruddy* means red and flushed.

3. A: Deduce. To *deduce* is to draw a logical conclusion or to infer.

4. B: Untoward. Something *untoward* is inconvenient and unexpected.

5. C: Any disorder of the nervous system that includes involuntary, jerky movements. It usually affects distal musculature and the face.

6. D: Itchiness. The intense itchiness of pruritis may be caused by dry skin, allergies, pregnancy, or other causes.

7. B: Ipsilateral. *Bilateral* is on both sides and *contralateral* is on opposite sides.

8. A: Excessive sweating. Causes of diaphoresis are varied and can include anxiety, medication side effects, malaria, and diabetes.

9. B: Sexually-transmitted. Syphilis and chlamydia are examples of venereal diseases.

10. C: Abjure. To *abjure* is to solemnly renounce a claim, belief, stance etc.

11. C: Harmful. Something *deleterious* causes damage or harm.

12. D: Anhedonia. *Hedonism* is the pursuit of pleasure. *Anhedonia* is often a sign of depression.

13. B: Subtle differences. *Nuances* are shades or subtle differences, particularly in tone, expression, or sound.

14. B: Distal means "situated away from." *Proximal* structures are closer to the trunk.

15. D: Phlegmatic. *Egregious* means appalling or shockingly bad. *Insolent* means rude and disrespectful. Something *impervious* does not allow fluid to penetrate or pass through.

16. C: Exogenous. Exogenous agents arise from outside the body.

17. C: From the Latin root *fortis*, *fortify* literally means to make strong. *Foster* has nothing to do with the term at all. *Undermine* is to weaken, so this is the opposite. While a *barricade* can be used to fortify something, it is a means of protection, not the action of protection, unless used as a verb.

18. D: Cachexia. *Catatonia* may occur with schizophrenia or other disorders and refers to an abnormality of behavior or movement. *Anorexia* refers to a loss of appetite or reduction of eating; it is often heard in association with the eating disorder anorexia nervosa. *Ataxia* refers to a loss of being able to fully control one's body parts.

19. C: To physically examine using touch. Medical professionals use their hands to palpate and feel an area of a patient's body to examine the physical structures using touch. They might detect lumps, areas of abnormal swelling, nodules, or other abnormalities.

20. D: Ancillary. Something *auxiliary* is ancillary or provides additional help or support. *Axillary* refers to the armpit.

21. A: Guileless. *Guileless* is to be without guile or deception, or to be innocent and childlike.

22. A: Inane. Someone described as *vacuous* lacks intelligence or thought. Something *vacuous* is inane or silly.

23. B: Dignity. *Gravitas* is dignity or seriousness of manner.

24. A: Adhesions. To *adhere* is to stick together, so adhesions are tissues sticking together.

25. B: Relating to the liver. The prefix *hepa-* relates to the liver.

26. D: The serous membrane lining the abdominal cavity. Choice *A* is referring to peristalsis. Choice *B* is referring to the perineum. Choice *C* is referring to the periosteum.

27. A: Ardent. *Vehement* means showing passionate feelings or being forceful.

28. A: Lumen. Arteries, blood vessels, and hollow organs have lumens.

29. C: Befuddled. *Lucid* means intelligible or expressed clearly, and *diffident* means modest or shy.

30. A: Decubitus ulcer. Bed sores are pressure ulcers or decubitus ulcers. They often occur in skin areas with underlying bony prominences, such as the heel or tailbone.

31. D: Afferent. Afferent nerves, for example, go from a receptor on the skin or other area of the body to the spinal cord. They relay sensory messages.

32. C: Dark scab. An eschar may result from a bad burn or from a mite bite or other causes.

33. C: Wan. *Pallor* means pale, lacking in color, or wan.

381

34. A: Nasal discharge. The prefix *rhin-* means nose or related to the nose, while the suffix *-rrhea* means flow or discharge. Menorrhea, for example, is menstrual flow.

35. B: Around the spinal cord. Baclofen, for spastic cerebral palsy, may have an intrathecal route of administration.

36. A: Verbally express grief. To *lament* is to mourn or verbally express sorrow or grief.

37. D: Harmful. Something noxious is poisonous, harmful, or very unpleasant.

38. C: An outward curvature of the thoracic spine. *Lordosis* is an exaggerated lumbar spine curve like swayback. *Scoliosis* is an abnormal lateral curvature of the spine.

39. D: The study of aging. The prefix *ger-* or *gero-* means old age as in geriatric.

40. B: Peptic ulcer. An endoscopy is a procedure that uses a flexible tube with a camera to visualize an internal structure.

41. A: Intransigent. *Complacent* means smug or self-satisfied. Something *inexplicable* cannot be accounted for or explained. *Confound* can mean to amaze or astonish, or to mix-up and cause difficulty distinguishing something.

42. B: Objective data. In SOAP notes, observable tests like blood pressure, weight, and pulse oximetry are recorded under the objective section.

43. A: One from which a patient will likely not recover. Examples of terminal illnesses are congestive heart failure, AIDs, and advanced kidney disease.

44. A: The knee. The shallow depression behind the knee is the popliteal fossa.

45. C: Paragon. A *parable* is like a fable or simple story, often with a moral lesson. A *paradox* is an apparent contradiction. *Paraphrase* can be a noun or a verb. As a noun, it is a rewording of something spoken or written, while as a verb, it means to use original language to reword what someone else wrote or said.

46. D: Clean and new. Something in pristine condition is unused or appears as it did when it was new.

47. A: Ringing in the ear. Tinnitus is a symptom of an underlying medical condition such as an ear injury or a circulation disturbance.

48. C: Inflammation. Tendonitis, conjunctivitis, and colitis are examples of medical conditions that are specific areas of inflammation.

49. C: Difficulty swallowing. The suffix *-phagia* usually refers to eating.

50. D: Hives. Urticaria may result from an allergic reaction to food, medicine, environmental trigger, or other allergen.

51. B: To *elucidate*, a light is figuratively shined on a previously unknown or confusing subject. This Latin root, "lux" meaning "light," prominently figures into the solution. *Enlighten* means to educate, or bring into the light.

382

52. D: Looking at the Latin word "veritas," meaning "truth," will yield a clue as to the meaning of verify. To *verify* is the act of finding or assessing the truthfulness of something. This usually means amassing evidence to substantiate a claim. *Substantiate,* of course, means to provide evidence to prove a point.

53. A: If someone is *inspired*, they are motivated to do something. Someone who is an inspiration motivates others to follow their example.

54. D: *Mendacious* describes dishonesty or lying in several ways. This is another word of classical lineage. *Mendacio* in Latin means "liar." While *liar* lacks the Latin root, the meanings fit.

55. A: *Mitigate* refers to easing tension or making less severe. *Focus, fiery,* and *conspire* do not relate. *Alleviate* is synonymous, meaning to make less severe. Note the ending *-ate*, which also indicates function. Both terms reflect the function of easing difficult circumstances.

Grammar

1. A: The clause *that is autographed* is essential to the sentence so the word *that* is appropriate. *Whom* is the object of the verb *belongs to,* so you would not use *who.* Choice *B* is incorrect because the clause *which is autographed* is not enclosed in commas, and you would not use *who* as the object in the sentence. Choice *C* is incorrect because you would not use *whom* as the subject of the sentence and the clause *which is autographed* is not enclosed in commas. Choice *D* is incorrect because you would not use *whom* as the subject of the sentence.

2. A: The correct spelling of this word is *caffeine.* This answer, along with Choices *B* and *C* are exceptions to the rule *i before e, except after c.* Choice *D* follows this rule because the letters *ie* follow the letter *c,* so the correct order would be *ei.*

3. B: Use the word *may* instead of *can* at the beginning of the sentence because it is asking for permission and *can* means "able to." Choice *A* is a proper sentence using the word *bring* (coming toward) and the word *take* (going away) correctly. Choice *C* is a proper sentence using the word *lend* as a verb and the word *loan* as a noun. Choice *D* is a proper sentence using the words *two* (the number), *to* (the infinitive) and *too* (meaning "very") in the correct placements.

4. A: *Badly* is an adverb describing how hurt and *good* is used with the sensory word *feels.* Choice *B* is incorrect because *bad* is an adjective not an adverb. Choice *C* is incorrect because *bad* is an adjective where an adverb is needed and *well* is an adverb where an adjective is needed. Choice *D* is incorrect because *badly* fits but *good* should be used instead of *well* because of the sensory word *feels.*

5. C: *Because the lion and tiger habitat was closed* is a dependent clause and needs a subject. Choice *A* is incorrect because the sentence is an independent clause with both a subject and a verb, therefore it creates a complete sentence. Choice *B* is incorrect because the sentence is also a complete independent clause. Choice *D* is incorrect because the sentence is a complete independent clause forming an interrogative sentence.

6. A: *I love to go water-skiing, I love alpine skiing,* and *I also love Nordic skiing* are all independent clauses and are not connected with coordinating conjunctions or separated with semi colons, colons, or dashes. This makes it a run-on sentence. Choice *B* is not a run-on sentence; it is a simple single independent clause. Choice *C* is incorrect; it is a complete independent clause with both a subject (*types*

383

of skiing) and a verb (*require*). Choice *D* is incorrect. It contains two independent clauses but a semicolon correctly separates them, therefore it is a complete compound sentence.

7. B: *Eating a large meal* cannot modify the word *food*. The food is not eating the meal. Choice *A* does not contain a dangling modifier. *Eating a large meal* modifies the pronoun *I*. Choice *C* does not contain a dangling modifier. It contains an incorrect preposition. The sentence should say, *"After eating a large meal, I was too full."* Choice *D* does not contain a dangling modifier. *Eating a large meal* correctly modifies the pronoun *I*. *I* ate the large meal.

8. C: The words *didn't* and *nothing* are both negatives. The sentence actually means a positive: *"They did like something I said."* Choice *A* is incorrect because it is a proper sentence with a single negative, *couldn't*. Choice *B* is incorrect because it is a proper sentence without any negatives. Choice *D* is incorrect because it is actually a triple negative; the words *cannot*, *don't*, and *disapprove* are all negatives. The sentence actually means: *"I disapprove of that."*

9. D: *Pulling heavy rope* is the subject complement for the word *helps*. Choice *A* is incorrect because *heavy rope* is the object complement for the word *pulling*. Choice *B* is incorrect because *muscles* is the object complement for the word *strengthen*. Choice *C* is incorrect because *strengthen* is the object complement for the word *helps*.

10. C: *I* needs to be capitalized because it begins a sentence and the pronoun *I* is always capitalized. The word *mother* needs to be capitalized because it is naming the name of a relative. The title of the book *All the Light We Cannot See* needs capitalization except for the article *the*. *Martha* needs to be capitalized because it is a proper noun. The word *she* needs to be capitalized because it is in the beginning of a sentence inside quotations. Choice *A* is incorrect because *I* at the beginning of the sentence needs to be capitalized and the words *favorite*, *book*, and *said* do not need capitalization because they are not proper nouns.

Choice *B* is incorrect because *Mother* needs to be capitalized as a relative's name. *Book* is a common noun and does not need to be capitalized. The word *the* in the title of the book does not need to be capitalized because it is an article. *Said* does not need to be capitalized because it does not begin the sentence, and the word *she* needs to be capitalized because it does begin a new sentence inside quotation marks. Choice *D* is incorrect because the title *ALL THE LIGHT WE CANNOT SEE* should not be in all caps; rather it should be italicized and the first letter of each word should capitalized except *the*. It should be: *All the Light We Cannot See.*

11. C: There needs to be a period after the letters of the abbreviation *P.M.* There needs to be a period after the abbreviation *Dr.* There needs to be a period at the end of the declarative sentence. Choice *A* is incorrect because the periods after *P.M.* are omitted as is the period after the abbreviation *Dr.* The period after the end of the declarative sentence is also omitted. Choice *B* is incorrect because there is no ending punctuation for the declarative sentence and the periods in the abbreviation *P.M.* are omitted. Choice *D* is incorrect because the period after the word *forgotten* is extraneous.

12. D: *"Didn't anybody take the garbage out?"* is an interrogative sentence requiring a question mark for end punctuation. Choice *A* is incorrect because, *"Can you please take the garbage out,"* is an imperative sentence requiring a period for end punctuation. Choice *B* is incorrect because, *"I wonder if anyone has taken the garbage out,"* is a declarative sentence requiring a period for end punctuation. Choice *C* is incorrect because, *"Miles asked Lisa if she'd taken the garbage out,"* is also a declarative sentence.

13. B: *"Yikes!"* is an interjection. *"That startled me!"* is an exclamatory sentence. Both are punctuated with an exclamation mark. Choice *A* is incorrect because, *"Can you eat more than one slice of pizza!"* is an interrogative sentence so the end punctuation should be a question mark. Choice *C* is incorrect because we do not use both a question mark and an exclamation mark on the same sentence. Choice *D* is incorrect because we should never use more than one exclamation point in a grammatically correct sentence.

14. B: *A humanitarian* is a phrase describing the noun *Mother Teresa*, therefore it gets commas on both sides. There is a comma after *said* because the remark that follows is a quotation. Choice *A* is incorrect because there are extraneous commas after the words *two* and *three*. There only needs to be commas between the items in the list. Choice *C* is incorrect because there is an extraneous comma after the word *been*. Choice *D* is incorrect because there should be a period after the word *food,* and the word *consequently* should start a new sentence. The comma after the word *consequently* would be correct. There would not need to be a comma between *stomachache* and *heartburn* because it is a list of only two items.

15. D: There is a colon at the end of the introduction, *"There are four people who are most important to me."* There are serial commas already in a list—*my husband, my daughter, my friend, and my sister*—separated by semicolons after the names of each person. Choice *A* is incorrect because there are only semicolons separating the introduction and the items in the list. Choice *B* is incorrect because there is an extraneous colon between *people* and *who* and because the items in the list are only separated by commas. Choice *C* is incorrect because a semicolon instead of a colon separates the introduction from the list, and colons instead of semicolons separate the names of the people. In other words, in Choice *C* the roles of the colon and semicolon are reversed.

16. A: There should be a comma after the introduction *Daniel said* because it is a short quote. Quotation marks belong before and after exactly what was said, *"I want to travel to Mars,"* and the period belongs inside the quotation marks. Choice *B* is incorrect because there is no comma after the introduction, and the period is outside the quotation marks. Choice *C* is incorrect because the quotes are not around the actual statement, just the fragment *travel to Mars;* also, the period is outside the quotation marks. Choice *D* is incorrect because the quotations are enclosing the entire sentence, not just what was said, and there is no comma after the introduction.

17. C: The *team* is a collective noun acting as one, and therefore a singular verb *competes* creates subject/verb agreement. Choice *A* is incorrect. *Teams* is a plural subject, and *competes* is a singular verb; they do not create subject/verb agreement. Choice *B* is incorrect. *Teams* is plural, and *wins* is singular; they do not create subject/verb agreement. Choice *D* is incorrect. *Team* is a collective noun acting as one and agrees with a singular verb, but *win* is plural.

18. A: The *professor* is the singular subject (*of physics* should be ignored) and *compliments* is a singular verb. Choice *B* is incorrect. *Professor* is the singular subject but *compliment* is a plural verb. Choice *C* is incorrect. *Professors* is a plural subject and *compliments* is a singular verb; they do not agree. Choice *D* is incorrect; adding the word *will* to *compliments* does not change the fact that *compliments* is a singular verb and does not agree with the plural subject *professors*.

19. A: It is necessary to put a comma between the date and the year and between the day of the week and the month. Choice *B* is incorrect because it is missing the comma between the day of the week and the month. Choice *C* is incorrect because it adds an unnecessary comma between the month and date. Choice *D* is missing the necessary comma between day of the week and month.

20. B: *Conscientious* and *judgment* are both spelled correctly in this sentence. These are both considered commonly misspelled words. One or both words are spelled incorrectly in all the other examples.

21. B: In this sentence, the word *stress* is a noun. While the word *stress* can also act as a verb, in this particular case, it functions as a noun as the subject of the sentence. The word *stress* cannot be used as an adjective or adverb, so these answers are also incorrect.

22. B: The correct answer is o*ctopi,* the plural form of the word *octopus*. Choice *A* is the incorrect spelling of the plural of *roof,* which should be *roofs.* Choice *C* is the incorrect spelling of the plural form of the word *potato*, which should be *potatoes.* Choice *D* is the incorrect plural form of the word *fish,* which remains the same in the singular and the plural, *fish.*

23. A: Quotation marks are used to indicate something someone has said. This is a direct quotation that interrupts, or breaks, the sentence in half. A comma is necessary before the quotation and after it, and inside the quotation marks, to set off the quote from the rest of the sentence. Choice *B* is incorrect because there is no comma at the end of the quotation. Choice *C* is incorrect because there is no comma before or after the quotation. Choice *D* is incorrect because the comma at the end of the quotation is placed outside the quotation marks.

24. C: In this sentence, the word *counter* functions as an adjective that modifies the word *argument*. Choice *A* is incorrect because the word *counter* functions as a noun. Choice *B* is incorrect because the word *counter* functions as a verb. Choice *D* is incorrect because the word *counter* functions as an adverb.

25. B: This sentence correctly uses the plural pronoun *their,* which agrees in number with its antecedent, *human beings*. Choice *A* is incorrect because *his* is a singular pronoun and does not agree in number with the antecedent. Choice *C* is incorrect because *its* is a singular pronoun and usually refers to an object. Choice *D* is incorrect because *her* is a singular pronoun and does not agree with the antecedent.

26. D: *Every single one of my mother's siblings, their spouses, and their children* is the complete subject because it includes who or what is doing the action in the sentence as well as the modifiers that go with it. The other answer choices are incorrect because they only include part of the complete subject.

27. C: Choice *C* is the one that incorrectly uses italics; quotation marks should be used for the title of a short work such as a poem, not italics. Choice *A* correctly italicizes the title of a novel. Choice *B* correctly italicizes the title of both musicals, and Choice *D* correctly italicizes the name of a work of art.

28. A: In this sentence, the commonly misused words *it's* and *than* are used correctly. *It's* is a contraction for the pronoun *it* and the verb *is*. The word *than* accurately shows comparison between two things. The other examples all contain some combination of the commonly misused words *then* and *its*. *Then* is an adverb that conveys time, and *its* is a possessive pronoun. Both are incorrectly used in the other examples.

29. C: This example is an imperative sentence because it gives a command and ends with a period. Choice *A* is a declarative sentence that states a fact and ends with a period. Choice *B* is an interrogative sentence that asks a question and ends with a question mark. Choice *D* is an exclamatory sentence that shows strong emotion and ends with an exclamation point.

30. D: This is a compound sentence because it joins two independent clauses, *Felix plays the guitar in my roommate's band* and *Alicia is the lead vocalist*, with a comma and the coordinating conjunction *and*. Choices *A* and *C* are simple sentences, each containing one independent clause with a complete subject and predicate. Choice *A* does contain a compound subject, *John and Adam*, and Choice *C* contains a compound predicate, *ran and went*, but they are still simple sentences that only contain one independent clause. Choice *B* is a complex sentence because it contains one dependent clause, *As I was leaving*, and one independent clause, *my dad called and needed to talk*. This sentence also contains a compound predicate, *called and needed*.

31. B: This answer includes all the words functioning as nouns in the sentence. Choice *A* is incorrect because it does not include the proper noun *Monday*. The word *he* makes Choice *C* incorrect because it is a pronoun. This example also includes the word *dorm*, which can function as a noun, but in this sentence, it functions as an adjective modifying the word *room*. Choice *D* is incorrect because it leaves out the proper noun *Jose*.

32. D: The simple subject of this sentence, *Everyone*, although it names a group, is a singular noun and therefore agrees with the singular verb form *has*. Choice *A* is incorrect because the simple subject *each* does not agree with the plural verb form *have*. In Choice *B*, the plural subject *players* does not agree with the singular verb form *was*. In Choice *C*, the plural subject *friends* does not agree with the singular verb form *has*.

33. A: In this sentence, the word *Mom* should not be capitalized because it is not functioning as a proper noun. If the possessive pronoun *My* was not there, then it would be considered a proper noun and would be capitalized. *East Coast* is correctly capitalized. Choice *B* correctly capitalizes the name of a specific college course, which is considered a proper noun. Choice *C* correctly capitalizes the name of a specific airline, which is a proper noun, and Choice *D* correctly capitalizes the proper nouns *Martha's Vineyard* and *New England*.

34. C: In this sentence, *exhilarating* is functioning as an adjective that modifies the word *morning*, which in turn, modifies the word *air*. The words *air* and *morning* are functioning as nouns, and the word *inspired* is functioning as a verb in this sentence. Other words functioning as adjectives in the sentence include, *beautiful, mountain, every*, and *lengthy*.

35. D: This is the correct answer because the pronouns *him* and *me* are in the objective case. *Him* and *me* are the indirect objects of the verb *gave*. Choice *A* is incorrect because the personal pronoun in this case, *me*, should always go last. Choices *B* and *C* are incorrect because they contain at least one subjective pronoun.

36. B: In this sentence, a colon is correctly used to introduce a series of items. Choice *A* incorrectly uses a semicolon to introduce the series of states. Choice *C* incorrectly uses a dash to introduce the series. Choice *D* is incorrect because it incorrectly uses a comma to introduce the series.

37. A: This sentence uses the correct form of the contraction *you are* as the subject of the sentence, and it uses the correct form of the possessive pronoun *your* to indicate ownership of the backpack. It also uses the correct form of the adverb *there*, indicating place and the possessive pronoun *their* indicating ownership. Choice *B* is incorrect because it reverses the possessive pronoun *your* and the contraction

387

you are. Choice *C* is incorrect because it reverses the adverb *there* and the possessive pronoun *their*. Choice *D* is incorrect because it reverses the contraction *you are* and the possessive pronoun *your* and the possessive pronoun *their* and the adverb *there*.

38. C: This sentence correctly places an apostrophe after the plural proper noun *Joneses* to show possession. When a proper name ends in *s*, it is necessary to add *–es* to make it plural, then an apostrophe to make the plural form possessive. In Choice *A*, to make the word *children* possessive, add an apostrophe and then *-s* since the word *children* is already plural. Choice *B* does not need an apostrophe because *Smiths* is plural, not possessive. Choice *D* incorrectly places an apostrophe after the *–s*. In this case, to make *people* possessive, it is necessary to add an apostrophe and then an *–s* since the word *people* is already plural.

39. A: When parallel structure is used, all parts of the sentence are grammatically consistent. Choice *A* uses incorrect parallel structure because *swimming* and *biking* are gerunds, whereas *a run* is an infinitive, so the structure is grammatically inconsistent. Choices *B*, *C*, and *D* all have lists that are grammatically consistent.

40. C: The original sentence states that despite the author being nervous, she was able to read with poise and confidence, which is stated in Choice *C*. Choice *A* changes the meaning by adding *because*; however, the author didn't read with confidence *because* she was nervous, but *despite* being nervous. Choice *B* is closer to the original meaning; however, it loses the emphasis of her succeeding *despite* her condition. Choice *D* adds the word *before*, which doesn't make much sense on its own, much less in relation to the original sentence.

41. D: The original sentence states that there was a storm surge and loss of electricity during the hurricane, making Choice *D* correct. Choices *A* and *B* arrange the storm surge and the loss of electricity within a cause and effect statement, which changes the meaning of the original sentence. Choice *C* changes *surge* from a noun into a verb and creates an entirely different situation.

42. B: The original sentence states that an elephant herd will help and support another herd member if it is sick, so Choice *B* is correct. Choice *A* is incorrect because it states the whole herd will be too sick and too tired to walk instead of a single elephant. Choice *C* is incorrect because the original sentence does not say that the herd gathers food when *they* are sick, but when a single member of the herd is sick. Although Choice *D* might be correct in a general sense, it does not relate to the meaning of the original sentence and is therefore incorrect.

43. A: The original sentence says that after a soccer game, they went out to eat. Choice *A* shows the same sequence: they finished the soccer game *then* went out to eat. Choice *B* is incorrect because it reverses the sequence of events. Choices *C* and *D* are incorrect because the words *so* and *because* change the meaning of the original sentence.

44. C: Choice *C* is the correct choice because the word "their" indicates possession, and the text is talking about "their students," or the students of someone. Choice *A* is not a word. Choice *B*, "they're," is a contraction and means "they are." Choice *D*, "there," means at a certain place and is incorrect.

45. B: Choice *B* uses all punctuation correctly in this sentence. Punctuation here should go inside the quotes, making Choice *A* incorrect. In American English, single quotes should only be used if they are quotes within a quote, making Choices *C* and *D* incorrect.

46. A: The correct choice for this sentence is that "they are . . . shaped by the influences." The prepositions "for," "to," and "with" do not make sense in this context. People are *shaped by*, not *shaped for, shaped to,* or *shaped with*.

47. D: Choice *D* is the best choice for this sentence. Choice *A* is incorrect because adding "was" to "spent" is incorrect verb usage in the sentence. Choice *B* is incorrect. Adding "to spend" to "he must" is grammatically incorrect. Choice *C* is incorrect because saying "he must spending" is also incorrect usage of the verb "spending."

48. D: There should be no change here. Both underlined sentences are complete and do not need changing. Choice *A* is incorrect. The underlined portion could *possibly* act with a colon. However, it's not the best choice, so omit Choice *A*. Choice *B* is incorrect because there is no punctuation between the two independent clauses; it is considered a run-on. Choice *C* is incorrect because placing a comma between two independent clauses creates a comma splice.

49. C: Choice *C* is correct because it uses the appropriate verb tense and usage. Choice *A* is incorrect. "When Ariana going off to college" is incorrect usage of the verb "to go." Choice *B* is incorrect because of the faulty subject/verb agreement. The verb "go" should be paired with a plural subject, and "Ariana" is singular. Choice *D* is incorrect. The verb agrees with the subject; however, the rest of the sentence is in past tense, so this verb should also be in past tense.

50. A: Choice *A* is correct because it connects a dependent clause (Although they were closed down) with an independent clause (they are open again after remodeling) with a comma. Choice *B* is a run-on sentence. Choice *C* creates a fragment beginning with "Although." Choice *D* puts a comma after the word "Although," which is incorrect.

51. C: Choice *C* correctly uses *from* to describe the fact that dogs are related to wolves. The word *through* is incorrectly used here, so Choices *A* is incorrect. Choice *B* makes no sense. Choice *D* unnecessarily changes the verb tense in addition to incorrectly using *through*.

52. B: Choice *B* is correct because the Oxford comma is applied, clearly separating the specific terms. Choice *A* lacks this clarity. Choice *C* is correct but too wordy since commas can be easily applied. Choice *D* doesn't flow with the sentence's structure.

53. C: Choice *C* is correct because it fixes the core issue with this sentence: the singular *has* should not describe the plural *scientists*. Thus, Choice *A* is incorrect. Choices *B* and *D* add unnecessary commas.

54. D: Choice *D* correctly applies a semicolon to introduce a new line of thought while remaining in a single sentence. The comma after *however* is also appropriately placed. Choice *A* is a run-on sentence. Choice *B* is also incorrect because the single comma is not enough to fix the sentence. Choice *C* adds commas around *uncertain* which are unnecessary.

55. A: Choice *A* is correct because the sentence contains no errors. The comma after *bias* successfully links the two halves of the sentence, and the use of *it's* is correct as a contraction of *it is*. Choice *B* creates a sentence fragment, while Choice *C* creates a run-on. Choice *D* incorrectly changes *it's* to *its*.

Biology

1. C: Molecules that are soluble in lipids, like fats, sterols, and vitamins (A, D, E and K), for example, are able to move in and out of a cell using passive transport. Water and oxygen are also able to move in and out of the cell without the use of cellular energy. Complex sugars and non-lipid-soluble molecules are too large to move through the cell membrane without relying on active transport mechanisms. Molecules naturally move from areas of high concentration to those of lower concentration. It requires active transport to move molecules in the opposite direction, as suggested by Choice *D*.

2. A: Both types of cells are enclosed by a cell membrane, which is selectively permeable. Selective permeability means essentially that it is a gatekeeper, allowing certain molecules and ions in and out, and keeping unwanted ones at bay, at least until they are ready for use. Prokaryotes contain a nucleoid and do not have organelles; eukaryotes contain a nucleus enclosed by a membrane, as well as organelles.

3. B: Diffusion and osmosis are examples of passive transport. Unlike active transport, passive transport does not require cellular energy. Diffusion is the movement of particles, such as ions, nutrients, or waste, from high concentration to low. Osmosis is the spontaneous movement of water from an area of high concentration to one of low concentration. Facilitated diffusion is another type of passive transport where particles move from high concentration to low concentration via a protein channel.

4. D: Meiosis has the same phases as mitosis, except that they occur twice—once in meiosis I and once in meiosis II. During meiosis I, the cell splits into two. Each cell contains two sets of chromosomes. Next, during meiosis II, the two intermediate daughter cells divide again, producing four total haploid cells that each contain one set of chromosomes.

5. D: Catabolism is the process of breaking large molecules into smaller molecules to release energy for work. Carbohydrates and fats are catabolized to provide energy for exercise and daily activities. Anabolism synthesizes larger molecules from smaller constituent building blocks. Bioenergetics and metabolism are more general terms involving overall energy production and usage.

6. B: Dominant alleles are considered to have stronger phenotypes and, when mixed with recessive alleles, will mask the recessive trait. The recessive trait would only appear as the phenotype when the allele combination is "aa" because a dominant allele is not present to mask it.

7. A: Mitochondria is described as the powerhouse of the cell. The nucleus, Choice *B*, contains the cell's DNA. The ribosomes, Choice *C*, build proteins. The cell wall, Choice *D*, maintains the shape of plant cells and protects its contents.

8. B: 1/8. Color blindness is a recessive, sex-linked trait. The Punnett square below shows the cross between a carrier female and a color-blind male. The two offspring in bold are color blind. The probability of having one child that is color blind is ½. The probability of having three color-blind children is ½ x ½ x ½ (law of multiplication) or 1/8.

	X^C	X^c
X^c	X^CX^c	X^cX^c
Y	X^CY	X^cY

9. A: Fungal cells have a cell wall, similar to plant cells; however, they use oxygen as a source of energy and cannot perform photosynthesis. Because they do not perform photosynthesis, fungal cells do not contain chloroplasts.

10. A: Roots are responsible for absorbing water and nutrients that will get transported up through the plant. They also anchor the plant to the ground. Photosynthesis occurs in leaves, stems transport materials through the plant and support the plant body, and phloem moves sugars downward to the leaves.

11. A: The correct answer is Choice A. Botanists study the field of botany, which is the study of plants. Neither the evolution of monkeys nor the genetic changes in human brain cancer, Choices B and C, involve studying plants. An ecologist would study how worker bees interact with a queen bee, Choice D, because that subdiscipline involves analyzing how organisms interact with each other.

12. C: The best answer is Choice C. Water molecules form a V-shape because of the uneven sharing of electrons between the atoms. The oxygen atom is slightly negatively charged, and the hydrogen atoms are slightly positively charged, so they pull away from each other and the molecule forms a V-shape.

13. B: The correct answer is Choice B. Nucleic acids include DNA and RNA, which store an organism's genetic information. Carbohydrates, Choice A, are used as an energy source for an organism. Proteins, Choice C, are important for the structure and function of organisms. Lipids, Choice D, are important for energy storage and insulation.

14. C: Chloroplasts are responsible for photosynthesis in plant cells, which is the process of converting sunlight energy to glucose energy. The cell wall helps maintain the cell's shape, Choice A. The nucleus contains the cell's DNA, Choice B. Ribosomes build proteins, Choice D.

15. D: The correct answer is Choice D. Enzymes increase the rate of the metabolic reaction. They do not change the starting or ending amount of free energy in the reactants or products, so Choices A and C are incorrect. The number of products also remains the same, so Choice B is incorrect.

16. B: The correct answer is Choice B. An animal cell is surrounded by a cell membrane. The cell membrane contains proteins that regulate which molecules are allowed in and out of the cell. Only plant cells are surrounded by a cell wall, so Choice A is incorrect. The nucleus, Choice C, is located in middle of the cell and would not be the first organelle that a molecule would encounter. The endoplasmic reticulum, Choice D, is located within the cytoplasm, inside the cell membrane.

391

17. A: The correct answer is Choice *A*. Oxidative phosphorylation is the final part of aerobic respiration and generates between 26 and 28 ATP molecules. In total, aerobic respiration generates between 30 and 32 ATP molecules, Choice *B*. Glycolysis and the citric acid cycle are the first parts of aerobic respiration and generate 4 ATP molecules, Choice *C*.

18. C: The correct answer is Choice *C*. On the right side of the chemical equation, O_2 is one of the products of the reaction. The left side of the equation contains the reactants. The reactants are CO_2, which is Choice *A*, and H_2O, which is Choice *B*. Solar energy, Choice *D*, joins the reactants to drive the reaction forward.

19. D: The correct answer is Choice *D*. In both mitosis and meiosis, DNA replication occurs during interphase. Mitosis has one cell division whereas meiosis has two cell divisions; therefore, Choice *A*, the number of divisions, is incorrect. Mitosis produces two daughter cells whereas meiosis produces four daughter cells; therefore, Choice *B* is incorrect. Synapsis of homologous chromosomes, Choice *C*, does not occur in mitosis.

20. C: mRNA is directly transcribed from DNA before being taken to the cytoplasm and translated by rRNA into a protein. tRNA transfers amino acids from the cytoplasm to the rRNA for use in building these proteins. siRNA is a special type of RNA which interferes with other strands of mRNA typically by causing them to get degraded by the cell rather than translated into protein.

21. B: Since the genotype is a depiction of the specific alleles that an organism's genes code for, it includes recessive genes that may or may not be otherwise expressed. The genotype does not have to name the proteins that its alleles code for; indeed, some of them may be unknown. The phenotype is the physical, visual manifestations of a gene, not the genotype. The genotype does not necessarily include any information about the organism's physical characters. Although some information about an organism's parents can be obtained from its genotype, its genotype does not actually show the parents' phenotypes.

22. C: One in four offspring (or 25%) will be short, so all four offspring cannot be tall. Although both of the parents are tall, they are hybrid or heterozygous tall, not homozygous. The mother's phenotype is for tall, not short. A Punnett square cannot determine if a short allele will die out. Although it may seem intuitive that the short allele will be expressed by lower numbers of the population than the tall allele, it still appears in 75% of the offspring (although its effects are masked in 2/3 of those). Besides, conditions could favor the recessive allele and kill off the tall offspring.

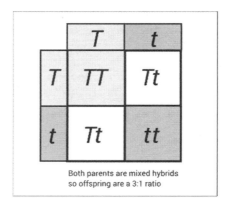

Both parents are mixed hybrids
so offspring are a 3:1 ratio

23. A: Human genes are strictly DNA and do not include proteins or amino acids. A human's genome and collection of genes will include even their recessive traits, mutations, and unused DNA.

24. A: The law of dominance states that dominant traits are always passed on and will be present in future generations, even if recessive alleles are inherited. Choice *B*, the law of similarity, is not one of Mendel's laws. The law of segregation, Choice *C*, states that the alleles of a gene are separated during meiosis. The law of independent assortment, Choice *D*, states that genes on the same chromosome are all independently and randomly sorted and assigned during the second division of meiosis.

25. B: The correct answer is Choice *B*. In DNA, adenine pairs only with thymine. Uracil, Choice *A*, is only found in RNA, not DNA. Guanine and cytosine, Choices *C* and *D*, pair with each other exclusively in DNA.

26. B: Looking at Figures 1 and 2, crossbreeding experiment #3 in round #1 produces plants that are completely recessive and would have white flowers. Choices *A* and *C*, crossbreeding experiments #1 and 2, respectively, only produce flowers with a dominant allele present, making red flowers. Choice *D* does not have any recessive alleles, so white flowers are not a possibility.

27. C: Looking at Figure 2, which represents the number of plants that were produced from each crossbreeding experiment, it can be seen that only 2 plants produced white flowers out of 12 plants total, 4 from each experiment. To find the percentage, divide 2 by 12 and multiply by 100. The result is 16.7%. Choice *A* is the total number of plants that were produced. Choice *B* represents the percentage of white flowers in experiment #3 alone.

28. B: In a Punnett Square, each box represents one allele from each of the parent's genes. To find the genetic makeup of the second parent, take out the allele that was contributed from the first parent. Here, the first parent contributed a recessive allele, a, to each offspring. In the top row, that leaves a dominant allele, A, and in the bottom row, that leaves a recessive allele, a. Therefore, the genetic makeup of the second parent is Aa.

29. D: Crossbreeding the plants with only recessive alleles will result in 100% white flowering plants. All four offspring have white flowering plants. Choice *B* gives 100% red flowering plants. Choice *C* gives 25%, 1 out of 4 plants, with white flowers.

30. A: The observation step of the scientific method involves using your senses to identify the results of the experiment. In this case, the experiment depended on identifying the color of the flowers. This was done using sight. If the experiment had involved different scents produced by the flowers, Choice *B* would have worked. If it has involved different textures of the flowers, Choice *C* would have worked. Flowers generally do not make any noise, so Choice *D* would not have been useful.

Chemistry

1. D: Nuclear reactions take place in the nucleus of certain unstable atoms. They involve a change in the structure of the nucleus, through some type of decomposition, and energy is released. Unlike in regular chemical reactions where mass is conserved, in nuclear reactions, there is a change in mass between the reactants and products.

2. A: A Lewis Dot diagram shows the alignment of the valence (outer) shell electrons and how readily they can pair or bond with the valence shell electrons of other atoms to form a compound. Choice *B* is incorrect because the Lewis Dot structure aids in understanding how likely an atom is to bond or not bond with another atom, so the inner shell would add no relevance to understanding this likelihood. The positioning of protons and neutrons concerns the nucleus of the atom, which again would not lend information to the likelihood of bonding.

3. B: A decomposition reaction breaks down a compound into its constituent elemental components. Choice *A* is incorrect because a synthesis reaction joins two or more elements into a single compound. Choice *C,* an organic reaction, is a type of reaction involving organic compounds, primarily those containing carbon and hydrogen. Choice *D,* oxidation/reduction (redox or half) reaction, is incorrect because it involves the loss of electrons from one species (oxidation) and the gain of electrons to the other species (reduction). There is no mention of this occurring within the given reaction, so it is incorrect.

4. C: The number of each element must be equal on both sides of the equation, so Choice *C* is the only correct option:

$$2Na + Cl_2 \rightarrow 2NaCl$$

2 Na + 2 Cl does equal 2 Na + 2 Cl (the number of sodium atoms and chlorine atoms match)

Choice *A:* $Na + Cl_2 \rightarrow NaCl$

1Na + 2Cl does not equal 1Na + 1Cl (the number of chlorine atoms do not match)

Choice *B:* $2Na + Cl_2 \rightarrow NaCl$

2Na + 2Cl does not equal 1Na + 1Cl (neither the number of sodium atoms nor chlorine atoms match)

Choice *D:* $2Na + 2Cl_2 \rightarrow 2NaCl$

2Na + 4Cl does not equal 2Na + 2Cl (the number of chlorine atoms do not match)

5. D: The naming of compounds focuses on the second element in a chemical compound. Elements from the non-metal category are written with an "ide" at the end. The compound CO has one carbon and one oxygen, so it is called carbon monoxide. Choice *B* represents that there are two oxygen atoms, and Choices *A, B,* and *C* incorrectly alter the name of the first element, which should remain as carbon.

6. B: To solve this, the number of moles of NaCl needs to be calculated:

First, to find the mass of NaCl, the mass of each of the molecule's atoms is added together as follows:

$$23.0 \text{ g Na} + 35.5 \text{ g Cl} = 58.5 \text{ g NaCl}$$

Next, the given mass of the substance is multiplied by one mole per total mass of the substance:

$$4.0 \text{ g NaCl} \times \frac{1 \text{ mol NaCl}}{58.5 \text{ g NaCl}} = 0.068 \text{ mol NaCl}$$

Finally, the moles are divided by the number of liters of the solution to find the molarity:

$$\frac{0.068 \text{ mol NaCl}}{0.120 \text{ L}} = 0.57 \text{ M NaCl}$$

7. C: According to the *ideal gas law* ($PV = nRT$), if volume is constant, the temperature is directly related to the pressure in a system. Therefore, if the pressure increases, the temperature will increase in direct proportion. Choice *A* would not be possible, since the system is closed and a change is occurring, so the temperature will change. Choice *B* incorrectly exhibits an inverse relationship between pressure and temperature, or $P = 1/T$. Choice *D* is incorrect because even without actual values for the variables, the relationship and proportions can be determined.

8. C: The correct answer choice is *C*. While the other three statements about proteins are true, it is not true that two amino acids bond together at their amine groups. Proteins are assembled when two or more amino acids combine through a condensation reaction. The reaction creates a $C - N$ covalent linkage (peptide bonds) between a carboxyl group ($-COOH$) and an amine group (NH_2) of two different molecules rather than the amine group of both amino acids.

9. C: 2:9:10:4. These are the coefficients that follow the law of conservation of matter. The coefficient times the subscript of each element should be the same on both sides of the equation.

10. C: A catalyst functions to increase reaction rates by decreasing the activation energy required for a reaction to take place. Inhibitors would increase the activation energy or otherwise stop the reactants from reacting. Although increasing the temperature usually increases a reaction's rate, this is not true in all cases, and most catalysts do not function in this manner.

11. D: Sublimation is a change in state from a solid to a gas. Evaporation is a change in state from a liquid to a gas, melting is a change in state from a solid to a liquid, and condensation is a change in state from a gas to a liquid.

12. A: Salts are formed from compounds that use ionic bonds. Disulfide bridges are special bonds in protein synthesis which hold the protein in their secondary and tertiary structures. Covalent bonds are strong bonds formed through the sharing of electrons between atoms and are typically found in organic molecules like carbohydrates and lipids. London dispersion forces are fleeting, momentary bonds which occur between atoms that have instantaneous dipoles but quickly disintegrate.

13. C: As in the last question, covalent bonds are special because they share electrons between multiple atoms. Most covalent bonds are formed between the elements H, F, N, O, S, and C, while hydrogen bonds are formed nearly exclusively between H and either O, N, or F of other molecules. Covalent bonds may inadvertently form dipoles, but this does not necessarily happen. With similarly electronegative atoms like carbon and hydrogen, dipoles do not form, for instance. Crystal solids are typically formed by substances with ionic bonds like the salts sodium iodide and potassium chloride.

14. A: Gases like air will move and expand to fill their container, so they are considered to have an indefinite shape and indefinite volume. Liquids like water will move and flow freely, so their shapes change constantly, but do not change volume or density on their own. Solids change neither shape nor volume without external forces acting on them, so they have definite shapes and volumes.

15. D: Evaporation takes place at the surface of a fluid while boiling takes place throughout the fluid. The liquid will boil when it reaches its boiling or vaporization temperature, but evaporation can happen due to a liquid's volatility. Volatile substances often coexist as a liquid and as a gas, depending on the pressure forced on them. The phase change from gas to liquid is condensation, and both evaporation and boiling take place in nature.

16. C: Water's polarity lends it to be extremely cohesive and adhesive; this cohesion keeps its atoms very close together. Because of this, it takes a large amount of energy to melt and boil its solid and liquid forms. Phospholipid bilayers are made of nonpolar lipids and water, a polar liquid, cannot easily flow through it. Cell membranes use proteins called aquaporins to solve this issue and let water flow in and out. Fish breathe by capturing dissolved oxygen through their gills. Water can self-ionize, wherein it decomposes into a hydrogen ion (H^+) and a hydroxide ion (OH^-), but it cannot self-hydrolyze.

17. D: An isotope of an element has an atomic number equal to its number of protons, but a different mass number because of the additional neutrons. Even though there are differences in the nucleus, the behavior and properties of isotopes of a given element are identical. Atoms with different atomic numbers also have different numbers of protons and are different elements, so they cannot be isotopes.

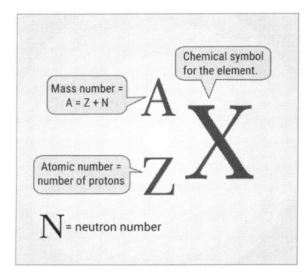

18. A: Choice *A* is correct. The mass of alpha particles is several times greater than the mass of a proton or neutron. It is several thousand times greater than the mass of a beta particle, so Choice *B* is wrong. Because they are so large, their tissue penetration power is quite low. In fact, just a thick sheet of paper or clothes are enough to stop them and protect the body from penetration; thus, Choice *C* is incorrect. It is beta particles, not alpha, that are high-energy electrons.

19. C: Neon, one of the noble gases, is chemically inert or not reactive because it contains eight valence electrons in the outermost shell. The atomic number is 10, with a 2.8 electron arrangement meaning that there are 2 electrons in the inner shell and the remaining 8 electrons in the outer shell. This is extremely stable for the atom, so it will not want to add or subtract any of its electrons and will not react under typical circumstances.

20. D: The law states that matter cannot be created or destroyed in a closed system. In this equation, there are the same number of molecules of each element on either side of the equation. Matter is not gained or lost, although a new compound is formed. As there are no ions on either side of the equation, no electrons are lost. The law prevents the hydrogen from losing mass and prevents oxygen atoms from being spontaneously spawned.

21. B: A solid produced during a reaction in solution is called a precipitate. In a neutralization reaction, the products (an acid and a base) react to form a salt and water. Choice *A*, an oxidation reaction, involves the transfer of an electron. Choice *C*, a synthesis reaction, involves the joining of two molecules to form a single molecule. Choice D, a decomposition reaction, involves the separation of a molecule into two other molecules.

22. A: The decimal point for this value is located after the final zero. Because the decimal is moved 12 places to the left in order to get it between the 8 and the 6, then the resulting exponent is positive, so Choice A is the correct answer. Choice B is false because the decimal has been moved in the wrong direction. Choice C is incorrect because the decimal has been moved an incorrect number of times. Choice D is false because the decimal needs to be moved to after the first non-zero number. This will always result in a significand which is less than 10.

$$8{,}600{,}000{,}000{,}000$$
$$12\ 11\ 10\ 9\quad 8\ 7\ 6\quad 5\ 4\quad 3\ 2\ 1$$

23. C: Choice C is the correct answer. Oxidation is always the loss of electrons, while reduction is the gain of one or more electrons. This fact, which must be memorized, eliminates Choices B and D. In this equation, Fe is oxidized (loses 2 electrons) to Fe^{2+} and acts as a reducing agent to Cu^{2+}. Cu^{2+} is reduced (gains two electrons) to form Cu.

24. D: Choice D is the correct answer. The following roadmap can be used to determine the produced amount of ammonia gas:

$$\text{Mass of } H_2 \rightarrow \text{Moles of } H_2 \rightarrow \text{Moles of } NH_3 \rightarrow \text{Mass of } NH_3$$

Setting up the equation:

$$500.\,\text{g } H_2 \times \left(\frac{1\text{ mol } H_2}{2.02\text{ g } H_2}\right) \times \left(\frac{2\text{ mol } NH_3}{3\text{ mol } H_2}\right) \times \left(\frac{17.0\text{ g } NH_3}{1\text{ mol } NH_3}\right) = 2805.28\text{ g } NH_3$$

$$2800\text{ g } NH_3$$

The molar masses are first obtained by using the periodic table. For example, the molar mass of H_2 is 2.02 grams (2×1.008); by summing the masses of each element in the compound, the molar mass of ammonia is found to be 17.0 g/mol. And finally, the answer is specific to three significant figures, which come from the initial amount of H_2 gas (500 g). Significant figures are not obtained from the unit type expressions. The final answer is rounded down to give 2,800 grams of NH_3.

25. B: Choice B is the correct answer. To find the molarity, first find the molar mass of glucose, which is about 180.2 grams/mole because $(6 \times 12.01\text{ amu}) + (12 \times 1.008\text{ amu}) + (6 \times 16.0\text{ amu}) = 180.2$ amu or grams/mole. The number of moles of glucose is calculated by dividing the mass of glucose over the molar mass of glucose. Applying dimensional analysis gives:

$$\frac{\text{g}}{\left(\frac{\text{g}}{\text{mol}}\right)} = \text{g} \cdot \text{g}^{-1} \cdot \text{mol} = \text{moles}$$

The mass of water is converted to liters of solution given that the density of water is 1 gram/milliliter.

The expression for molarity is:

$$Molarity = \frac{Moles\ of\ solute}{Liters\ of\ solution}$$

$$\frac{150\ \text{Grams glucose} \times \left(\frac{1\ \text{Mole glucose}}{180.2\ (\text{Grams} \cdot \text{mole}^{-1})\text{glucose}}\right)}{1{,}400\ \text{Grams of water} \times \left(\frac{1\ \text{mL of water}}{1\ \text{Gram of water}}\right) \times \left(\frac{1\ \text{L of water}}{1{,}000\ \text{mL of water}}\right)} = 0.595\ M$$

26. B: Choice *B* is the correct answer because it is the only one that contains an incorrect statement about the properties of water. When it acts as an acid, it donates a proton to the molecule it is reacting with, Choice *A*, and then becomes hydroxide ions and acts as a conjugate base, Choice *C*. When it acts like a base, it accepts a proton, Choice *D*, and becomes hydronium ions, which act as a conjugate acid. When water acts as a base, it does not donate a proton, making Choice *B* the correct answer.

27. A: In redox reactions, exactly two elements must experience a change in oxidation number. Iodine starts with an oxidation number of +5 and ends with an oxidation number of 0. Carbon starts with an oxidation number of -2 and ends with an oxidation number of +4. Oxygen keeps an oxidation number of -2 throughout the reaction. Therefore, Choice *A* is the correct answer and Choices *B* and *C* are incorrect. Oxidation numbers are assigned to individual elements and not whole molecules, so Choice *D* is incorrect.

28. D: Chemical properties of a substance describe how they react with another substance, whereas physical properties describe the appearance of the substance by itself. Choice *D* is the correct answer because it describes how the substance reacts while burning and interacting with oxygen molecules. It is flammable because it does burn. The physical properties of color, density, and fragility are described by Choices *A*, *B*, and *C* respectively.

29. B: Recall that chemical changes involve changes to the molecular structure, whereas physical changes have to do with the appearance of the substance.

For Choice *A*, the condensation of water is represented by:

$$H_2O(g) \leftrightarrow H_2O(l)$$

This process is considered a physical change because there is no change in the identity of the substance. The process is reversible and is a common occurrence. The water vapor, or humidity, in the air tends to condense around cooler objects. If you are wearing glasses and walking from a cold building or car to the outside where it's warm, your glasses will quickly fog up due to condensation. When a glass mason jar is broken, which is the same as a glass cup, there are chemical bonds that break; however, the nature of the substance (glass, or SiO_2) is still the same. In other words, the glass is still glass. Therefore, this process is characterized as a physical change. In Choice *D*, mixing sand in water will not change the chemical structure of sand.

The process is reversible if you were to evaporate out the water, leaving only sand. In Choice *B*, baking is considered a chemical process for many reasons. For example, most people have smelled the aroma that is associated with baking brownies or a cake. There is also a color change in the batter (eggs, flour, butter, chocolate chips) as its heated. This process is not reversible, which is a key characteristic of a chemical change, because once we make the brownies, there is no way to get the eggs or butter back.

New chemical bonds form as the mixture is heated, e.g., the flaky crust and slightly burnt edges around the brownie.

30. C: Conjugate acid-base pairs are formed from one molecule donating a proton and another accepting it or one molecule accepting a proton and another donating it. The base accepts a proton, whereas the acid donates the proton. In this reaction, the ammonia molecule, NH_3, accepts a proton and becomes NH_4^+. Therefore, the NH_3 is the base and the NH_4^+ is the conjugate acid, making Choice *C* correct. Choices *A, B,* and *D* do not form acid-base pairs.

Anatomy and Physiology

1. B: Proximal tubule → Loop of Henle → Collecting duct is correct. Kidneys filter blood using nephrons that span the outer renal cortex and inner renal medulla. The inner kidneys are composed of the renal pelvis, which collects urine and sends it to the bladder via the ureters. Filtrate first enters the filtering tube of the nephron via the glomerulus, a bundle of capillaries where blood fluid (but not cells) diffuses into the Bowman's capsule, the entryway into the kidney filtration canal. Bowman's capsule collects fluid, but the nephron actually starts filtering blood in the proximal tubule where necessary ions, nutrients, wastes, and (depending on blood osmolarity) water are absorbed or released. Also, blood pH is regulated, here, as the proximal tubule fine-tunes pH by utilizing the blood buffering system, adjusting amounts of hydrogen ions, bicarbonate, and ammonia in the filtrate. Down the loop of Henle in the renal medulla, the filtrate becomes more concentrated as water exits, while on the way back up the loop of Henle, ion concentration is regulated with ion channels. The distal tubule continues to regulate ion and water concentrations, and the collecting duct delivers the filtrate to the renal pelvis.

2. A: Motor neurons transmit signals from the CNS to effector tissues and organs, such as skeletal muscle and glands. Sensory neurons carry impulses from receptors in the extremities to the CNS. Interneurons relay impulses from neuron to neuron.

3. A: When activated, B cells create antibodies against specific antigens. White blood cells are generated in yellow bone marrow, not cartilage. Platelets are not a type of white blood cell, and are typically cell fragments produced by megakaryocytes. White blood cells are active throughout nearly all of one's life, and have not been shown to specially activate or deactivate because of life events like puberty or menopause.

4. A: The exocrine portion of the pancreas (the majority of it) is an accessory organ to the digestive system (meaning that food never touches it—it is not part of the alimentary canal). It secretes bicarbonate to neutralize stomach acid and enzymes to aid in digestion. It also regulates blood sugar levels through the complementary action of insulin and glucagon that are located in the Islets of Langerhans (endocrine portion). *A* is incorrect because it is not the growth hormone that stimulates insulin secretion, but rather blood sugar levels.

5. D: The lymphatic system is composed of one-way vessels, lymph, and organs and is designed to filter pathogens and debris from the blood, return nutrients that have leaked from the blood, and maintain, and even stimulate, the immune system if necessary. It circulates lymph, a clear fluid filled with blood plasma that has leaked from capillary beds. The lymphatic system delivers lymph, a clear, colorless fluid, to the neck. It has several organs:

- Lymph nodes, which remove debris from lymph and forms lymphocytes
- The thymus, which develops lymphocytes
- The spleen, which removes pathogens from blood and makes lymphocytes
- Tonsils, which collect debris

The lymphatic system also absorbs lipids and fat-soluble vitamins from the gut and returns them to the circulatory system.

6. C: ADH secretion is correct. Antidiuretic hormone controls water reabsorption. In its presence, water is reabsorbed, and urine is more concentrated. When absent, water is excreted, and urine is dilute. It is a regulator of blood volume, not pH. The other choices do affect blood pH.

7. D: The gland that regulates blood calcium levels is the parathyroid gland. Humans have four parathyroid glands located by the thyroid on each side of the neck, just below the larynx. Typical with the endocrine system, the parathyroid glands operate via feedback loops. If calcium in the blood is low, the parathyroid glands produce parathyroid hormone, which circulates to the bones and removes calcium. If calcium is high, they turn off parathyroid hormone production.

8. D: The hypothalamus is the link between the nervous and endocrine system. It receives information from the brain and sends signals to the pituitary gland, instructing it to release or inhibit release of hormones. Aside from its endocrine function, it controls body temperature, hunger, sleep, circadian rhythms, and is part of the limbic system.

9. C: When muscles contract, they pull bones together. They cannot push apart though, so they work in antagonistic pairs where they are on opposite sides of the bone.

When the bicep contracts, the arm bends and the tricep is relaxed; on the other hand, when the tricep contracts, the arm opens, and the bicep relaxes.

The quadriceps on the thigh straighten the knee; the hamstrings behind the thigh bend the knee.

The trapezius, rhomboid major, and rhomboid minor are muscles on the upper back that pull the shoulders back. The pectoralis major and minor (pecs) are on the chest and allow movement of the shoulder (throwing, lifting, rotating).

The gluteus maximus is the buttocks muscle and extends to the hip. It is the major of the glutes and is responsible for large movements like jumping. The gluteus medius and minimus stabilize the pelvis. The antagonist muscle to the gluteus maximus is the iliopsoas, the flexor muscles. Therefore, Choice *C* is correct since the glutes are not antagonistic muscles.

10. C: During muscle contractions, myosin cross-bridges attach via their globular heads to actin, then they swivel and detach from actin filaments, causing the ends of the sarcomere to be pulled closer together. Choice *A* is incorrect because it is essentially the opposite of this. Actin (the thin filament) does

400

not attach to myosin (the thick filament). Choice *B* is incorrect because the action potential is initiated when calcium leaves—rather than enters—the sarcoplasmic reticulum. Choice *D* is incorrect because fibers do not physically shorten. They slide past one another, shortening the distance between the origin and insertion of the muscle.

11. C: The red bone marrow is the active site for production of stem cells, which are converted to WBCs to combat infection. The system does protect the spleen, store calcium, and make new bone tissue; however, these activities are not associated with the function of the immune system. Therefore, Choices *A, B,* and *D* are incorrect.

12. C: The transverse plane, also called an axial plane, is a horizontal line that divides the body into upper and lower sections. The sagittal plane is a vertical line, not a horizontal line, that divides the body into right and left sections, therefore Choice *A* is incorrect. Choice *B* is the definition of the sagittal plane, and since the caudal plane does not exist, Choice *B* is incorrect. The coronal plane is a vertical line that divides the body into dorsal and ventral halves; therefore, Choice *D* is incorrect.

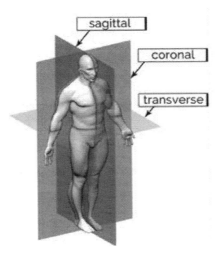

13. D: Passive range of motion assesses the non-contractile joint structures, such as ligaments, capsules, and fascia. Active range of motion would also assess the contractile elements, such as muscles and tendons, in addition to the non-contractile elements. Therefore, the specific muscles involved in knee flexion were not applicable to this question.

14. A: The renal pelvis acts like a funnel by delivering the urine from the millions of the collecting tubules to the ureters. It is the most central part of the kidney. The renal cortex is the outer layer of the kidney, while the renal medulla is the inner layer. The renal medulla contains the functional units of the kidneys—nephrons—which function to filter the blood. Choice *D,* Bowman's capsule, is the name for the structure that covers the glomeruli.

15. B: The smallest unit of a muscle fiber, a sarcomere, contains the actin and myosin proteins responsible for the mechanical process of muscle contractions. Located between two Z-lines, the actin and myosin filaments are configured in parallel, end-to-end, along the entire length of the myofibril. The sarcomere consists of four segments: the A-band, H-zone, I-band, and Z-line. The D-line is fictitious and is not a component of a sarcomere.

16. D: The autonomic nervous system (ANS), a division of the PNS, controls involuntary functions such as breathing, heart rate, blood pressure, digestion, and body temperature via the antagonistic parasympathetic and sympathetic nerves. Choices *A*, *B*, and *C* are incorrect because they describe characteristics of the somatic nervous system, which is the other division of the PNS. It controls skeletal muscles via afferent and efferent neurons. Afferent neurons carry sensory messages from skeletal muscles, skin, or sensory organs to the CNS, while Efferent neurons relay motor messages from the CNS to skeletal muscles, skin, or sensory organs. While skeletal muscle movement is under voluntary control, the somatic nervous system also plays a role in the involuntary reflex arc.

17. B: Epithelial tissue includes epithelia, which are the layers of cells that cover exposed surfaces of the body and line internal cavities, passageways, and glands. Epithelia do not contain blood vessels. This tissue can regenerate quickly to replace damaged and dead cells. The cells in epithelial tissue are tightly packed together, while in connective tissue they are sparser and scattered throughout the extracellular matrix.

18. B: The endocrine system's organs are glands which are spread throughout the body. The endocrine system itself does not connect the organs or transport the hormones they secrete. Rather, the various glands secrete the hormone into the bloodstream and lets the cardiovascular system pump it throughout the body. The other three body systems each include a network throughout the body:

- Cardiovascular system: veins and arteries
- Immune system: lymphatic vessels (it does also use the circulatory system)
- Nervous system: nerve networks

19. C: Elbow extension and wrist flexion are movements that both take place in the sagittal plane (the sagittal plane cuts through the middle of the body dividing the body into right and left regions). Shoulder abduction and neck left tilt movements both occur in the frontal plane.

20. B: Antagonists are muscles that oppose the action of the agonist—the primary muscle causing a motion. Hamstrings are the primary knee flexors—the agonists—and the quadriceps fire in opposition. The gastrocnemius does cross the knee joint, so it is a knee flexor, although secondary to the hamstrings. Tibialis anterior is on the shin and is involved in dorsiflexion.

21. B: The respiratory system mediates the exchange of gas between the air and the circulating blood, mainly by the act of breathing. It filters, warms, and humidifies the air that gets breathed in and then passes it into the blood stream. The digestive system transforms food and liquids into energy and helps excrete waste from the body. Eliminating waste via the kidneys and bladder is a function of the urinary system.

22. A: The skeletal system consists of the 206 bones that make up the skeleton, as well as the cartilage, ligaments, and other connective tissues that stabilize the bones. The skeletal system provides structural support for the entire body, a framework for the soft tissues and organs to attach to, and acts as a protective barrier for some organs, such as the ribs protecting the heart and lungs, and the vertebrae protecting the spinal cord. The muscular system includes skeletal muscles, cardiac muscle, and the smooth muscles found on the inside of blood vessels. The endocrine system uses ductless glands to produce hormones that help maintain hemostasis, and the reproductive system is responsible for the production of egg and sperm cells.

23. B: The best answer is Choice *B*. Choice *A* would describe foot pain. Choice *C* would describe pain in the arms. Choice *D* would describe pain in a person's head.

24. D: The correct answer is Choice *D*. The skeletal system provides protection for the delicate organs of the body. The brain is located in the head; the cranium—also called the skull—is the bony structure that provides protection to the head. The pelvic girdle, Choice *A*, supports the hips and protects the inner organs. The ribs, Choice *B*, protect the lungs and heart in the chest. The vertebrae, Choice *C*, protect the spinal cord.

25. D: The outermost layer of the skin, the epidermis, consists of *epithelial* cells. This layer of skin is dead, as it has no blood vessels. *Osteoclasts* are cells that make up bones. Notice the prefix *Osteo-* which means bone. *Connective* tissue macrophage cells can be found in a variety of places, and *dendritic* cells are part of the lymphatic system.

26. A: All three joint types given are synovial joints, allowing for a fair amount of movement (compared with fibrous and cartilaginous joints). Of the three given, hinge joints, such as the elbow, permit the least motion because they are uniaxial and permit movement in only one plane. Saddle joints and condyloid joints both have reciprocating surfaces that mate with one another and allow a variety of motions in numerous planes, but saddle joints, such as the thumb carpal-metacarpal joint, allow more motion than condyloid joints. In saddle joints, two concave surfaces articulate, and in a condyloid joint, such as the wrist, a concave surface articulates with a convex surface, allowing motion in mainly two planes.

27. D: Muscle fibers, also called muscle cells (i.e., myocytes), are long, striated, cylindrical cells that are approximately the diameter of a human hair (50 to 100 μm); have many nuclei dispersed on the outside of the cell; and are covered by a fibrous membrane called the sarcolemma. Myofibrils, one of the smaller functional units within a myocyte, consist of long, thin (approximately 1 μm) chains of proteins. The smallest unit of a muscle fiber, a sarcomere, contains the actin and myosin proteins responsible for the mechanical process of muscle contractions.

28. A: The sarcoplasmic reticulum is a network of tubular channels and vesicles that together provide structural integrity to the muscle fiber. The sarcoplasmic reticulum also acts as a calcium ion pump, moving Ca^{2+} ions from the sarcoplasm into the muscle fiber when the action potential reaches the cell. The Ca^{2+} binds with troponin, which causes the tropomyosin to move further into the double helix groove, allowing rapid binding of actin and myosin filaments and the power stroke that pulls the actin toward the center of the sarcomere, resulting in a contraction.

29. B: Choices *I*, II, and IV are correct. Here are examples of correct matches:

    Fibrous: sutures in skull
    Plane: intercarpal
    Saddle: thumb
    Hinge: elbow
    Condyloid: wrist
    Pivot: radial head on ulna
    Cartilaginous: pubic symphysis

30. A: It is most likely asthma. Any of the answer choices listed can cause heavy breathing. A blood clot in the lung (*B*) could cause this, but this would be very uncommon for a child. Choices *C* and *D* can both

403

be ruled out because the question mentions that it occurs even when the patient is relaxing. Hyperventilation is usually caused by a panic attack or some sort of physical activity. Asthma often develops during childhood. It would stand to reason then that the child may have not yet been diagnosed. While asthma attacks can be caused by exercise they can also occur when a person is not exerting themselves.

Physics

1. A: Potential energy represents the energy possessed by an object by virtue of its position. An object's gravitational potential energy can be found as a simple function of its height or by what distance it drops. In all of the answer choices, Choice *A* has the pendulum at its highest point. Choice *B* demonstrates when the pendulum has the most kinetic energy. Choice *C* has more potential energy than Choice *B* but less than Choice *A*. Choice *D* is incorrect, because the height of the pendulum changes during its swing, therefore its potential energy is changing.

2. A: Using Newton's equation for motion, $F = ma$, and substituting gravity in for acceleration (a), the weight, or force could be calculated for an object having mass (m). Weight is a force, mass is the amount of a substance, and acceleration and gravity are rate of speed over time.

3. C: The force that opposes motion is called *friction*. It also provides the resistance necessary for walking, running, braking, etc. In order for something to slide down a ramp, it must be acted upon by a force stronger than that of friction. Choices *A* and *B* are not actual terms, and Choice *D* is the measure of mass multiplied by velocity ($p = mv$).

4. A: The ends (or poles) of a straight magnet are different charges. One end is positive and one end is negative. Therefore, the positive end of magnet #1 would attract the negative end of magnet #2 and repel magnet #2's positive end.

5. D: Sir Isaac Newton simplified the laws of motion into three basic rules, based upon his observations in experimentation and advanced mathematical calculations. Albert Einstein was known for his theories involving electricity and magnetism, relativity, energy, light, and gravitational waves. Stephen Hawking is known for his theories and studies of space, dark matter, black holes, and relativity. Copernicus was known for his observations and theories regarding the movements of the planets in our universe; specifically, that the sun was the center of our solar system, not earth.

6. D: The weight of an object is equal to the mass of the object multiplied by gravity. According to Newton's Second Law of Motion, $F = m \times a$. Weight is the force resulting from a given situation, so the mass of the object needs to be multiplied by the acceleration of gravity on Earth: $W = m \times g$. Choice *A* is incorrect because, according to Newton's first law, all objects exert some force on each other, based on their distance from each other and their masses. This is seen in planets, which affect each other's paths and those of their moons. Choice *B* is incorrect because an object in motion or at rest can have inertia; inertia is the resistance of a physical object to change its state of motion. Choice *C* is incorrect because the mass of an object is a measurement of how much substance of there is to the object, while the weight is gravity's effect of the mass.

7. B: In a parallel circuit, more charges will seek the path with least resistance. Because of this, more current passes through circuit paths with lower resistance. If the resistance is the same in both paths, then the same amount of current passes through each resistor. An important feature of parallel circuits is that the voltage is the same across each resistor; it does not drop as it does in series circuits. In series circuits, voltage drops after each resistor, and current is constant, and in parallel circuits, voltage stays the same after each resistor, and current increases. The total current can be calculated as the sum of the electric current in each branch of the parallel circuit.

8. A: An object moving in a circular motion also has momentum; it is called *angular momentum* and it is determined by the amount of rotational inertia, rotational velocity, and the distance of the mass from the axis of rotation. Objects exhibiting circular motion also demonstrate the conservation of angular momentum. This means that the angular momentum of a system is always constant, regardless of the placement of the mass. Rotational inertia can be affected by the distance of the mass of the object from the center of rotation (axis of rotation). The farther the mass is from the center of rotation, the slower the rotational velocity. While Choices *B, C,* and *D* are all conserved, none of them deal directly with circular motion, so they would not apply to the question.

9. B: The ice skater is demonstrating the conservation of angular momentum. This means that the amount of momentum for the situation will remain the same. If the skater is redistributing the mass (their arms), then the angular speed will compensate for that alteration. In this case, the mass is extended out away from the axis of rotation, so the rate of rotation is slowed down. If their arms were brought back in near their body, then the rate of rotation would increase, making the skater spin faster.

10. C: Review the following:

$$a = \frac{\Delta v}{\Delta t}$$

$$a = \frac{15\frac{m}{s} - 0\frac{m}{s}}{5.0\ s - 0\ s} = \frac{15\frac{m}{s}}{5.0\ s}$$

$$a = 3.0\frac{m}{s^2}$$

Choices *A* and *B* have the wrong units for acceleration; they are labeled with the units for velocity. Choices *B* and *D* integrate a miscalculation with the formula — multiplying, rather than dividing, 15 and 5.

11. C: The answer is $10\ kg \times 2\ m \times 9.81\ m/s^2$. This must also be read carefully. Choice *D* is incorrect because it isn't necessary to know the ground elevation. The potential energy is measured *with respect to the ground* and the ground (or datum elevation) can be set to any arbitrary value.

12. B: The answer is 1 centimeter. Remember that the force (F) required to stretch a spring a certain amount (d) is given by the equation $F = kd$. Therefore, $k = F/d = 10\ N/0.5\ cm = 20\ N/cm$. Doubling the weight to 20 N gives the deflection:

$$d = \frac{F}{k} = \frac{20\ N}{20\frac{N}{cm}} = 1\ cm$$

All of the calculations can be bypassed by remembering that the relation between force and deflection is linear. This means that doubling the force doubles the deflection, as long as the spring isn't loaded past its elastic limit.

13. A: The answer is 981 N. The start-up and sliding friction forces are calculated in the same way: normal force (or weight) times the friction coefficient. The difference between the two coefficients is 0.1, so the difference in forces is $0.1 \times 1000 \times 9.81 = 981$ N.

14. C: The answer is 1.6 m^2. The pressure created by the load is:

$$\frac{50 \text{ N}}{0.1 \text{ m}^2} = 500 \frac{\text{N}}{\text{m}^2}$$

This pressure acts throughout the jack, including the large cylinder. Force is pressure times area, so the area equals pressure divided by force:

$$\frac{800 \text{ N}}{500 \frac{\text{N}}{\text{m}^2}} = 1.6 \text{ m}^2$$

15. D: The answer is $\frac{F}{A} \times (V_2 - V_1)$. Remember that the work for a piston expanding is pressure multiplied by change in volume: $W = P \times \Delta V$. Because pressure is equal to force over an area, $P = \frac{F}{A}$, and change in volume is $V_2 - V_1$, the resulting equation for the work done is $\frac{F}{A} \times (V_2 - V_1)$.

16. C: The answer is 500 J/s. Choice *A* is incorrect because kg $\times$ m/s^2 is an expression of force, not power. Choice *B* is incorrect because N $\cdot$ m is an expression of work, not power. That leaves Choices *C* and *D,* both of which are expressed in units of power: watts or joules/second. Using an approximate calculation (as suggested):

$$1,000 \text{ kg} \times 10 \frac{\text{m}}{\text{s}^2} \times 30 \text{ m} = 300,000 \text{ N} \cdot \text{m}$$

Dividing the total work done by 10 minutes, or 600 seconds, gives the approximate power expended:

$$\frac{300,000 \text{ N} \cdot \text{m}}{600 \text{ s}} = 500 \text{ watts} = 500 \text{ J/s}$$

17. B: The answer is 12,000 Pa. The top of the block is under 12 meters of water:

$$P = 1,000 \frac{\text{N}}{\text{m}^3} \times 12 \text{ meters} = 12,000 \frac{\text{N}}{\text{m}^2} = 12,000 \text{ Pa}$$

There are two "red herrings" here: Choice *C* of 14,000 Pa is the pressure acting on the *bottom* of the block (perhaps through the sand on the bottom of the bay). Choice *D* (that it can't be calculated without knowing the top area of the block) is also incorrect. The top area is needed to calculate the total *force* acting on the top of the block, not the pressure.

18. B: The answer is that the water level rises in B but not in A. Why? Because ice is not as dense as water, so a given mass of water has more volume in a solid state than in a liquid state. Thus, it floats. As the mass of ice in Basin A melts, its volume (as a liquid) is reduced. In the end, the water level doesn't change. The ice in Basin B isn't floating. It's perched on high ground in the center of the basin. When it melts, water is added to the basin and the water level rises.

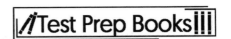

19. B: The answer is 5,000 seconds. The volume is $3 \times 25 \times 50 = 3750$ m^3. The volume divided by the flow rate gives the time. Since the pump capacity is given in liters per second, it's easier to convert the volume to liters. One thousand liters equals a cubic meter:

$$t = \frac{3{,}750{,}000 \text{ L}}{750 \text{ L/s}} = 5{,}000 \text{ s}$$

20. A: The answer is 30 m^3/s. One of the few equations that must be memorized is $Q = v \times A$. The area of flow is 1 m $\times$ 10 m because only half the depth of the channel is full of water.

Mathematics

1. Add 5,089 + 10,323
    a. 15,402
    b. 15,412
    c. 5,234
    d. 15,234

2. Add 103,678 + 487
    a. 103,191
    b. 103,550
    c. 104,265
    d. 104,165

3. Add 1.001 + 5.629
    a. 6.630
    b. 4.628
    c. 5.630
    d. 6.628

4. Add 143.77 + 5.2
    a. 138.57
    b. 148.97
    c. 138.97
    d. 148.57

5. Add and express in reduced form $\frac{5}{12} + \frac{4}{9}$.
    a. $\frac{9}{17}$
    b. $\frac{1}{3}$
    c. $\frac{31}{36}$
    d. $\frac{3}{5}$

6. Add and express in reduced form $\frac{14}{33} + \frac{10}{11}$.
    a. $\frac{2}{11}$
    b. $\frac{6}{11}$
    c. $\frac{4}{3}$
    d. $\frac{44}{33}$

7. Subtract 9,576 − 891.
   a. 10,467
   b. 9,685
   c. 8,325
   d. 8,685

8. Subtract 112,076 − 1,243.
   a. 110,833
   b. 113,319
   c. 113,833
   d. 110,319

9. Subtract 50.888 − 13.091.
   a. 37.797
   b. 63.979
   c. 37.979
   d. 33,817

10. Subtract 701.1 − 52.33.
   a. 753.43
   b. 648.77
   c. 652.77
   d. 638.43

11. Subtract and express in reduced form $\frac{23}{24} - \frac{1}{6}$.
   a. $\frac{22}{18}$
   b. $\frac{11}{9}$
   c. $\frac{19}{24}$
   d. $\frac{4}{5}$

12. Subtract and express in reduced form $\frac{43}{45} - \frac{11}{15}$.
   a. $\frac{10}{45}$
   b. $\frac{16}{15}$
   c. $\frac{32}{30}$
   d. $\frac{2}{9}$

13. Multiply 578 × 15.
   a. 8,770
   b. 8,760
   c. 8,660
   d. 8,670

409

14. Multiply $13,114 \times 191$.
    a. 2,504,774
    b. 250,477
    c. 150,474
    d. 2,514,774

15. Multiply 12.4×0.2.
    a. 12.6
    b. 2.48
    c. 12.48
    d. 2.6

16. Multiply $1,987 \times 0.05$.
    a. 9.935
    b. 99.35
    c. 993.5
    d. 999.35

17. Multiply and reduce $\frac{15}{23} \times \frac{54}{127}$.
    a. $\frac{810}{2,921}$
    b. $\frac{81}{292}$
    c. $\frac{69}{150}$
    d. $\frac{810}{2,929}$

18. Multiply and reduce $54/55 \times 5/9$.
    a. 59/64
    b. 270/495
    c. 6/11
    d. 5/9

19. Divide, express with a remainder $1,202 \div 44$.
    a. 27 and 2/7
    b. 2 and 7/22
    c. 7 and 2/7
    d. 27 and 7/22

20. Divide, express with a remainder $188 \div 16$.
    a. 1 and 3/4
    b. 111 and 3/4
    c. 10 and 3/4
    d. 11 and 3/4

21. Divide $702 \div 2.6$.
    a. 27
    b. 207
    c. 2.7
    d. 270

22. Divide $1,015 \div 1.4$.
    a. 7,250
    b. 725
    c. 7.25
    d. 72.50

23. Divide and reduce $\frac{26}{55} \div \frac{26}{11}$.
    a. $\frac{52}{11}$
    b. $\frac{26}{11}$
    c. $\frac{1}{5}$
    d. $\frac{2}{5}$

24. Divide and reduce $\frac{4}{13} \div \frac{27}{169}$.
    a. $\frac{52}{27}$
    b. $\frac{51}{27}$
    c. $\frac{52}{29}$
    d. $\frac{51}{29}$

25. What number is MCDXXXII?
    a. 142
    b. 1642
    c. 1632
    d. 1432

26. What number is CCLI?
    a. 1111
    b. 1151
    c. 151
    d. 251

27. Express 111 in Roman numerals.
    a. CCI
    b. CXI
    c. DDI
    d. DXI

28. Express 515 in Roman numerals.
   a. CVI
   b. DCV
   c. DXV
   d. VDV

29. Convert 1300 hours into a 12-hour clock time.
   a. 1:00 p.m.
   b. 11:00 a.m.
   c. 1:00 a.m.
   d. 11:00 p.m.

30. Convert 0830 hours into a 12-hour clock time.
   a. 8:30 p.m.
   b. 8:30 a.m.
   c. 11:30 a.m.
   d. 11:30 p.m.

31. What time is 5:00 p.m. in military (24-hour clock) time?
   a. 1500 hours
   b. 1700 hours
   c. 0500 hours
   d. 0700 hours

32. What time is 11:00am in military (24-hour clock) time?
   a. 0100 hours
   b. 1100 hours
   c. 1200 hours
   d. 0200 hours

33. The hospital has a nurse-to-patient ratio of 1:25. If there is a maximum of 325 patients admitted at a time, how many nurses are there?
   a. 13 nurses
   b. 25 nurses
   c. 325 nurses
   d. 12 nurses

34. A hospital has a bed to room ratio of 2: 1. If there are 145 rooms, how many beds are there?
   a. 145 beds
   b. 2 beds
   c. 90 beds
   d. 290 beds

35. Solve for x: $\frac{2x}{5} - 1 = 59$
   a. 60
   b. 145
   c. 150
   d. 115

412

36. A National Hockey League store in the state of Michigan advertises 50% off all items. Sales tax in Michigan is 6%. How much would a hat originally priced at $32.99 and a jersey originally priced at $64.99 cost during this sale? Round to the nearest penny.
   a. $97.98
   b. $103.86
   c. $51.93
   d. $48.99

37. Store brand coffee beans cost $1.23 per pound. A local coffee bean roaster charges $1.98 per 1 ½ pounds. How much more would 5 pounds from the local roaster cost than 5 pounds of the store brand?
   a. $0.55
   b. $1.55
   c. $1.45
   d. $0.45

38. Paint Inc. charges $2,000 for painting the first 1,800 feet of trim on a house and $1.00 per foot for each foot after. How much would it cost to paint a house with 3,125 feet of trim?
   a. $3125
   b. $2000
   c. $5125
   d. $3325

39. A bucket can hold 11.4 liters of water. A kiddie pool needs 35 gallons of water to be full. How many times will the bucket need to be filled to fill the kiddie pool?
   a. 12
   b. 35
   c. 11
   d. 45

40. In Jim's school, there are 3 girls for every 2 boys. There are 650 students in total. Using this information, how many students are girls?
   a. 260
   b. 130
   c. 65
   d. 390

41. Convert 0.351 to a percentage.
   a. 3.51%

   b. 35.1%

   c. $\frac{351}{100}$

   d. 0.00351%

42. Convert $\frac{2}{9}$ to a percentage.
    a. 22%
    b. 4.5%
    c. 450%
    d. 0.22%

43. Convert 57% to a decimal.
    a. 570
    b. 5.70
    c. 0.06
    d. 0.57

44. What is 3 out of 8 expressed as a percent?
    a. 37.5%
    b. 37%
    c. 26.7%
    d. 2.67%

45. What is 39% of 164?
    a. 63.96
    b. 23.78
    c. 6,396
    d. 2.38

46. 32 is 25% of what number?
    a. 64
    b. 128
    c. 12.65
    d. 8

47. Convert $\frac{5}{8}$ to a decimal to the nearest hundredth.
    a. 0.62
    b. 1.05
    c. 0.63
    d. 1.60

48. Change $3\frac{3}{5}$ to a decimal.
    a. 3.6
    b. 4.67
    c. 5.3
    d. 0.28

49. Change 0.56 to a fraction.
    a. 5.6/100
    b. 14/25
    c. 56/1000
    d. 56/10

50. Change 9.3 to a fraction.

    a. $9\frac{3}{7}$

    b. $\frac{903}{1000}$

    c. $\frac{9.03}{100}$

    d. $9\frac{3}{10}$

51. A rectangle was formed out of pipe cleaner. Its length was $\frac{1}{2}$ feet and its width was $\frac{11}{2}$ inches. What is its area in square inches?

    a. $\frac{11}{4}$ inch^2

    b. $\frac{11}{2}$ inch^2

    c. 22 inch^2

    d. 33 inch^2

52. What is the perimeter of the figure below? Note that the solid outer line is the perimeter.

    a. 48.565 in
    b. 36.565 in
    c. 39.78 in
    d. 39.565 in

53. What is the slope of this line?

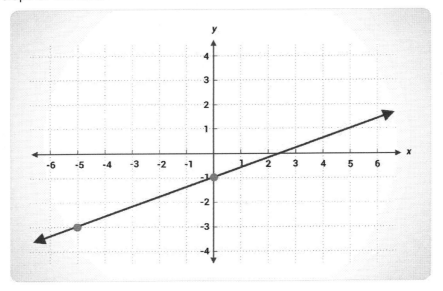

    a. 2

    b. $\frac{5}{2}$

    c. $\frac{1}{2}$

    d. $\frac{2}{5}$

54. Write the expression for three times the sum of twice a number and one minus 6.
    a. $2x + 1 - 6$
    b. $3x + 1 - 6$
    c. $3(x + 1) - 6$
    d. $3(2x + 1) - 6$

55. Two cards are drawn from a shuffled deck of 52 cards. What's the probability that both cards are kings if the first card isn't replaced after it's drawn?

    a. $\frac{1}{169}$

    b. $\frac{1}{221}$

    c. $\frac{1}{13}$

    d. $\frac{4}{13}$

Reading Comprehension

Questions 1-6 are based on the following passage:

When researchers and engineers undertake a large-scale scientific project, they may end up making discoveries and developing technologies that have far wider uses than originally intended. This is especially true in NASA, one of the most influential and innovative scientific organizations in America. NASA *spinoff technology* refers to innovations originally developed for NASA space projects that are now used in a wide range of different commercial fields. Many consumers are unaware that products they are buying are based on NASA research! Spinoff technology proves that it is worthwhile to invest in science research because it could enrich people's lives in unexpected ways.

The first spinoff technology worth mentioning is baby food. In space, where astronauts have limited access to fresh food and fewer options about their daily meals, malnutrition is a serious concern. Consequently, NASA researchers were looking for ways to enhance the nutritional value of astronauts' food. Scientists found that a certain type of algae could be added to food, improving the food's neurological benefits. When experts in the commercial food industry learned of this algae's potential to boost brain health, they were quick to begin their own research. The nutritional substance from algae then developed into a product called life's DHA, which can be found in over 90% of infant food sold in America.

Another intriguing example of a spinoff technology can be found in fashion. People who are always dropping their sunglasses may have invested in a pair of sunglasses with scratch resistant lenses—that is, it's impossible to scratch the glass, even if the glasses are dropped on an abrasive surface. This innovation is incredibly advantageous for people who are clumsy, but most shoppers don't know that this technology was originally developed by NASA. Scientists first created scratch resistant glass to help protect costly and crucial equipment from getting scratched in space, especially the helmet visors in space suits. However, sunglasses companies later realized that this technology could be profitable for their products, and they licensed the technology from NASA.

1. What is the main purpose of this article?
   a. To advise consumers to do more research before making a purchase
   b. To persuade readers to support NASA research
   c. To tell a narrative about the history of space technology
   d. To define and describe instances of spinoff technology

2. What is the organizational structure of this article?
   a. A general definition followed by more specific examples
   b. A general opinion followed by supporting arguments
   c. An important moment in history followed by chronological details
   d. A popular misconception followed by counterevidence

3. Why did NASA scientists research algae?
   a. They already knew algae was healthy for babies.
   b. They were interested in how to grow food in space.
   c. They were looking for ways to add health benefits to food.
   d. They hoped to use it to protect expensive research equipment.

417

4. What does the word "neurological" mean in the second paragraph?
   a. Related to the body
   b. Related to the brain
   c. Related to vitamins
   d. Related to technology

5. Why does the author mention space suit helmets?
   a. To give an example of astronaut fashion
   b. To explain where sunglasses got their shape
   c. To explain how astronauts protect their eyes
   d. To give an example of valuable space equipment

6. Which statement would the author probably NOT agree with?
   a. Consumers don't always know the history of the products they are buying.
   b. Sometimes new innovations have unexpected applications.
   c. It is difficult to make money from scientific research.
   d. Space equipment is often very expensive.

Questions 7-13 are based on the following passage:

People who argue that William Shakespeare is not responsible for the plays attributed to his name are known as anti-Stratfordians (from the name of Shakespeare's birthplace, Stratford-upon-Avon). The most common anti-Stratfordian claim is that William Shakespeare simply was not educated enough or from a high enough social class to have written plays overflowing with references to such a wide range of subjects like history, the classics, religion, and international culture. William Shakespeare was the son of a glove-maker, he only had a basic grade school education, and he never set foot outside of England—so how could he have produced plays of such sophistication and imagination? How could he have written in such detail about historical figures and events, or about different cultures and locations around Europe? According to anti-Stratfordians, the depth of knowledge contained in Shakespeare's plays suggests a well-traveled writer from a wealthy background with a university education, not a countryside writer like Shakespeare. But in fact, there is not much substance to such speculation, and most anti-Stratfordian arguments can be refuted with a little background about Shakespeare's time and upbringing.

First of all, those who doubt Shakespeare's authorship often point to his common birth and brief education as stumbling blocks to his writerly genius. Although it is true that Shakespeare did not come from a noble class, his father was a very *successful* glove-maker and his mother was from a very wealthy landowning family—so while Shakespeare may have had a country upbringing, he was certainly from a well-off family and would have been educated accordingly. Also, even though he did not attend university, grade school education in Shakespeare's time was actually quite rigorous and exposed students to classic drama through writers like Seneca and Ovid. It is not unreasonable to believe that Shakespeare received a very solid foundation in poetry and literature from his early schooling.

Next, anti-Stratfordians tend to question how Shakespeare could write so extensively about countries and cultures he had never visited before (for instance, several of his most famous works like *Romeo and Juliet* and *The Merchant of Venice* were set in Italy, on the opposite side of Europe!). But again, this criticism does not hold up under scrutiny. For one thing, Shakespeare was living in London, a bustling metropolis of international trade, the most populous city in England, and a political and cultural hub of

Europe. In the daily crowds of people, Shakespeare would certainly have been able to meet travelers from other countries and hear firsthand accounts of life in their home country. And, in addition to the influx of information from world travelers, this was also the age of the printing press, a jump in technology that made it possible to print and circulate books much more easily than in the past. This also allowed for a freer flow of information across different countries, allowing people to read about life and ideas from throughout Europe. One needn't travel the continent in order to learn and write about its culture.

7. What is the main purpose of this article?
    a. To explain two sides of an argument and allow readers to choose which side they agree with
    b. To encourage readers to be skeptical about the authorship of famous poems and plays
    c. To give historical background about an important literary figure
    d. To criticize a theory by presenting counterevidence

8. Which sentence contains the author's thesis?
    a. People who argue that William Shakespeare is not responsible for the plays attributed to his name are known as anti-Stratfordians.
    b. But in fact, there is not much substance to such speculation, and most anti-Stratfordian arguments can be refuted with a little background about Shakespeare's time and upbringing.
    c. It is not unreasonable to believe that Shakespeare received a very solid foundation in poetry and literature from his early schooling.
    d. Next, anti-Stratfordians tend to question how Shakespeare could write so extensively about countries and cultures he had never visited before.

9. How does the author respond to the claim that Shakespeare was not well-educated because he did not attend university?
    a. By insisting upon Shakespeare's natural genius
    b. By explaining grade school curriculum in Shakespeare's time
    c. By comparing Shakespeare with other uneducated writers of his time
    d. By pointing out that Shakespeare's wealthy parents probably paid for private tutors

10. What does the word "bustling" in the third paragraph most nearly mean?
    a. Busy
    b. Foreign
    c. Expensive
    d. Undeveloped

11. What can be inferred from the article?
    a. Shakespeare's peers were jealous of his success and wanted to attack his reputation.
    b. Until recently, classic drama was only taught in universities.
    c. International travel was extremely rare in Shakespeare's time.
    d. In Shakespeare's time, glove-makers were not part of the upper class.

12. Why does the author mention *Romeo and Juliet*?
    a. It is Shakespeare's most famous play.
    b. It was inspired by Shakespeare's trip to Italy.
    c. It is an example of a play set outside of England.
    d. It was unpopular when Shakespeare first wrote it.

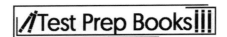

13. Which statement would the author probably agree with?
    a. It is possible to learn things from reading rather than from firsthand experience.
    b. If you want to be truly cultured, you need to travel the world
    c. People never become successful without a university education.
    d. All of the world's great art comes from Italy.

Questions 14-17 are based on the following passage which is adapted from Abraham Lincoln's Address Delivered at the Dedication of the Cemetery at Gettysburg, November 19, 1863:

Four score and seven years ago our fathers brought forth on this continent, a new nation, conceived in liberty, and dedicated to the proposition that all men are created equal.

Now we are engaged in a great civil war, testing whether that nation, or any nation so conceived and so dedicated, can long endure. We are met on a great battlefield of that war. We have come to dedicate a portion of that field, as a final resting place for those who here gave their lives that this nation might live. It is altogether fitting and proper that we should do this.

But, in a larger sense, we cannot dedicate --- we cannot consecrate that we cannot hallow --- this ground. The brave men, living and dead, who struggled here, have consecrated it, far above our poor power to add or detract. The world will little note, nor long remember what we say here, but it can never forget what they did here. It is for us the living, rather, to be dedicated here to the unfinished work which they who fought here have thus far so nobly advanced. It is rather for us to be here and dedicated to the great task remaining before us--- that from these honored dead we take increased devotion to that cause for which they gave the last full measure of devotion --- that we here highly resolve that these dead shall not have died in vain --- that this nation, under God, shall have a new birth of freedom--- and that government of people, by the people, for the people, shall not perish from the earth.

14. The best description for the phrase "Four score and seven years ago" is?
    a. A unit of measurement
    b. A period of time
    c. A literary movement
    d. A statement of political reform

15. Which war is Abraham Lincoln referring to in the following passage:

    "Now we are engaged in a great civil war, testing whether that nation, or any nation so conceived and so dedicated, can long endure."

    a. World War I
    b. The War of Spanish Succession
    c. World War II
    d. The American Civil War

420

16. What message is the author trying to convey through this address?
    a. The audience should perpetuate the ideals of freedom that the soldiers died fighting for.
    b. The audience should honor the dead by establishing an annual memorial service.
    c. The audience should form a militia that would overturn the current political structure.
    d. The audience should forget the lives that were lost and discredit the soldiers.

17. What is the effect of Lincoln's statement in the following passage:

"But, in a larger sense, we cannot dedicate --- we cannot consecrate that we cannot hallow --- this ground. The brave men, living and dead, who struggled here, have consecrated it, far above our poor power to add or detract."

    a. His comparison emphasizes the great sacrifice of the soldiers who fought in the war.
    b. His comparison serves as a reminder of the inadequacies of his audience.
    c. His comparison serves as a catalyst for guilt and shame among audience members.
    d. His comparison attempts to illuminate the great differences between soldiers and civilians.

Questions 18-20 are based on the following passage, which is an adaptation of Robert Louis Stevenson's The Strange Case of Dr. Jekyll and Mr. Hyde:

"Did you ever come across a protégé of his—one Hyde?" He asked.

"Hyde?" repeated Lanyon. "No. Never heard of him. Since my time."

That was the amount of information that the lawyer carried back with him to the great, dark bed on which he tossed to and fro until the small hours of the morning began to grow large. It was a night of little ease to his toiling mind, toiling in mere darkness and besieged by questions.

Six o'clock struck on the bells of the church that was so conveniently near to Mr. Utterson's dwelling, and still he was digging at the problem. Hitherto it had touched him on the intellectual side alone; but now his imagination also was engaged, or rather enslaved; and as he lay and tossed in the gross darkness of the night in the curtained room, Mr. Enfield's tale went by before his mind in a scroll of lighted pictures. He would be aware of the great field of lamps in a nocturnal city; then of the figure of a man walking swiftly; then of a child running from the doctor's; and then these met, and that human Juggernaut trod the child down and passed on regardless of her screams. Or else he would see a room in a rich house, where his friend lay asleep, dreaming and smiling at his dreams; and then the door of that room would be opened, the curtains of the bed plucked apart, the sleeper recalled, and, lo! There would stand by his side a figure to whom power was given, and even at that dead hour he must rise and do its bidding. The figure in these two phrases haunted the lawyer all night; and if at anytime he dozed over, it was but to see it glide more stealthily through sleeping houses, or move the more swiftly, and still the more smoothly, even to dizziness, through wider labyrinths of lamplighted city, and at every street corner crush a child and leave her screaming. And still the figure had no face by which he might know it; even in his dreams it had no face, or one that baffled him and melted before his eyes; and thus there it was that there sprung up and grew apace in the lawyer's mind a singularly

421

strong, almost an inordinate, curiosity to behold the features of the real Mr. Hyde. If he could but once set eyes on him, he thought the mystery would lighten and perhaps roll altogether away, as was the habit of mysterious things when well examined. He might see a reason for his friend's strange preference or bondage, and even for the startling clauses of the will. And at least it would be a face worth seeing: the face of a man who was without bowels of mercy: a face which had but to show itself to raise up, in the mind of the unimpressionable Enfield, a spirit of enduring hatred.

From that time forward, Mr. Utterson began to haunt the door in the by-street of shops. In the morning before office hours, at noon when business was plenty of time scarce, at night under the face of the full city moon, by all lights and at all hours of solitude or concourse, the lawyer was to be found on his chosen post.

"If he be Mr. Hyde," he had thought, "I should be Mr. Seek."

18. What can one infer about the meaning of the word "Juggernaut" from the author's use of it in the passage?
    a. It is an apparition that appears at daybreak.
    b. It scares children.
    c. It is associated with space travel.
    d. Mr. Utterson finds it soothing.

19. What is the definition of the word *haunt* in the following passage?

    From that time forward, Mr. Utterson began to haunt the door in the by-street of shops. In the morning before office hours, at noon when business was plenty of time scarce, at night under the face of the full city moon, by all lights and at all hours of solitude or concourse, the lawyer was to be found on his chosen post.

    a. To levitate
    b. To constantly visit
    c. To terrorize
    d. To daunt

20. What can one reasonably conclude from the final comment of this passage:

    "If he be Mr. Hyde," he had thought, "I should be Mr. Seek."

    a. The speaker is considering a name change.
    b. The speaker is experiencing an identity crisis.
    c. The speaker has mistakenly been looking for the wrong person.
    d. The speaker intends to continue to look for Hyde.

Questions 21-25 are based on the following passage:

    Dana Gioia argues in his article that poetry is dying, now little more than a limited art form confined to academic and college settings. Of course, poetry remains healthy in the academic setting, but the idea of poetry being limited to this academic subculture is a stretch. New technology and social networking alone have contributed to poets and other writers' work being shared across the world. YouTube has emerged to be a major asset to poets, allowing live performances to be streamed to billions of users. Even now, poetry continues to grow and voice topics that are relevant to the culture of our time. Poetry is not in the spotlight as it may have been in earlier times, but it's still a relevant art form that continues to expand in scope and appeal.

Furthermore, Gioia's argument does not account for live performances of poetry. Not everyone has taken a poetry class or enrolled in university—but most everyone is online. The Internet is a perfect launching point to get all creative work out there. An example of this was the performance of Buddy Wakefield's *Hurling Crowbirds at Mockingbars*. Wakefield is a well-known poet who has published several collections of contemporary poetry. One of my favorite works by Wakefield is *Crowbirds*, specifically his performance at New York University in 2009. Although his reading was a campus event, views of his performance online number in the thousands. His poetry attracted people outside of the university setting.

Naturally, the poem's popularity can be attributed both to Wakefield's performance and the quality of his writing. *Crowbirds* touches on themes of core human concepts such as faith, personal loss, and growth. These are not ideas that only poets or students of literature understand, but all human beings: "You acted like I was hurling crowbirds at mockingbars / and abandoned me for not making sense. / Evidently, I don't experience things as rationally as you do" (Wakefield 15-17). Wakefield weaves together a complex description of the perplexed and hurt emotions of the speaker undergoing a separation from a romantic interest. The line "You acted like I was hurling crowbirds at mockingbars" conjures up an image of someone confused, seemingly out of their mind . . . or in the case of the speaker, passionately trying to grasp at a relationship that is fading. The speaker is looking back and finding the words that described how he wasn't making sense. This poem is particularly human and gripping in its message, but the entire effect of the poem is enhanced through the physical performance.

At its core, poetry is about addressing issues/ideas in the world. Part of this is also addressing the perspectives that are exiguously considered. Although the platform may look different, poetry continues to have a steady audience due to the emotional connection the poet shares with the audience.

21. Which one of the following best explains how the passage is organized?
    a. The author begins with a long definition of the main topic, and then proceeds to prove how that definition has changed over the course of modernity.
    b. The author presents a puzzling phenomenon and uses the rest of the passage to showcase personal experiences in order to explain it.
    c. The author contrasts two different viewpoints, then builds a case showing preference for one over the other.
    d. The passage is an analysis of another theory that the author has no stake in.

22. The author of the passage would likely agree most with which of the following?
    a. Buddy Wakefield is a genius and is considered at the forefront of modern poetry.
    b. Poetry is not irrelevant; it is an art form that adapts to the changing time while containing its core elements.
    c. Spoken word is the zenith of poetic forms and the premier style of poetry in this decade.
    d. Poetry is on the verge of vanishing from our cultural consciousness.

23. Which one of the following words, if substituted for the word *exiguously* in the last paragraph, would LEAST change the meaning of the sentence?
    a. Indolently
    b. Inaudibly
    c. Interminably
    d. Infrequently

24. Which of the following is most closely analogous to the author's opinion of Buddy Wakefield's performance in relation to modern poetry?
    a. Someone's refusal to accept that the Higgs Boson will validate the Standard Model.
    b. An individual's belief that soccer will lose popularity within the next fifty years.
    c. A professor's opinion that poetry contains the language of the heart, while fiction contains the language of the mind.
    d. A student's insistence that psychoanalysis is a subset of modern psychology.

25. What is the primary purpose of the passage?
    a. To educate readers on the development of poetry and describe the historical implications of poetry in media.
    b. To disprove Dana Gioia's stance that poetry is becoming irrelevant and is only appreciated in academia.
    c. To inform readers of the brilliance of Buddy Wakefield and to introduce them to other poets that have influenced contemporary poetry.
    d. To prove that Gioia's article does have some truth to it and to shed light on its relevance to modern poetry.

Questions 26-29 are based upon the following passage, which is an **adaptation from** Mineralogy --- Encyclopedia International, *Grolier*

Mineralogy is the science of minerals, which are the naturally occurring elements and compounds that make up the solid parts of the universe. Mineralogy is usually considered in terms of materials in the Earth, but meteorites provide samples of minerals from outside the Earth.

A mineral may be defined as a naturally occurring, homogeneous solid, inorganically formed, with a definite chemical composition and an ordered atomic arrangement. The qualification *naturally occurring* is essential because it is possible to reproduce most minerals in the laboratory. For example, evaporating a solution of sodium chloride produces crystal indistinguishable from those of the mineral halite, but such laboratory-produced crystals are not minerals.

A *homogeneous solid* is one consisting of a single kind of material that cannot be separated into simpler compounds by any physical method. The requirement that a mineral be solid eliminates gases and liquids from consideration. Thus ice is a mineral (a very common one, especially at high altitudes and

424

latitudes) but water is not. Some mineralogists dispute this restriction and would consider both water and native mercury (also a liquid) as minerals.

The restriction of minerals to *inorganically formed* substances eliminates those homogenous solids produced by animals and plants. Thus, the shell of an oyster and the pearl inside, though both consist of calcium carbonate indistinguishable chemically or physically from the mineral aragonite, are not usually considered minerals.

The requirement of a *definite chemical composition* implies that a mineral is a chemical compound, and the composition of a chemical compound is readily expressed by a formula. Mineral formulas may be simple or complex, depending upon the number of elements present and the proportions in which they are combined.

Minerals are crystalline solids, and the presence of an *ordered atomic arrangement* is the criterion of the crystalline state. Under favorable conditions of formation the ordered atomic arrangement is expressed in the external crystal form. In fact, the presence of an ordered atomic arrangement and crystalline solids was deduced from the external regularity of crystals by a French mineralogist, Abbé R. Haüy, early in the 19th century.

26. According to the text, an object or substance must have all of the following criteria to be considered a mineral except for?
    a. Be naturally occurring
    b. Be a homogeneous solid
    c. Be organically formed
    d. Have a definite chemical composition

27. One can deduce that French mineralogist Abbé R. Haüy specialized in what field of study?
    a. Geology
    b. Psychology
    c. Biology
    d. Botany

28. What is the definition of the word "homogeneous" as it appears in the following passage?

    "A homogeneous solid is one consisting of a single kind of material that cannot be separated into simpler compounds by any physical method."

    a. Made of similar substances
    b. Differing in some areas
    c. Having a higher atomic mass
    d. Lacking necessary properties

29. The suffix -logy refers to:
    a. The properties of
    b. The chemical makeup of
    c. The study of
    d. The classification of

Questions 30-33 are based upon the following passage:

This excerpt is an adaptation from *Our Vanishing Wildlife,* by William T. Hornaday

> Three years ago, I think there were not many bird-lovers in the United States who believed it possible to prevent the total extinction of both egrets from our fauna. All the known rookeries accessible to plume-hunters had been totally destroyed. Two years ago, the secret discovery of several small, hidden colonies prompted William Dutcher, President of the National Association of Audubon Societies, and Mr. T. Gilbert Pearson, Secretary, to attempt the protection of those colonies. With a fund contributed for the purpose, wardens were hired and duly commissioned. As previously stated, one of those wardens was shot dead in cold blood by a plume hunter. The task of guarding swamp rookeries from the attacks of money-hungry desperadoes to whom the accursed plumes were worth their weight in gold, is a very chancy proceeding. There is now one warden in Florida who says that "before they get my rookery they will first have to get me."

> Thus far the protective work of the Audubon Association has been successful. Now there are twenty colonies, which contain all told, about 5,000 egrets and about 120,000 herons and ibises which are guarded by the Audubon wardens. One of the most important is on Bird Island, a mile out in Orange Lake, central Florida, and it is ably defended by Oscar E. Baynard. To-day, the plume hunters who do not dare to raid the guarded rookeries are trying to study out the lines of flight of the birds, to and from their feeding-grounds, and shoot them in transit. Their motto is—"Anything to beat the law, and get the plumes." It is there that the state of Florida should take part in the war.

> The success of this campaign is attested by the fact that last year a number of egrets were seen in eastern Massachusetts—for the first time in many years. And so to-day the question is, can the wardens continue to hold the plume-hunters at bay?

30. What is the meaning of the word *rookeries* in the following text?

To-day, the plume hunters who do not dare to raid the guarded rookeries are trying to study out the lines of flight of the birds, to and from their feeding-grounds, and shoot them in transit.

    a. Houses in a slum area
    b. A place where hunters gather to trade tools
    c. A place where wardens go to trade stories
    d. A colony of breeding birds

31. What is on Bird Island?
    a. Hunters selling plumes
    b. An important bird colony
    c. Bird Island Battle between the hunters and the wardens
    d. An important egret with unique plumes

32. What is the main purpose of the passage?
     a. To persuade the audience to act in preservation of the bird colonies
     b. To show the effect hunting egrets has had on the environment
     c. To argue that the preservation of bird colonies has had a negative impact on the environment
     d. To demonstrate the success of the protective work of the Audubon Association

33. Why are hunters trying to study the lines of flight of the birds?
     a. To study ornithology, one must know the lines of flight that birds take.
     b. To help wardens preserve the lives of the birds
     c. To have a better opportunity to hunt the birds
     d. To build their homes under the lines of flight because they believe it brings good luck

Questions 34-39 are based upon the following passage:

The Myth of Head Heat Loss

It has recently been brought to my attention that most people believe that 75% of your body heat is lost through your head. I had certainly heard this before, and am not going to attempt to say I didn't believe it when I first heard it. It is natural to be gullible to anything said with enough authority. But the "fact" that the majority of your body heat is lost through your head is a lie.

Let me explain. Heat loss is proportional to surface area exposed. An elephant loses a great deal more heat than an anteater because it has a much greater surface area than an anteater. Each cell has mitochondria that produce energy in the form of heat, and it takes a lot more energy to run an elephant than an anteater.

So, each part of your body loses its proportional amount of heat in accordance with its surface area. The human torso probably loses the most heat, though the legs lose a significant amount as well. Some people have asked, "Why does it feel so much warmer when you cover your head than when you don't?" Well, that's because your head, because it is not clothed, is losing a lot of heat while the clothing on the rest of your body provides insulation. If you went outside with a hat and pants but no shirt, not only would you look stupid but your heat loss would be significantly greater because so much more of you would be exposed. So, if given the choice to cover your chest or your head in the cold, choose the chest. It could save your life.

34. What is the primary purpose of this passage?
     a. To provide evidence that disproves a myth
     b. To compare elephants and anteaters
     c. To explain why it is appropriate to wear clothes in winter
     d. To show how people are gullible

35. Which of the following best describes the main idea of the passage?
     a. It is better to wear a shirt than a hat
     b. Heat loss is proportional to surface area exposed
     c. It is natural to be gullible
     d. The human chest loses the most heat

427

36. Why does the author compare elephants and anteaters?
    a. To express an opinion
    b. To give an example that helps clarify the main point
    c. To show the differences between them
    d. To persuade why one is better than the other

37. The statement, "If you went outside with a hat and pants but no shirt, not only would you look stupid but your heat loss would be significantly greater because so much more of you would be exposed" is which of the following?
    a. An opinion
    b. A fact
    c. An opinion within a fact
    d. Neither

38. Which of the following best describes the tone of the passage?
    a. Harsh
    b. Angry
    c. Casual
    d. Indifferent

39. Which of the following sentences provides the best evidence to support the main idea?
    a. "It is natural to be gullible to anything said with enough authority."
    b. "Each part of your body loses its proportional amount of heat in accordance with its surface area."
    c. "If given the choice to cover your chest or your head in the cold, choose the chest."
    d. "But the 'fact' that the majority of your body heat is lost through your head is a lie."

Questions 40-47 are based upon the following passage:

The Global Water Crisis

For decades, the world's water supply has been decreasing. At least ten percent of the world population, or over 780 million people, do not have access to potable water. They have to walk for miles, carrying heavy buckets in intense heat in order to obtain the essential life source that comes freely from our faucets.

We are in a global water crisis. Only 2.5% of the water on Earth is suitable for drinking, and over seventy percent of this water is frozen in the polar ice caps, while much of the rest is located deep underground. This leaves a very small percentage available for drinking, yet we see millions of gallons of water wasted on watering huge lawns in deserts like Arizona, or on running dishwashers that are only half-full, or on filling all the personal pools in Los Angeles, meanwhile people in Africa are dying of thirst.

In order to reduce water waste, Americans and citizens of other first world countries should adhere to the following guidelines: run the dishwasher only when it is full, do only full loads of laundry, wash the car with a bucket and not with a hose, take showers only when necessary, swim in public pools, and just be cognizant of how much water they are using in general. Our planet is getting thirstier by the year, and if we do not solve this problem, our species will surely perish.

40. Which of the following best supports the assertion that we need to limit our water usage?
    a. People are wasting water on superfluous things.
    b. There is very little water on earth suitable for drinking.
    c. At least ten percent of the world population does not have access to drinking water.
    d. There is plenty of drinking water in first world countries, but not anywhere else.

41. How is the content in the selection organized?
    a. In chronological order
    b. Compare and contrast
    c. As a set of problems and solutions
    d. As a series of descriptions

42. Which of the following, if true, would challenge the assertion that we are in a global water crisis?
    a. There are abundant water stores on earth that scientists are not reporting.
    b. Much of the water we drink comes from rain.
    c. People in Africa only have to walk less than a mile to get water.
    d. Most Americans only run the dishwasher when it is full.

43. The selection is written in which of the following styles?
    a. As a narrative
    b. In a persuasive manner
    c. As an informative piece
    d. As a series of descriptions

44. Which of the following is implicitly stated within the following sentence:

    "This leaves a very small percentage available for drinking, yet we see millions of gallons of water wasted on watering huge lawns in deserts like Arizona, or on running dishwashers that are only half-full, or on filling all the personal pools in Los Angeles, meanwhile people in Africa are dying of thirst."

    a. People run dishwashers that are not full.
    b. People in Africa are dying of thirst.
    c. People take water for granted.
    d. People should stop watering their lawns.

45. Why does the author mention that people have to walk for miles in intense heat to get water?
    a. To inform the reader on the hardships of living in a third world country.
    b. To inspire compassion in the reader.
    c. To show that water is only available in first world countries.
    d. To persuade the reader to reduce their water usage.

46. What is meant by the word <u>cognizant</u>?
    a. To be interested
    b. To be amused
    c. To be mindful
    d. To be accepting

429

47. What is the main idea of the passage?
    a. People should reduce their water usage.
    b. There is very little drinking water on earth.
    c. People take their access to water for granted.
    d. People should swim in public pools.

Directions for questions 48–55: Read the statement or passage and then choose the best answer to the question. Answer the question based on what is stated or implied in the statement or passage.

48. There are two major kinds of cameras on the market right now for amateur photographers. Camera enthusiasts can either purchase a digital single-lens reflex camera (DSLR) camera or a compact system camera (CSC). The main difference between a DSLR and a CSC is that the DSLR has a full-sized sensor, which means it fits in a much larger body. The CSC uses a mirrorless system, which makes for a lighter, smaller camera. While both take quality pictures, the DSLR generally has better picture quality due to the larger sensor. CSCs still take very good quality pictures and are more convenient to carry than a DSLR. This makes the CSC an ideal choice for the amateur photographer looking to step up from a point-and-shoot camera.

    What is the main difference between the DSLR and CSC?

    a. The picture quality is better in the DSLR.
    b. The CSC is less expensive than the DSLR.
    c. The DSLR is a better choice for amateur photographers.
    d. The DSLR's larger sensor makes it a bigger camera than the CSC.

49. When selecting a career path, it's important to explore the various options available. Many students entering college may shy away from a major because they don't know much about it. For example, many students won't opt for a career as an actuary, because they aren't exactly sure what it entails. They would be missing out on a career that is very lucrative and in high demand. Actuaries work in the insurance field and assess risks and premiums. The average salary of an actuary is $100,000 per year. Another career option students may avoid, due to lack of knowledge of the field, is a hospitalist. This is a physician that specializes in the care of patients in a hospital, as opposed to those seen in private practices. The average salary of a hospitalist is upwards of $200,000. It pays to do some digging and find out more about these lesser-known career fields.

    What is an actuary?

    a. A doctor who works in a hospital
    b. The same as a hospitalist
    c. An insurance agent who works in a hospital
    d. A person who assesses insurance risks and premiums

50. Hard water occurs when rainwater mixes with minerals from rock and soil. Hard water has a high mineral count, including calcium and magnesium. The mineral deposits from hard water can stain hard surfaces in bathrooms and kitchens as well as clog pipes. Hard water can stain dishes, ruin clothes, and reduce the life of any appliances it touches, such as hot water heaters, washing machines, and humidifiers.

One solution is to install a water softener to reduce the mineral content of water, but this can be costly. Running vinegar through pipes and appliances and using vinegar to clean hard surfaces can also help with mineral deposits.

From this passage, what can be concluded?

a. Hard water can cause a lot of problems for homeowners.
b. Calcium is good for pipes and hard surfaces.
c. Water softeners are easy to install.
d. Vinegar is the only solution to hard water problems.

51. Coaches of kids' sports teams are increasingly concerned about the behavior of parents at games. Parents are screaming and cursing at coaches, officials, players, and other parents. Physical fights have even broken out at games. Parents need to be reminded that coaches are volunteers, giving up their time and energy to help kids develop in their chosen sport. The goal of kids' sports teams is to learn and develop skills, but it's also to have fun. When parents are out of control at games and practices, it takes the fun out of the sport.

From this passage, what can be concluded?

a. Coaches are modeling good behavior for kids.
b. Organized sports are not good for kids.
c. Parents' behavior at their kids' games needs to change.
d. Parents and coaches need to work together.

52. While scientists aren't entirely certain why tornadoes form, they have some clues into the process. Tornadoes are dangerous funnel clouds that occur during a large thunderstorm. When warm, humid air near the ground meets cold, dry air from above, a column of the warm air can be drawn up into the clouds. Winds at different altitudes blowing at different speeds make the column of air rotate. As the spinning column of air picks up speed, a funnel cloud is formed. This funnel cloud moves rapidly and haphazardly. Rain and hail inside the cloud cause it to touch down, creating a tornado. Tornadoes move in a rapid and unpredictable pattern, making them extremely destructive and dangerous. Scientists continue to study tornadoes to improve radar detection and warning times.

The main purpose of this passage is to do which of the following?

a. Show why tornadoes are dangerous.
b. Explain how a tornado forms.
c. Compare thunderstorms to tornadoes.
d. Explain what to do in the event of a tornado.

431

53. Many people are unsure of exactly how the digestive system works. Digestion begins in the mouth where teeth grind up food and saliva break it down, making it easier for the body to absorb. Next, the food moves to the esophagus, and it is pushed into the stomach. The stomach is where food is stored and broken down further by acids and digestive enzymes, preparing it for passage into the intestines. The small intestine is where the nutrients are taken from food and passed into the blood stream. Other essential organs like the liver, gall bladder, and pancreas aid the stomach in breaking down food and absorbing nutrients. Finally, food waste is passed into the large intestine where it is eliminated by the body.

The purpose of this passage is to do which of the following?

a. Explain how the liver works.
b. Show why it is important to eat healthy foods.
c. Explain how the digestive system works.
d. Show how nutrients are absorbed by the small intestine.

54. Osteoporosis is a medical condition that occurs when the body loses bone or makes too little bone. This can lead to brittle, fragile bones that easily break. Bones are already porous, and when osteoporosis sets in, the spaces in bones become much larger, causing them to weaken. Both men and women can contract osteoporosis, though it is most common in women over age 50. Loss of bone can be silent and progressive, so it is important to be proactive in prevention of the disease.

The main purpose of this passage is to do which of the following?

a. Discuss some of the ways people contract osteoporosis.
b. Describe different treatment options for those with osteoporosis.
c. Explain how to prevent osteoporosis.
d. Define osteoporosis.

55. Vacationers looking for a perfect experience should opt out of Disney parks and try a trip on Disney Cruise Lines. While a park offers rides, characters, and show experiences, it also includes long lines, often very hot weather, and enormous crowds. A Disney Cruise, on the other hand, is a relaxing, luxurious vacation that includes many of the same experiences as the parks, minus the crowds and lines. The cruise has top-notch food, maid service, water slides, multiple pools, Broadway-quality shows, and daily character experiences for kids. There are also many activities, such as bingo, trivia contests, and dance parties that can entertain guests of all ages. The cruise even stops at Disney's private island for a beach barbecue with characters, waterslides, and water sports. Those looking for the Disney experience without the hassle should book a Disney cruise.

The main purpose of this passage is to do which of the following?

a. Explain how to book a Disney cruise.
b. Show what Disney parks have to offer.
c. Show why Disney parks are expensive.
d. Compare Disney parks to a Disney cruise.

Vocabulary

1. Which of the following words is most synonymous with the underlined word in the sentence below?

"I promise, I did not <u>instigate</u> the fight."

a. Begin
b. Ponder
c. Swim
d. Overwhelm

2. A patient has been vocal in the past about not needing to change anything about his lifestyle. The patient feels angry and frustrated by his conversation with the doctor. The patient is very agitated when the nurse aide comes to collect vital signs and tells her that he thinks she is lazy. What kind of defense mechanism is the patient displaying?
a. Intellectualization
b. Undoing
c. Reaction formation
d. Displacement

3. *Altitude* most nearly means
a. Behavior
b. Outlook
c. Haughtiness
d. Height

4. The nurse aide walks into the room where the patient is clutching his chest, sweating, and appears short of breath. He reports that he is experiencing chest pain that is crushing and severe, with some pain in his left arm as well. Which type of chest pain is this most likely associated with?
a. Myocardial infarction
b. Gastroesophageal reflux
c. Pneumonia
d. Pleuritis

5. Which of the following is the best definition of *reconnaissance?*
a. Preliminary surveying
b. Capturing
c. Proliferation and growth
d. Ingenuity

6. What does *ineffable* mean?
a. Insincere
b. Inefficient
c. Indescribable
d. Inexperienced

7. What does *gregarious* most nearly mean?
   a. Monstrous
   b. Meek
   c. Sociable
   d. Impressive

8. What word is a synonym for *caustic*?
   a. Sarcastic
   b. Luxurious
   c. Expensive
   d. Uncooperative

9. The patient violently convulses with rigid muscles. The patient is completely unconscious. What kind of seizure is this?
   a. Myoclonic
   b. Absence
   c. Grand Mal
   d. Tonic

10. The patient is having trouble forming thoughts into sentences, and one side of his face appears to be drooping. What emergency condition is likely occurring in the patient?
   a. Meningitis
   b. Migraine
   c. Seizure
   d. Cerebrovascular accident

11. A patient with diabetes has been off the floor all morning for a test and returns just as the lunch trays are being picked up. The patient was NPO for their test so did not receive his breakfast either. What does the nurse notice this patient is at risk for?
   a. Hypoglycemia
   b. Diabetic ketoacidosis
   c. Diabetic coma
   d. Hyperglycemia

12. What is a synonym for *obtuse*?
   a. Slow-witted
   b. Large
   c. Gluttonous
   d. Stretched

13. Which of the following words is most synonymous with the underlined word in the sentence below?

   The toddler, who had just learned to speak, seemed rather loquacious.

   a. Verbose
   b. Humorous
   c. Silent
   d. Cranky

434

14. A patient who has been admitted with tuberculosis begins to cough up blood in their sputum. What is the medical term for this condition?
  a. Hematopoiesis
  b. Hemoptysis
  c. Hematemesis
  d. Hematochezia

15. What word means *sordid*?
  a. Semantic
  b. Surly
  c. Vile
  d. Basic

16. _____ may present with vague signs which may mimic chest pain, depression, or other physical illnesses.
  a. Bereavement
  b. Stroke
  c. Anorexia Nervosa
  d. Myocardial Infarction

17. _____ have a side effect causing excessive thirst.
  a. Antidepressants
  b. Antibiotics
  c. Antispasmodics
  d. Anti-inflammatories

18. What does *solicit* mean?
  a. Ask
  b. Donate
  c. Perturb
  d. Solace

19. What kind of ulcer is most commonly found between the knees and ankles?
  a. Arterial
  b. Neuropathic
  c. Venous
  d. Stage IV

20. What type of strength exercise is performed without moving the joint using resistance?
  a. Isometric
  b. Isotonic
  c. Isokinetic
  d. Plyometric

21. Select the best meaning of the italicized word in the following sentence:

Given his rude comments, her reaction seemed *plausible*.
a. Conceivable
b. Skeptical
c. Diurnal
d. Erudite

22. *Discourse* most nearly means
a. Praise
b. Disagreement
c. Speech
d. Path

23. Select the best meaning of the italicized word in the following sentence:

The young boy seemed to be capable of nothing, other than his uncanny ability to *exasperate* his babysitter.

a. Annoy
b. Breathe
c. Disappoint
d. Stifle

24. Which of the following is the best definition for *genicular?*
a. Relating to aging
b. Relating to the knee
c. Relating to sperm
d. Relating to the genitals

25. Based on the words *transfer, transact, translation, transport*, what is the meaning of the prefix *trans*?
a. Separation
b. All, everywhere
c. Forward
d. Across, beyond, over

26. The term *cubital* refers to what body region?
a. The skin
b. The fingertips
c. The elbow
d. The shoulder

27. Mitigate most nearly means which of the following?
a. Alleviate
b. Focus
c. Fiery
d. Conspire

28. _____ is a structural protein and the primary constituent of things like hair and nails.
    a. Keratin
    b. Antigens
    c. Channel proteins
    d. Actin

29. Which word best fits in the following sentence:

    The dermis is _____ relative to the epidermis.

    a. Superficial
    b. Deep
    c. Superior
    d. Inferior

30. Select the correct meaning of the underlined word in the following sentence:

    The student wanted to become a phlebotomist.

    a. A professional who takes x-rays
    b. A professional who makes artificial limbs
    c. A professional who draws blood
    d. A professional who counsels patients

31. What word meaning "to return to an earlier state" best fits in the following sentence:

    The child seemed to emotionally _____ when he felt sick.

    a. Rescind
    b. Digress
    c. Regress
    d. Diverge

32. Where is the acromion process located?
    a. The spine
    b. The skull
    c. The shoulder
    d. The sternum

33. Select the correct meaning of the underlined word in the following sentence:

    The patient's eyes appeared glassy.

    a. Sad
    b. Expressionless
    c. Emotional
    d. Blind

437

34. What word meaning "to be in alignment such that there is a continuous plane" best fits in the following sentence:

It is important that the brace remains _____ with the skin to avoid skin irritation.

a. Flush
b. Flesh
c. Articulated
d. Adjacent

35. What is the meaning of the word *innervate*?
a. To attach a muscle to a bone
b. To shorten a muscle
c. To supply nerves to
d. To conduct a nerve impulse

36. What is a potential complication of gangrene?
a. Amputation
b. Ulcer
c. Parasites
d. Diabetes

37. What word meaning "urgent" best fits in the following sentence:

The _____ demands of the supervising physician made it difficult to complete paperwork in a timely manner.

a. Lenient
b. Extoll
c. Exigent
d. Lackadaisical

38. Select the correct meaning of the underlined word in the following sentence:

The patient had aphasia after his stroke.

a. Memory loss
b. Droopy face
c. Impairment in facial recognition
d. Language impairment

39. What does the abbreviation NPO mean?
a. Not per orders
b. Do not resuscitate
c. Nothing by mouth
d. Nothing by orders

40. Select the correct meaning of the underlined word in the following sentence:

The professor was notorious for his <u>jejune</u> lectures.

a. Dull
b. Stimulating
c. Interactive
d. Expert

41. What word meaning "shortage" best fits in the following sentence:

The salary hike for all unionized workers increased the hospital's budgetary _____.

a. Deficit
b. Diffident
c. Dearth
d. Defiant

42. What is the best definition of the word *paradox*?
a. Sensation
b. Hypothesis
c. Insinuation
d. Contradiction

43. What word meaning "agile" best fits in the following sentence:

The _____ dancer was graceful and beautiful to watch.

a. Lithe
b. Ballerina
c. Unwieldly
d. Chivalrous

44. What word meaning "a bluish discoloration of the skin caused by lack of oxygen" best fits in the following sentence:

It is not uncommon for a chocking or drowning child to exhibit _____.

a. Flushing
b. Cyanosis
c. Listless
d. Rall

45. What is the best definition of the word *venerate*?
a. Respect
b. Reject
c. Expect
d. Deserve

439

46. What word meaning "a fungal infection or disease" best fits in the following sentence:

Ringworm is considered a type of _____.

a. Lichen
b. Mycosis
c. Virus
d. Pustule

47. What word meaning "blood in the urine" best fits in the following sentence:

A common sign of a kidney infection is _____.

a. Anuria
b. Nocturia
c. Uremia
d. Polyurea

48. What is the best definition of the word *tetanus*?
a. A muscle twitch
b. A sustained muscle contraction
c. A muscle spasm
d. Muscle paralysis

49. Select the correct meaning of the underlined word in the following sentence:

The patient had a difficulty with <u>proprioception.</u>

a. Spatial awareness of the body
b. Balance and agility
c. Pain detection
d. Sensory integration

50. The charge nurse used the word "archetype" in a handoff report. Which of the following words is closest in meaning to that word?
a. Ancestor
b. Literature
c. Policy
d. Model

51. What is the best definition of the word *retort*?
a. Conversation
b. Jest
c. Counter
d. Flexible

440

52. What is the best definition of the word *subliminal*?
    a. Subconscious
    b. Transportation
    c. Underground
    d. Substitute

53. What is the best definition of the word *incite*?
    a. Understanding
    b. Illumination
    c. Rally
    d. Judgment

54. What is the best definition of the word *sustain*?
    a. strength
    b. invigorate
    c. embolden
    d. expedite

55. What is the best definition of the word *malevolent*?
    a. Evil
    b. Concerned
    c. Maximum
    d. Cautious

Grammar

1. Which of the following sentences has an error in capitalization?
    a. The East Coast has experienced very unpredictable weather this year.
    b. My Uncle owns a home in Florida, where he lives in the winter.
    c. I am taking English Composition II on campus this fall.
    d. There are several nice beaches we can visit on our trip to the Jersey Shore this summer.

2. Julia Robinson, an avid photographer in her spare time, was able to capture stunning shots of the local wildlife on her last business trip to Australia.

   Which of the following is an adjective in the preceding sentence?

    a. Time
    b. Capture
    c. Avid
    d. Photographer

3. Which of the following sentences uses correct punctuation?
    a. Carole is not currently working; her focus is on her children at the moment.
    b. Carole is not currently working and her focus is on her children at the moment.
    c. Carole is not currently working, her focus is on her children at the moment.
    d. Carole is not currently working her focus is on her children at the moment.

441

4. Which of these examples is a compound sentence?
    a. Alex and Shane spent the morning coloring and later took a walk down to the park.
    b. After coloring all morning, Alex and Shane spent the afternoon at the park.
    c. Alex and Shane spent the morning coloring, and then they took a walk down to the park.
    d. After coloring all morning and spending part of the day at the park, Alex and Shane took a nap.

5. Which of these examples shows incorrect use of subject-verb agreement?
    a. Neither of the cars are parked on the street.
    b. Both of my kids are going to camp this summer.
    c. Any of your friends are welcome to join us on the trip in November.
    d. Each of the clothing options is appropriate for the job interview.

6. When it gets warm in the spring, _____ and _____ like to go fishing at Cobbs Creek.

    Which of the following word pairs should be used in the blanks above?

    a. me, him
    b. he, I
    c. him, I
    d. he, me

Select the best version of the underlined part of the sentence. If you think the original sentence is best, choose the first answer.

7. Since <u>none of the furniture were delivered</u> on time, we have to move in at a later date.
    a. none of the furniture were delivered
    b. none of the furniture was delivered
    c. all of the furniture were delivered
    d. all of the furniture was delivered

8. <u>An important issues stemming from this meeting</u> is that we won't have enough time to meet all of the objectives.
    a. An important issues stemming from this meeting
    b. Important issue stemming from this meeting
    c. An important issue stemming from this meeting
    d. Important issues stemming from this meeting

9. There were many questions <u>about what causes the case to have gone cold</u>, but the detective wasn't willing to discuss it with reporters.
    a. about what causes the case to have gone cold
    b. about why the case is cold
    c. about what causes the case to go cold
    d. about why the case went cold

Directions for questions 10-14: Select the best version of the underlined part of the sentence. The first choice is the same as the original sentence. If you think the original sentence is best, choose the first answer.

10. The fact <u>the train set only includes four cars and one small track was a big disappointment</u> to my son.
    a. the train set only includes four cars and one small track was a big disappointment
    b. that the trains set only include four cars and one small track was a big disappointment
    c. that the train set only includes four cars and one small track was a big disappointment
    d. that the train set only includes four cars and one small track were a big disappointment

11. The rising popularity of the clean eating movement can be attributed <u>to the fact that experts say added sugars and chemicals in our food are to blame for the obesity epidemic.</u>
    a. to the fact that experts say added sugars and chemicals in our food are to blame for the obesity epidemic.
    b. in the facts that experts say added sugars and chemicals in our food are to blame for the obesity epidemic.
    c. to the fact that experts saying added sugars and chemicals in our food are to blame for the obesity epidemic.
    d. with the facts that experts say added sugars and chemicals in our food are to blame for the obesity epidemic.

12. She's looking for a suitcase that can fit all of her <u>clothes, shoes, accessory, and makeup.</u>
    a. clothes, shoes, accessory, and makeup.
    b. clothes, shoes, accessories, and makeup.
    c. clothes, shoes, accessories, and makeups.
    d. clothes, shoe, accessory, and makeup.

13. Shawn started taking guitar lessons <u>while he wanted to become a better musician.</u>
    a. while he wanted to become a better musician.
    b. because he wants to become a better musician.
    c. even though he wanted to become a better musician.
    d. because he wanted to become a better musician.

14. <u>Considering the recent rains we have had, it's a wonder</u> the plants haven't drowned.
    a. Considering the recent rains we have had, it's a wonder
    b. Consider the recent rains we have had, it's a wonder
    c. Considering for how much recent rain we have had, it's a wonder
    d. Considering, the recent rains we have had, it's a wonder

15. Which of the following is an imperative sentence?
    a. Pennsylvania's state flag includes two draft horses and an eagle.
    b. Go down to the basement and check the hot water heater for signs of a leak.
    c. You must be so excited to have a new baby on the way!
    d. How many countries speak Spanish?

16. Which of the following examples is a compound sentence?
    a. Shawn and Jerome played soccer in the backyard for two hours.
    b. Marissa last saw Elena and talked to her this morning.
    c. The baby was sick, so I decided to stay home from work.
    d. Denise, Kurt, and Eric went for a run after dinner.

17. Which of the following sentences uses correct subject-verb agreement?
    a. There is two constellations that can be seen from the back of the house.
    b. At least four of the sheep needs to be sheared before the end of summer.
    c. Lots of people were auditioning for the singing competition on Saturday.
    d. Everyone in the group have completed the assignment on time.

18. Philadelphia is home to some excellent walking tours where visitors can learn more about the culture and rich history of the city of brotherly love.

    What are the adjectives in the preceding sentence?

    a. Philadelphia, tours, visitors, culture, history, city, love
    b. Excellent, walking, rich, brotherly
    c. Is, can, learn
    d. To, about, of

19. The realtor showed _____ and _____ a house on Wednesday afternoon.

    Which of the following pronoun pairs should be used in the blanks above?

    a. She, I
    b. She, me
    c. Me, her
    d. Her, me

20. Which of the following examples uses correct punctuation?
    a. Recommended supplies for the hunting trip include the following: rain gear, large backpack, hiking boots, flashlight, and non-perishable foods.
    b. I left the store, because I forgot my wallet.
    c. As soon as the team checked into the hotel; they met in the lobby for a group photo.
    d. None of the furniture came in on time: so they weren't able to move in to the new apartment.

21. Which of the following sentences shows correct word usage?
    a. Your going to have to put you're jacket over their.
    b. You're going to have to put your jacket over there.
    c. Your going to have to put you're jacket over they're.
    d. You're going to have to put your jacket over their.

22. A teacher notices that, when students are talking to each other between classes, they are using their own unique vocabulary words and expressions to talk about their daily lives. When the teacher hears these non-standard words that are specific to one age or cultural group, what type of language is she listening to?
    a. Slang
    b. Jargon
    c. Dialect
    d. Vernacular

23. A teacher wants to counsel a student about using the word *ain't* in a research paper for a high school English class. What advice should the teacher give?

    a. *Ain't* is not in the dictionary, so it isn't a word.

    b. Because the student isn't in college yet, *ain't* is an appropriate expression for a high school writer.

    c. *Ain't* is incorrect English and should not be part of a serious student's vocabulary because it sounds uneducated.

    d. *Ain't* is a colloquial expression, and while it may be appropriate in a conversational setting, it is not standard in academic writing.

24. What is the structure of the following sentence:

    The restaurant is unconventional because it serves both Chicago style pizza and New York style pizza.

    a. Simple

    b. Compound

    c. Complex

    d. Compound-complex

25. The following sentence contains what kind of error:

    This summer, I'm planning to travel to Italy, take a Mediterranean cruise, going to Pompeii, and eat a lot of Italian food.

    a. Parallelism

    b. Sentence fragment

    c. Misplaced modifier

    d. Subject-verb agreement

26. The following sentence contains what kind of error:

    Forgetting that he was supposed to meet his girlfriend for dinner, Anita was mad when Fred showed up late.

    a. Parallelism

    b. Run-on sentence

    c. Misplaced modifier

    d. Subject-verb agreement

27. The following sentence contains what kind of error:

    Some workers use all their sick leave, other workers cash out their leave.

    a. Parallelism

    b. Comma splice

    c. Sentence fragment

    d. Subject-verb agreement

445

28. A student writes the following in an essay:

> Protestors filled the streets of the city. Because they were dissatisfied with the government's leadership.

Which of the following is an appropriately-punctuated correction for this sentence?

a. Protestors filled the streets of the city, because they were dissatisfied with the government's leadership.

b. Protesters, filled the streets of the city, because they were dissatisfied with the government's leadership.

c. Because they were dissatisfied with the government's leadership protestors filled the streets of the city.

d. Protestors filled the streets of the city because they were dissatisfied with the government's leadership.

29. What is the part of speech of the underlined word in the sentence:

We need to come up with a fresh <u>approach</u> to this problem.

a. Noun
b. Verb
c. Adverb
d. Adjective

30. What is the part of speech of the underlined word in the sentence:

Investigators conducted an <u>exhaustive</u> inquiry into the accusations of corruption.

a. Noun
b. Verb
c. Adverb
d. Adjective

31. The underlined portion of the sentence is an example of which sentence component:

New students should report <u>to the student center</u>.

a. Dependent clause
b. Adverbial phrase
c. Adjective clause
d. Noun phrase

32. Which word choices will correctly complete the sentence:

Increasing the price of bus fares has had a greater [affect / effect] on ridership [then / than] expected.

a. affect; then
b. affect; than
c. effect; then
d. effect; than

33. The following is an example of what type of sentence:

Although I wished it were summer, I accepted the change of seasons, and I started to appreciate the fall.

a. Compound
b. Simple
c. Complex
d. Compound-Complex

34. A student reads the following sentence:

A hundred years ago, automobiles were rare, but now cars are ubiquitous.

However, she doesn't know what the word *ubiquitous* means. Which key context clue is essential to decipher the word's meaning?

a. Ago
b. Cars
c. Now
d. Rare

35. Which word in the following sentence is a proper noun:

People think the Statue of Liberty is an awesome sight.

a. People
b. Statue of Liberty
c. Awesome
d. Sight

36. Which word in the following sentence is a plural noun:

The black kitten was the girl's choice from the litter of kittens.

a. Kitten
b. Girl's
c. Choice
d. Kittens

447

37. Which pronoun makes the following sentence grammatically correct:

_____ ordered the flowers?

a. Whose
b. Whom
c. Who
d. Who've

38. Which pronoun makes the following sentence grammatically correct:

The giraffe nudged _____ baby.

a. it's
b. hers
c. their
d. its

39. What is the word *several* in the following sentence called:

Several are laughing loudly on the bus.

a. Singular indefinite pronoun
b. Plural indefinite pronoun
c. Singular objective pronoun
d. Indefinite adjective

40. Which word in the following sentence is an adjective:

The connoisseur slowly enjoyed the delectable meal.

a. Delectable
b. Connoisseur
c. Slowly
d. Enjoyed

41. Which choice identifies all of the prepositions in the following sentence:

We went down by the water, near the lake, before dawn, to see the pretty sunrise.

a. Went, to see, pretty
b. By, near, before
c. Water, lake, dawn, sunrise
d. We, down, the, pretty

42. Which sentence has an interjection?
    a. The cookie was full of chocolaty goodness.
    b. Well, Carrie didn't like the cookie.
    c. Can't you see that cookie is broken?
    d. That's too bad, but I'll still eat it!

43. Identify the complete subject in the following sentence:

    The heaviest green bike is mine.

    a. bike
    b. green bike
    c. The heaviest green bike
    d. is mine

44. Identify the complete predicate in the following sentence:

    My house is the yellow one at the end of the street.

    a. My house
    b. is the yellow one
    c. at the end of the street.
    d. is the yellow one at the end of the street.

45. Which sentence shows incorrect subject/verb agreement?
    a. All of the kittens in the litter show their courage.
    b. The black kitten pounce on the ball of yarn.
    c. The calico kitten eats voraciously.
    d. My favorite kitten snuggles with its mother.

46. What is the indirect object in the following sentence:

    Calysta brought her mother the beautiful stained-glass lamp.

    a. Stained-glass lamp
    b. Brought
    c. Her mother
    d. Beautiful

47. Which sentence is grammatically correct?
    a. They're on their way to New Jersey but there not there yet.
    b. Their on their way to New Jersey but they're not there yet.
    c. They're on their way to New Jersey but they're not there yet.
    d. They're on their way to New Jersey but there not their yet.

48. Identify the prepositional phrase in the following sentence:

For the longest time, I have wanted to learn to roller skate.

    a. I have wanted
    b. wanted to learn
    c. learn to roller skate
    d. For the longest time

49. Identify the sentence structure of the following sentence:

The weight of the world was on his shoulders, so he took a long walk.

    a. Simple sentence
    b. Compound sentence
    c. Complex sentence
    d. Compound-complex sentence

50. Identify the sentence structure of the following sentence:

The last thing she wanted to do was see the Eiffel Tower before the flight.

    a. Simple sentence
    b. Compound sentence
    c. Complex sentence
    d. Compound-complex sentence

Directions for questions 51–55

Select the best version of the underlined part of the sentence. The first choice is the same as the original sentence. If you think the original sentence is best, choose the first answer.

51. Besides the novel's engaging <u>writing style the story's central theme</u> remains highly relevant in a world of constant discovery and moral dilemmas.
    a. writing style the story's central theme
    b. writing style the central theme of the story
    c. writing style, the story's central theme
    d. the story's central theme's writing style

52. Looking deeper into the myth of Prometheus sheds light not only on the character of Frankenstein <u>but also poses a psychological dilemma to the audience</u>.
    a. but also poses a psychological dilemma to the audience
    b. but also poses a psychological dilemma with the audience
    c. but also poses a psychological dilemma for the audience
    d. but also poses a psychological dilemma there before the audience

53. There are many things to consider when addressing <u>this question but the chief factor</u> is whether there is credible evidence.
   a. this question but the chief factor
   b. this question, but the chief factor
   c. this question however the chief factor
   d. this question; but the chief factor

54. <u>For science to formally recognize that such a species exists, there needs to be physical proof.</u>
   a. For science to formally recognize that such a species exists, there needs to be physical proof.
   b. Physical proof are needed in order for science to formally recognize that such a species exists.
   c. For science to formally recognize that such a species exists there needs to be physical proof.
   d. For science, to formally recognize that such a species exists, there needs to be physical proof.

55. Today, laws prohibit the <u>use of unnecessary force in self-defense; these serve to eliminate</u> beating someone to a pulp once they have been neutralized.
   a. use of unnecessary force in self-defense; these serve to eliminate
   b. use of unnecessary force in self-defense serving to eliminate
   c. use of unnecessary force, in self-defense, these serve to eliminate
   d. use of unnecessary force. In self-defense, these serve to eliminate

Biology

1. A scientist is trying to determine how much poison will kill a rat the fastest. Which of the following statements is an example of an appropriate hypothesis?
   a. Rats that are given lots of poison seem to die quickly.
   b. Does the amount of poison affect how quickly the rat dies?
   c. The more poison a rat is given, the quicker it will die.
   d. Poison is fatal to rats.

2. Which of the following is NOT a unique property of water?
   a. High cohesion and adhesion
   b. High surface tension
   c. High density upon melting
   d. High freezing point

3. What is a metabolic reaction that releases energy called?
   a. Catabolic
   b. Carbolic
   c. Anabolic
   d. Endothermic

4. What organic compounds facilitate chemical reactions by lowering activation energy?
   a. Carbohydrates
   b. Lipids
   c. Enzymes
   d. Nucleotides

5. Which structure is exclusively in eukaryotic cells?
    a. Cell wall
    b. Nucleus
    c. Cell membrane
    d. Vacuole

6. Which of these is NOT found in the cell nucleus?
    a. Golgi complex
    b. Chromosomes
    c. Nucleolus
    d. Chromatin

7. Which is the cellular organelle used for digestion to recycle materials?
    a. Golgi apparatus
    b. Lysosome
    c. Centriole
    d. Mitochondria

8. What are the energy-generating structures of the cell called?
    a. Nucleoplasms
    b. Mitochondria
    c. Golgi Apparatus
    d. Ribosomes

9. Which is a component of plant cells not found in animal cells?
    a. Nucleus
    b. Plastid
    c. Cell membrane
    d. Lysosome

10. What is the LAST phase of mitosis?
    a. Prophase
    b. Telophase
    c. Anaphase
    d. Metaphase

11. The combination of alleles of an organism, when expressed, manifests as the organism's _____.
    a. genotype.
    b. phenotype.
    c. gender.
    d. karyotype.

12. Which of the choices below are the reproductive cells produced by meiosis?
    a. Zygotes
    b. Germ cells
    c. Blastocyst
    d. Gametes

13. What is the process of cell division in somatic (most body) cells called?
    a. Mitosis
    b. Meiosis
    c. Respiration
    d. Cytogenesis

14. Water has many unique properties due to its unique structure. Which of the following does not play a role in water's unique properties?
    a. Hydrogen bonding between molecules
    b. Polarity within one molecule
    c. Molecules held apart in solid state
    d. Equal sharing of electrons

15. Which function below is NOT one of lipids?
    a. Provides cellular instructions
    b. Can be chemical messages
    c. Provides energy
    d. Composes cell membranes

16. What is an alteration in the normal gene sequence called?
    a. Mutation
    b. Gene migration
    c. Polygenetic inheritance
    d. Incomplete dominance

17. Blood type is a trait determined by multiple alleles, and two of them are co-dominant: I^A codes for A blood and I^B codes for B blood. The i allele codes for O blood and is recessive to both. If an A individual and an O individual have a child, what is the probably that the child will have A blood?
    a. 25%
    b. 50%
    c. 75%
    d. 100%

18. What are the building blocks of DNA referred to as?
    a. Helices
    b. Proteins
    c. Genes
    d. Nucleotides

19. Which statement is NOT true about DNA?
    a. It has guanine.
    b. DNA enables living organisms to pass on their genetic information.
    c. It contains uracil.
    d. DNA replication happens in interphase.

453

20. Which of the following is true about an endergonic reaction?
    a. The reaction results in a negative delta G (−ΔG).
    b. The reaction is considered spontaneous.
    c. The reaction absorbs energy.
    d. The reaction releases energy.

21. What is the term used for the set of metabolic reactions that convert chemical bonds to energy in the form of ATP?
    a. Photosynthesis
    b. Reproduction
    c. Active transport
    d. Cellular respiration

22. Which level of protein structure is defined by the folds and coils of the protein's polypeptide backbone?
    a. Primary
    b. Secondary
    c. Tertiary
    d. Quaternary

23. What is the broadest, or LEAST specialized, classification of the Linnaean taxonomic system?
    a. Species
    b. Family
    c. Domain
    d. Phylum

24. Which of the following is NOT a function of lipids?
    a. Provides cellular instructions
    b. Can be chemical messages
    c. Provides energy
    d. Composes cell membranes

25. What is the cell structure responsible for protein synthesis called?
    a. DNA
    b. Golgi Apparatus
    c. Nucleus
    d. Ribosome

Questions 26–30 pertain to the passage:

Scientists often use an assay called an enzyme-linked immunosorbent assay, or ELISA, to quantify specific substances within a larger sample. An ELISA works based on the specificity of an antibody to an antigen. One type of ELISA is called a sandwich ELISA. In this type of ELISA, a plate is coated with a capture antibody that adheres the antigen in the sample when it is added. Then the primary antibody is added and sticks to any antigen bound to the capture antibody. Next, a secondary antibody is added. Once it attaches to the primary antibody, it releases a colored tag that can be detected by a piece of laboratory equipment. If more color is released, it is indicative of more antigen having been present in the sample.

Figure 1 below describes how a sandwich ELISA works.

The cytokine protein IL-1β is a marker of inflammation in the body. Scientist A took samples from different locations within the body to find out where there was elevated inflammation in a patient.

Figure 2 below is a picture of the ELISA plate from Scientist A's experiment.

Figure 3 below is a graph of the results of Scientist A's experiment.

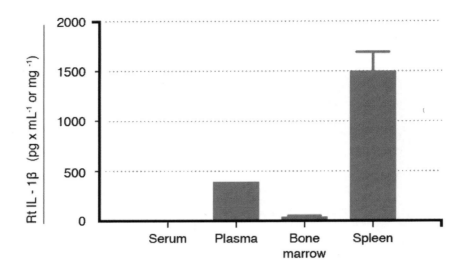

26. Which step of the ELISA allows for the color to be released for detection of the antigen?
    a. Addition of the antigen
    b. Addition of the primary antibody
    c. The presence of the capture antibody
    d. Addition of the secondary antibody

27. According to Figure 2, which row had the largest amount of antigen in the sample?
    a. Row 2
    b. Row 1
    c. Row 5
    d. Row 3

28. According to the ELISA results in Figure 3, which area of the body had the most inflammation?
    a. Serum
    b. Plasma
    c. Spleen
    d. Bone marrow

29. Which two antibodies sandwich the antigen in a sandwich ELISA?
    a. Capture antibody and secondary antibody
    b. Capture antibody and primary antibody
    c. Primary antibody and secondary antibody
    d. Two units of the secondary antibody

30. What is the purpose of an ELISA?
    a. Quantify specific substances within a larger sample
    b. Quantify all substances within a larger sample
    c. To create a colorful pattern with the samples
    d. To develop different antibodies

Chemistry

1. What is 45 °C converted to °F?
    a. 113 °F
    b. 135 °F
    c. 57 °F
    d. 88 °F

2. What is the electrical charge of the nucleus?
    a. A nucleus always has a positive charge.
    b. A stable nucleus has a positive charge, but a radioactive nucleus may have no charge and instead be neutral.
    c. A nucleus always has no charge and is instead neutral.
    d. A stable nucleus has no charge and is instead neutral, but a radioactive nucleus may have a charge.

3. What is the temperature in Fahrenheit when it is 35°C outside?
    a. 67°F
    b. 95°F
    c. 63°F
    d. 75°F

4. How are a sodium atom and a sodium isotope different?
    a. The isotope has a different number of protons.
    b. The isotope has a different number of neutrons.
    c. The isotope has a different number of electrons.
    d. The isotope has a different atomic number.

5. Which statement is true about nonmetals?
    a. They form cations.
    b. They form covalent bonds.
    c. They are mostly absent from organic compounds.
    d. They are all diatomic.

6. What is the basic unit of matter?
    a. Elementary particle
    b. Atom
    c. Molecule
    d. Photon

457

7. Which particle is responsible for all chemical reactions?
    a. Electrons
    b. Neutrons
    c. Protons
    d. Orbitals

8. Which of these give atoms a negative charge?
    a. Electrons
    b. Neutrons
    c. Protons
    d. Orbital

9. How are similar chemical properties of elements grouped on the periodic table?
    a. In rows according to their total configuration of electrons
    b. In columns according to the electron configuration in their outer shells
    c. In rows according to the electron configuration in their outer shells
    d. In columns according to their total configurations of electrons

10. In a chemical equation, the reactants are on which side of the arrow?
    a. Right
    b. Left
    c. Neither right nor left
    d. Both right and left

11. What does the law of conservation of mass state?
    a. All matter is equally created.
    b. Matter changes but is not created.
    c. Matter can be changed, and new matter can be created
    d. Matter can be created, but not changed.

12. Which factor decreases the solubility of solids?
    a. Heating
    b. Agitation
    c. Large Surface area
    d. Decreasing solvent

13. What information is used to calculate the quantity of solute in a solution?
    a. Molarity of the solution
    b. Equivalence point
    c. Limiting reactant
    d. Theoretical yield

14. How does adding salt to water affect its boiling point?
    a. It increases it.
    b. It has no effect.
    c. It decreases it.
    d. It prevents it from boiling.

458

15. What is the effect of pressure on a liquid solution?
   a. It decreases solubility.
   b. It increases solubility.
   c. It has little effect on solubility.
   d. It has the same effect as with a gaseous solution.

16. Nonpolar molecules must have what kind of regions?
   a. Hydrophilic
   b. Hydrophobic
   c. Hydrolytic
   d. Hydrochloric

17. Which of these is a substance that increases the rate of a chemical reaction?
   a. Catalyst
   b. Brine
   c. Solvent
   d. Inhibitor

18. Which of the following are composed of chains of amino acids?
   a. Lipids
   b. Nucleic Acids
   c. Proteins
   d. Carbohydrates

19. What is the balance of the following combustion equation?

$$\_C_2 H_{10+}\_O_2 \rightarrow \_H_2O+\_CO_2$$

   a. 1:5:5:2
   b. 1:9:5:2
   c. 2:9:10:4
   d. 2:5:10:4

20. Which type of bonding results from transferring electrons between atoms?
   a. Ionic bonding
   b. Covalent bonding
   c. Hydrogen bonding
   d. Dipole interactions

21. Which substance is oxidized in the following reaction?

$$4Fe+3O_2 \rightarrow 2Fe_2O_3$$

   a. Fe
   b. O
   c. O_2
   d. Fe_2O_3

22. Which statements are true regarding nuclear fission?

  I. Splitting of heavy nuclei
  II. Utilized in power plants
  III. Occurs on the sun

 a. I only
 b. II and III only
 c. I and II only
 d. III only

23. Which type of nuclear decay is occurring in the equation below?

$$U_{92}^{236} \rightarrow He_2^4 + Th_{90}^{232}$$

 a. Alpha
 b. Beta
 c. Gamma
 d. Delta

24. Which statement is true about the pH of a solution?
 a. A solution cannot have a pH less than 1.
 b. The more hydroxide ions there are in the solution, the higher the pH will be.
 c. If an acid has a pH of greater than -1, it is considered a weak acid.
 d. A solution with a pH of 2 has ten times more hydrogen ions than a solution with a pH of 1.

25. Which radioactive particle is the most penetrating and damaging and is used to treat cancer in radiation?
 a. Alpha
 b. Beta
 c. Gamma
 d. Delta

Questions 26–30 pertain to the passage:

In chemistry, a titration is a method that is used to determine the concentration of an unknown solution. Generally, a known volume of a solution of known concentration is mixed with the unknown solution. Once the reaction of the two solutions has been completed, the concentration of the unknown solution can be calculated. When acids and bases are titrated, the progress of the reaction is monitored by changes in the pH of the known solution. The equivalence point is when just enough of the unknown solution has been added to neutralize the known solution. A color reaction may also occur so that with the drop of solution that causes complete neutralization, the solution turns bright pink, for example. For acids that only have one proton, usually a hydrogen atom, the halfway point between the beginning of the curve and the equivalence point is where the amount of acid and base are equal in the solution. At this point, the pH is equal to the pK_a, or the acid dissociation constant.

Figure 1 below shows a general titration curve of a strong acid with a strong base.

Volume NaOH added

Figure 2 below shows the chemical reaction of a strong acid with a strong base.

Figure 3 shows the titration curve for acetic acid.

Titration Curve of Acetic Acid

26. How much NaOH is added to the HCl solution to reach the equivalence point in Figure 1?
    a. 10
    b. 40
    c. 50
    d. 25

27. What is the acid dissociation constant of the titration curve in the Figure 3?
    a. 4.21
    b. 3.50
    c. 4.76
    d. 6.52

28. What is the pH of the acetic acid before the titration has started in Figure 3?
    a. 2
    b. 4.76
    c. 7
    d. 6

29. What is one of the products of the chemical equation in Figure 2?
    a. HCl
    b. NaCl
    c. NaOH
    d. Cl⁻

30. How would you describe the solution at the equivalence point in Figure 1?
    a. Neutral
    b. Acidic
    c. Basic
    d. Unknown

Anatomy and Physiology

1. Why do arteries have valves?
    a. They have valves to maintain high blood pressure so that capillaries diffuse nutrients properly.
    b. Their valves are designed to prevent backflow due to their low blood pressure.
    c. The valves have no known purpose and thus appear to be unnecessary.
    d. They do not have valves, but veins do.

2. Which locations in the digestive system are sites of chemical digestion?

    I. Mouth
    II. Stomach
    III. Small Intestine

    a. II only
    b. III only
    c. II and III only
    d. I, II, and III

3. Which of the following are functions of the urinary system?

    I. Synthesizing calcitriol and secreting erythropoietin
    II. Regulating the concentrations of sodium, potassium, chloride, calcium, and other ions
    III. Reabsorbing or secreting hydrogen ions and bicarbonate
    IV. Detecting reductions in blood volume and pressure

    a. I, II, and III
    b. II and III
    c. II, III, and IV
    d. All of the above

463

4. If the pressure in the pulmonary artery is increased above normal, which chamber of the heart will be affected first?
    a. The right atrium
    b. The left atrium
    c. The right ventricle
    d. The left ventricle

5. What is the purpose of sodium bicarbonate when released into the lumen of the small intestine?
    a. It works to chemically digest fats in the chyme.
    b. It decreases the pH of the chyme so as to prevent harm to the intestine.
    c. It works to chemically digest proteins in the chyme.
    d. It increases the pH of the chyme so as to prevent harm to the intestine.

6. Which of the following describes a reflex arc?
    a. The storage and recall of memory
    b. The maintenance of visual and auditory acuity
    c. The autoregulation of heart rate and blood pressure
    d. A stimulus and response controlled by the spinal cord

7. Ligaments connect what?
    a. Muscle to muscle
    b. Bone to bone
    c. Bone to muscle
    d. Muscle to tendon

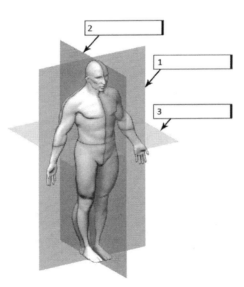

8. Identify the correct sequence of the 3 primary body planes as numbered 1, 2, and 3 in the above image.
    a. Plane 1 is coronal, plane 2 is sagittal, and plane 3 is transverse.
    b. Plane 1 is sagittal, plane 2 is coronal, and plane 3 is medial.
    c. Plane 1 is coronal, plane 2 is sagittal, and plane 3 is medial.
    d. Plane 1 is sagittal, plane 2 is coronal, and plane 3 is transverse.

9. Which of the following is NOT a major function of the respiratory system in humans?
    a. It provides a large surface area for gas exchange of oxygen and carbon dioxide.
    b. It helps regulate the blood's pH.
    c. It helps cushion the heart against jarring motions.
    d. It is responsible for vocalization.

10. Which of the following is NOT a function of the forebrain?
    a. To regulate blood pressure and heart rate
    b. To perceive and interpret emotional responses like fear and anger
    c. To perceive and interpret visual input from the eyes
    d. To integrate voluntary movement

11. A patient's body is not properly filtering blood. Which of the following body parts is most likely malfunctioning?
    a. Medulla
    b. Heart
    c. Nephrons
    d. Renal cortex

12. A pediatrician notes that an infant's cartilage is disappearing and being replaced by bone. What process has the doctor observed?
    a. Mineralization
    b. Ossification
    c. Osteoporosis
    d. Calcification

13. Which of the following creates sperm?
    a. Prostate gland
    b. Seminal vesicles
    c. Scrotum
    d. Seminiferous tubules

14. Which of the following functions corresponds to the parasympathetic nervous system?
    a. It stimulates the fight-or-flight response.
    b. It increases heart rate.
    c. It stimulates digestion.
    d. It increases bronchiole dilation.

15. Which of the following is the gland that helps regulate calcium levels?
    a. Osteotoid gland
    b. Pineal gland
    c. Parathyroid glands
    d. Thymus gland

16. What makes bone resistant to shattering?
    a. The calcium salts deposited in the bone
    b. The collagen fibers
    c. The bone marrow and network of blood vessels
    d. The intricate balance of minerals and collagen fibers

17. What type of vessel carries oxygen-rich blood from the heart to other tissues of the body?
    a. Veins
    b. Intestines
    c. Bronchioles
    d. Arteries

18. The somatic nervous system is responsible for which of the following?
    a. Breathing
    b. Thought
    c. Movement
    d. Fear

19. Which blood component is chiefly responsible for clotting?
    a. Platelets
    b. Red blood cells
    c. Antigens
    d. Plasma cells

20. What is the function of the sinuses?
    a. To trap the many airborne pathogens
    b. To direct air down the trachea rather than the esophagus
    c. To warm, humidify, and filter air
    d. To sweep away pathogens and direct them toward the top of the trachea

21. During which step of digestion do the teeth tear up food that has entered the mouth?
    a. Secretion
    b. Absorption
    c. Excretion
    d. Mechanical processing

22. A cluster of capillaries that functions as the main filter of the blood entering the kidney is known as which of the following?
    a. The Bowman's capsule
    b. The Loop of Henle
    c. The glomerulus
    d. The nephron

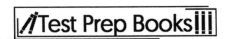

23. What is the name for the sac-shaped structures in which carbon dioxide and oxygen exchange takes place?
    a. Kidneys
    b. Medulla oblongata
    c. Alveoli
    d. Bronchioles

24. The muscular tube that connects the outer surface to the cervix in a woman's birth canal is referred to as which of the following?
    a. The uterus
    b. The cervix
    c. The vagina
    d. The ovaries

25. Which of the following organs functions both as an endocrine and exocrine gland?
    a. The kidney
    b. The spleen
    c. The pancreas
    d. The stomach

26. Which of the following correctly identifies a difference between the primary and secondary immune response?
    a. In the secondary response, macrophages migrate to the lymph nodes to present the foreign microorganism to helped T lymphocytes.
    b. The humeral immunity that characterizes the primary response is coordinated by T lymphocytes.
    c. The primary response is quicker and more powerful than the secondary response.
    d. Suppressor T cells activate in the secondary response to prevent an overactive immune response.

27. High blood sugar stimulates the kidneys to do which of the following?
    a. Produce less urine
    b. Concentrate the urine
    c. Retain more sodium
    d. Produce more urine

28. A patient experiencing itching related to an allergic reaction likely has the substance histamine being secreted by which white blood cell?
    a. Eosinophils
    b. Basophils
    c. Neutrophils
    d. Monocytes

29. Which structure of the brain is responsible for producing cerebral spinal fluid?
    a. Pons
    b. Ventricle
    c. Thalamus
    d. Corpus callosum

30. Which of the following statements is true?
    a. As fluid levels decrease, electrolyte levels increase.
    b. As fluid levels increase, electrolyte levels increase.
    c. As fluid levels osmose, electrolyte levels diffuse.
    d. As fluid levels homogenize, electrolyte levels dissipate.

Physics

1. Velocity is a measure of which of the following?
    a. Speed with direction
    b. The change in speed over the change in time
    c. Acceleration with direction
    d. All of the above

2. What is the definition of acceleration?
    a. The rate at which an object moves
    b. The rate of change in velocity
    c. Speed in a given direction
    d. The velocity of an object multiplied by its mass

3. Which of the following is NOT one of Newton's three laws of motion?
    a. An object a rest tends to stay at rest, and an object in motion tends to stay in motion
    b. $E=mc^2$
    c. For every action, there is an equal and opposite reaction
    d. $F=ma$

4. For circular motion, what is the name of the actual force pulling toward the axis of rotation?
    a. Centrifugal force
    b. Gravity
    c. Centripetal force
    d. No force is acting

5. The energy of motion is also referred to as what?
    a. Potential energy
    b. Kinetic energy
    c. Electric energy
    d. Electromagnetic energy

6. What is the purpose of a wave?
    a. To carry matter
    b. To transfer energy
    c. To do work
    d. To slow down matter

7. What is the term for when a wave bends?
   a. Refraction
   b. Diffraction
   c. Reflection
   d. Convection

8. Which of the following reside in the nucleus of an atom?
   a. Protons and neutrons
   b. Neutrons and electrons
   c. Electrons and ions
   d. Ions and protons

9. How does electrical energy flow?
   a. From objects with lesser potential energy to objects with greater potential energy
   b. Equally between objects with equal potential energy
   c. From objects with greater potential energy to objects with lesser potential energy
   d. From objects with greater magnetic energy to objects with greater electrical energy

10. Which of the following is true regarding electromagnetism?
   a. Opposite charges attract
   b. Like charges attract
   c. Opposite charge are neutral towards one another
   d. Like charges are neutral towards one another

11. A 150-kilogram mass is placed on the left side of the lever as shown. What force must be exerted on the right side (in the location shown by the arrow) to balance the weight of this mass?

   a. 675 kg·m
   b. 735.75 N
   c. 1471.5 N
   d. 2207.25 N·m

12. For the wheel and axle assembly shown, the shaft radius is 20 millimeters and the wheel radius is 300 millimeters. What's the required effort to lift a 600 N load?

a. 10 N
b. 20 N
c. 30 N
d. 40 N

13. The driver gear (Gear A) turns clockwise at a rate of 60 RPM. In what direction does Gear B turn and at what rotational speed?

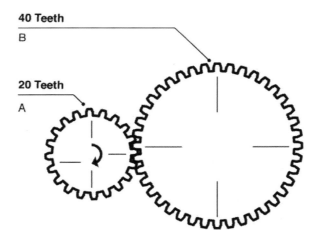

a. Clockwise at 120 RPM
b. Counterclockwise at 120 RPM
c. Clockwise at 30 RPM
d. Counterclockwise at 30 RPM

14. The three steel wheels shown are connected by rubber belts. The two wheels at the top have the same diameter, while the wheel below is twice their diameter. If the driver wheel at the upper left is turning clockwise at 60 RPM, at what speed and in which direction is the large bottom wheel turning?

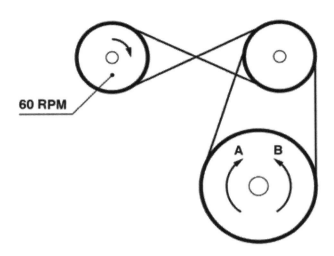

60 RPM

a. 30 RPM, clockwise (A)
b. 30 RPM, counterclockwise (B)
c. 120 RPM, clockwise (A)
d. 120 RPM, counterclockwise (B)

15. In case (a), both blocks are fixed. In case (b), the load is hung from a moveable block. Ignoring friction, what is the required force to move the blocks in both cases?

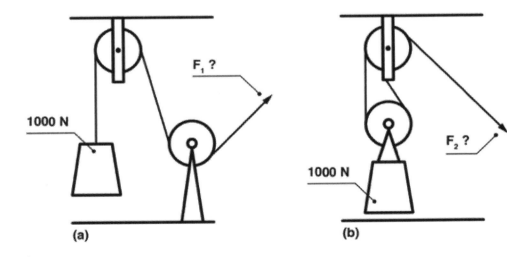

F_1 ?

1000 N

1000 N

F_2 ?

(a)

(b)

a. $F_1 = 500$ N; $F_2 = 500$ N
b. $F_1 = 500$ N; $F_2 = 1000$ N
c. $F_1 = 1000$ N; $F_2 = 500$ N
d. $F_1 = 1000$ N; $F_2 = 1000$ N

16. What is the total mechanical energy of a system?
   a. The total potential energy
   b. The total kinetic energy
   c. Kinetic energy plus potential energy
   d. Kinetic energy minus potential energy

17. What is the name of the scale used in sound level meters to measure the intensity of sound waves?
   a. Doppler
   b. Electron
   c. Watt
   d. Decibel

18. What effect changes the oscillations of a wave and can alter the appearance of light waves?
   a. Reflection
   b. Refraction
   c. Dispersion
   d. Polarization

19. What is the primary difference between an elastic and inelastic collision?
   a. In an elastic collision, the objects collide and then travel in different directions; in an inelastic collision, the objects collide and then stick together in their final direction of travel.
   b. In an elastic collision, the objects collide and then stick together in their final direction of travel; in an inelastic collision, the objects collide and then travel in different directions.
   c. An elastic collision adheres to the principle of the conservation of linear momentum while an inelastic collision does not.
   d. An inelastic collision adheres to the principle of the conservation of linear momentum while an elastic collision does not.

20. How is mechanical advantage calculated?
   a. The force input divided by the force output
   b. The force input multiplied by the force output
   c. The force output divided by 100
   d. The force output divided by the force input

Answer Explanations #3

Mathematics

1. B: 15,412

Set up the problem and add each column, starting on the far right (ones). Add, carrying anything over 9 into the next column to the left. Solve from right to left.

2. D: 104,165

Set up the problem and add each column, starting on the far right (ones). Add, carrying anything over 9 into the next column to the left. Solve from right to left.

3. A: 6.630

Set up the problem, with the larger number on top and numbers lined up at the decimal. Add, carrying anything over 9 into the next column to the left. Solve from right to left.

4. B: 148.97

Set up the problem, with the larger number on top and numbers lined up at the decimal. Insert 0 in any blank spots to the right of the decimal as placeholders. Add, carrying anything over 9 into the next column to the left.

5. C: $\frac{31}{36}$

Set up the problem and find a common denominator for both fractions.

$$\frac{5}{12} + \frac{4}{9}$$

Multiply each fraction across by 1 to convert to a common denominator.

$$\frac{5}{12} \times \frac{3}{3} + \frac{4}{9} \times \frac{4}{4}$$

Once over the same denominator, add across the top. The total is over the common denominator.

$$\frac{15 + 16}{36} = \frac{31}{36}$$

6. C: 4/3

Set up the problem and find a common denominator for both fractions.

$$\frac{14}{33} + \frac{10}{11}$$

473

Multiply each fraction across by 1 to convert to a common denominator

$$\frac{14}{33} \times \frac{1}{1} + \frac{10}{11} \times \frac{3}{3}$$

Once over the same denominator, add across the top. The total is over the common denominator.

$$\frac{14 + 30}{33} = \frac{44}{33}$$

Reduce by dividing both numerator and denominator by 11.

$$\frac{44 \div 11}{33 \div 11} = \frac{4}{3}$$

7. D: 8,685

Set up the problem, with the larger number on top. Begin subtracting with the far-right column (ones). Borrow 10 from the column to the left, when necessary.

8. A: 110,833

Set up the problem, with the larger number on top. Begin subtracting with the far-right column (ones). Borrow 10 from the column to the left, when necessary.

9. A: 37.797

Set up the problem, larger number on top and numbers lined up at the decimal. Begin subtracting with the far-right column. Borrow 10 from the column to the left, when necessary.

10. B: 648.77

Set up the problem, with the larger number on top and numbers lined up at the decimal. Insert 0 in any blank spots to the right of the decimal as placeholders. Begin subtracting with the far-right column. Borrow 10 from the column to the left, when necessary.

11. C: 19/24

Set up the problem and find a common denominator for both fractions.

$$\frac{23}{24} - \frac{1}{6}$$

Multiply each fraction across by 1 to convert to a common denominator.

$$\frac{23}{24} \times \frac{1}{1} - \frac{1}{6} \times \frac{4}{4}$$

Once over the same denominator, subtract across the top.

$$\frac{23 - 4}{24} = \frac{19}{24}$$

12. D: $2/9$

Set up the problem and find a common denominator for both fractions.

$$\frac{43}{45} - \frac{11}{15}$$

Multiply each fraction across by 1 to convert to a common denominator.

$$\frac{43}{45} \times \frac{1}{1} - \frac{11}{15} \times \frac{3}{3}$$

Once over the same denominator, subtract across the top.

$$\frac{43 - 33}{45} = \frac{10}{45}$$

Reduce:

$$\frac{10 \div 5}{45 \div 5} = \frac{2}{9}$$

13. D: 8670

Begin with the far-right digit on top and the far-right digit on the bottom (8×5).

Move one column left on top and multiply by the far-right column on the bottom. Remember to add the carry over after you multiply.

Starting on the far-right column, on top, repeat this pattern for the next number left on the bottom. Write the answers below the first line of answers. Remember to begin with a zero placeholder.

Continue the pattern.

Add the answer rows together, making sure they are still lined up correctly.

14. A: 2,504,774

Line up the numbers (the number with the most digits on top) to multiply. Begin with the right column on top and the right column on bottom.

Move one column left on top and multiply by the far-right column on the bottom. Remember to add the carry over after you multiply. Continue that pattern for each of the numbers on the top row.

Starting on the far-right column on top repeat this pattern for the next number left on the bottom. Write the answers below the first line of answers; remember to begin with a zero placeholder. Continue for each number in the top row.

Starting on the far-right column on top, repeat this pattern for the next number left on the bottom. Write the answers below the first line of answers. Remember to begin with zero placeholders.

475

Once completed, ensure the answer rows are lined up correctly, then add.

15. B: 2.48

Set up the problem, with the larger number on top. Multiply as if there are no decimal places. Add the answer rows together. Count the number of decimal places that were in the original numbers ($1 + 1 = 2$).

Place the decimal 2 places to the right for the final solution.

16. B: 99.35

Set up the problem, with the larger number on top. Multiply as if there are no decimal places. Add the answer rows together. Count the number of decimal places that were in the original numbers (2).

Place the decimal in that many spots from the right for the final solution.

17. A: $\frac{810}{2,921}$

Line up the fractions.

$$\frac{15}{23} \times \frac{54}{127}$$

Multiply across the top and across the bottom.

$$\frac{15 \times 54}{23 \times 127} = \frac{810}{2,921}$$

18. C: $\frac{6}{11}$

Line up the fractions.

$$\frac{54}{55} \times \frac{5}{9}$$

Reduce fractions through cross-canceling.

$$\frac{6}{11} \times \frac{1}{1}$$

Multiply across the top and across the bottom.

$$\frac{6 \times 1}{11 \times 1} = \frac{6}{11}$$

19. D: 27 and $\frac{7}{22}$

Set up the division problem.

$$44\overline{)1202}$$

44 does not go into 1 or 12 but will go into 120 so start there.

$$
\begin{array}{r}
27 \\
44\overline{)1202} \\
-88 \\
\hline
322 \\
-308 \\
\hline
14
\end{array}
$$

The answer is 27 and $\frac{7}{22}$.

Reduce the fraction for the final answer: 27 and $\frac{7}{22}$

20. D: 11 and 3/4

Set up the division problem.

$$16\overline{)188}$$

16 does not go into 1 but does go into 18 so start there.

$$
\begin{array}{r}
11 \\
16\overline{)188} \\
-16 \\
\hline
28 \\
-16 \\
\hline
12
\end{array}
$$

The result is 11 and 12/16

Reduce the fraction for the final answer: 11 and $\frac{3}{4}$

21. D: 270

Set up the division problem.

$$2.6\overline{)702}$$

Move the decimal over one place to the right in both numbers.

$$26\overline{)7020}$$

26 does not go into 7 but does go into 70 so start there.

$$
\begin{array}{r}
270 \\
26\overline{)7020} \\
-52 \\
\hline
182 \\
-182 \\
\hline
0
\end{array}
$$

The result is 270

22. B: 725

Set up the division problem.

$$1.4\overline{)1015}$$

Move the decimal over one place to the right in both numbers.

$$14\overline{)10150}$$

14 does not go into 1 or 10 but does go into 101 so start there.

$$
\begin{array}{r}
725 \\
14\overline{)10150} \\
-98 \\
\hline
35 \\
-28 \\
\hline
70 \\
-70 \\
\hline
0
\end{array}
$$

The result is 725.

23. C: $\frac{1}{5}$

Set up the division problem.

$$\frac{26}{55} \div \frac{26}{11}$$

Flip the second fraction and multiply.

$$\frac{26}{55} \times \frac{11}{26}$$

Simplify and reduce with cross multiplication.

$$\frac{1}{5} \times \frac{1}{1}$$

Multiply across the top and across the bottom.

$$\frac{1 \times 1}{5 \times 1} = \frac{1}{5}$$

24. A: $\frac{52}{27}$

Set up the division problem.

$$\frac{4}{13} \div \frac{27}{169}$$

Flip the second fraction and multiply.

$$\frac{4}{13} \times \frac{169}{27}$$

Simplify the fractions before multiplying to make numbers simpler to work with.

$$\frac{4}{1} \times \frac{13}{27}$$

Multiply across the top and across the bottom to solve.

$$\frac{4 \times 13}{1 \times 27} = \frac{52}{27}$$

25. D: 1,432

Break down the roman numerals into parts.

MCDXXXII

M is equal to 1000.

C is before D and is smaller than D, so it means $D - C$.

$$CD = 500 - 100 = 400$$

Add the following:

$$XXX = 10 + 10 + 10 = 30$$

$$II = 1 + 1 = 2$$

Add all parts:

$$1,000 + 400 + 30 + 2 = 1432$$

26. D: 251

Break down the roman numerals into parts.

CCLI

Add the following:

$$CC = 100 + 100 = 200$$

$$L = 50$$

$$I = 1$$

Add all parts:

$$200 + 50 + 1 = 251$$

27. B: CXI

Break down the number into parts.

$$111 = 100 + 10 + 1$$

100 is represented by C or $100 = C$.

10 is represented by X or $10 = X$.

1 is represented by 1 or $1 = I$.

Combine the Roman numerals.

CXI

28. C: DXV

Break down the number into parts.

$$515 = 500 + 10 + 5$$

500 is represented by D or $500 = D$.

10 is represented by X or $10 = X$.

5 is represented by V or $5 = V$.

Combine the Roman numerals.

DXV

29. A: 1:00 p.m.

Since military time starts with 0100 at 1:00 a.m., add 12 to get to 1300 hours, or 1:00 p.m.

30. B: 8:30 a.m.

Anything before 1200 would be in the a.m. hours of a 12-hour clock, so 0830 hours is 8:30 a.m.

31. B: 1700 hours

To convert 5:00 p.m. into 24-hour time, add 12 to 5.

32. B: 1100 hours

Anything before noon converts into its a.m. value.

33. A: 13 nurses

Using the given information of 1 nurse to 25 patients and 325 patients, set up an equation to solve for number of nurses (N):

$$\frac{N}{325} = \frac{1}{25}$$

Multiply both sides by 325 to get N by itself on one side.

$$\frac{N}{1} = \frac{325}{25} = 13 \text{ nurses}$$

34. D: 290 beds

Using the given information of 2 beds to 1 room and 145 rooms, set up an equation to solve for number of beds (B):

$$\frac{B}{145} = \frac{2}{1}$$

Multiply both sides by 145 to get B by itself on one side.

$$\frac{B}{1} = \frac{290}{1} = 290 \text{ beds}$$

35. C: $X = 150$

Set up the initial equation:

$$\frac{2X}{5} - 1 = 59$$

Add 1 to both sides:

$$\frac{2X}{5} - 1 + 1 = 59 + 1$$

Multiply both sides by $\frac{5}{2}$:

$$\frac{2X}{5} \times \frac{5}{2} = 60 \times \frac{5}{2} = 150$$

$$X = 150$$

36. C: $51.93

List the givens.

$$Tax = 6.0\% = 0.06$$

$$Sale = 50\% = 0.5$$

$$Hat = \$32.99$$

$$Jersey = \$64.99$$

Calculate the sales prices.

$$Hat\ Sale = 0.5\ (32.99) = 16.495$$

$$Jersey\ Sale = 0.5\ (64.99) = 32.495$$

Total the sales prices.

$$Hat\ sale + jersey\ sale = 16.495 + 32.495 = 48.99$$

Calculate the tax and add it to the total sales prices.

$$Total\ after\ tax = 48.99 + (48.99 \times 0.06) = \$51.93$$

37. D: $0.45

List the givens.

$$Store\ coffee = \$1.23/\text{lbs}$$

$$Local\ roaster\ coffee = \$1.98/1.5\ \text{lbs}$$

Calculate the cost for 5 lbs of store brand.

$$\frac{\$1.23}{1\ \text{lbs}} \times 5\ \text{lbs} = \$6.15$$

Calculate the cost for 5 lbs of the local roaster.

$$\frac{\$1.98}{1.5\ \text{lbs}} \times 5\ \text{lbs} = \$6.60$$

482

Subtract to find the difference in price for 5 lbs.

$$\begin{array}{r} \$6.60 \\ -\$6.15 \\ \hline \$0.45 \end{array}$$

38. D: $3,325

List the givens.

$$1,800 \, ft = \$2,000$$

$$Cost \, after \, 1,800 \, ft = \$1.00/ft$$

Find how many feet left after the first 1,800 ft.

$$\begin{array}{r} 3,125 \text{ ft} \\ - \quad 1,800 \text{ ft} \\ \hline 1,325 \text{ ft} \end{array}$$

Calculate the cost for the feet over 1,800 ft.

$$1,325 \text{ ft.} \times \frac{\$1.00}{1 \text{ ft}} = \$1,325$$

Add these together to find the total for the entire cost.

$$\$2,000 + \$1,325 = \$3,325$$

39. A: 12

Calculate how many gallons the bucket holds.

$$11.4 \text{ L} \times \frac{1 \text{ gal}}{3.8 \text{ L}} = 3 \text{ gal}$$

Next, calculate how many buckets are needed to fill the 35-gallon pool.

$$\frac{35}{3} = 11.67$$

Since the amount is more than 11 but less than 12, we must fill the bucket 12 times.

40. D: Three girls for every two boys can be expressed as a ratio: 3:2. This can be visualized as splitting the school into 5 groups: 3 girl groups and 2 boy groups. The number of students that are in each group can be found by dividing the total number of students by 5:

$$\frac{650 \text{ students}}{5 \text{ groups}} = \frac{130 \text{ students}}{\text{group}}$$

To find the total number of girls, multiply the number of students per group (130) by the number of girl groups in the school (3). This equals 390, Choice *D*.

41. B: 35.1%

To convert from a decimal to a percentage, the decimal needs to be moved two places to right. In this case, that makes 0.351 become 35.1%.

42. A: 22%

Converting from a fraction to a percentage generally involves two steps. First, the fraction needs to be converted to a decimal.

Divide 2 by 9 which results in $0.\overline{22}$. The top line indicates that the decimal actually goes on forever with an endless amount of 2's.

Second, the decimal needs to be moved two places to the right:

$$22\%$$

43. D: 0.57

To convert from a percentage to a decimal, or vice versa, you always need to move the decimal two places. A percentage like 57% has an invisible decimal after the 7, like this:

$$57.\%$$

That decimal then needs to be moved two places to the left to get:

$$0.57$$

44. A: 37.5%

Solve this by setting up the percent formula:

$$\frac{3}{8} = \frac{\%}{100}$$

Multiply 3 by 100 to get 300. Then, divide 300 by 8:

$$300 \div 8 = 37.5\%$$

Note that with the percent formula, 37.5 is automatically a percentage and does not need to have any further conversions.

45. A: 63.96

This question involves the percent formula. Since we're beginning with a percent, also known as a number over 100, we'll put 39 on the right side of the equation:

$$\frac{x}{164} = \frac{39}{100}$$

Now, multiply 164 and 39 to get 6,396, which then needs to be divided by 100.

$$6,396 \div 100 = 63.96$$

484

46. B: 128

This question involves the percent formula.

$$\frac{32}{x} = \frac{25}{100}$$

We multiply the diagonal numbers, 32 and 100, to get 3,200. Dividing by the remaining number, 25, gives us 128.

The percent formula does not have to be used for a question like this. Since 25% is $\frac{1}{4}$ of 100, you know that 32 needs to be multiplied by 4, which yields 128.

47. C: 0.63

Divide 5 by 8, which results in 0.625. This rounds up to 0.63.

48. A: 3.6

Divide 3 by 5 to get 0.6 and add that to the whole number 3, to get 3.6. An alternative is to incorporate the whole number 3 earlier on by creating an improper fraction: $\frac{18}{5}$. Then dividing 18 by 5 to get 3.6.

49. B: $\frac{14}{25}$

Since 0.56 goes to the hundredths place, it can be placed over 100:

$$\frac{56}{100}$$

Essentially, the way we got there is by multiplying the numerator and denominator by 100:

$$\frac{0.56}{1} \times \frac{100}{100} = \frac{56}{100}$$

Then, the fraction can be simplified down to $\frac{14}{25}$:

$$\frac{56}{100} \div \frac{4}{4} = \frac{14}{25}$$

50. D: $9\frac{3}{10}$

To convert a decimal to a fraction, remember that any number to the left of the decimal point will be a whole number. Then, since 0.3 goes to the tenths place, it can be placed over 10.

51. D: Recall the formula for area of a rectangle, area = length × width. The answer must be in square inches, so all values must be converted to inches. Half of a foot is equal to 6 inches. Therefore, the area of the rectangle is equal to:

$$6 \text{ in} \times \frac{11}{2} \text{ in} = \frac{66}{2} \text{ in}^2 = 33 \text{ in}^2$$

485

52. B: The figure is composed of three sides of a square and a semicircle. The sides of the square are simply added: $8 + 8 + 8 = 24$ inches. The circumference of a circle is found by the equation $C = 2\pi r$. The radius is 4 in, so the circumference of the circle is 25.13 in. Only half of the circle makes up the outer border of the figure (part of the perimeter) so half of 25.13 in is 12.565 in. Therefore, the total perimeter is: 24 in + 12.565 in = 36.565 in. The other answer choices use the incorrect formula or fail to include all of the necessary sides.

53. D: The slope is given by the change in y divided by the change in x. Specifically, it's:

$$slope = \frac{y_2 - y_1}{x_2 - x_1}$$

The first point is $(-5, -3)$, and the second point is $(0, -1)$. Work from left to right when identifying coordinates. Thus, the point on the left is point 1 $(-5, -3)$ and the point on the right is point 2 $(0, -1)$.

Now we need to just plug those numbers into the equation:

$$slope = \frac{-1 - (-3)}{0 - (-5)}$$

It can be simplified to:

$$slope = \frac{-1 + 3}{0 + 5}$$

$$slope = \frac{2}{5}$$

54. D: The expression is three times the sum of twice a number and 1, which is $3(2x + 1)$. Then, 6 is subtracted from this expression.

55. B: For the first card drawn, the probability of a king being pulled is $\frac{4}{52}$. Since this card isn't replaced, if a king is drawn first, the probability of a king being drawn second is $\frac{3}{51}$. The probability of a king being drawn in both the first and second draw is the product of the two probabilities:

$$\frac{4}{52} \times \frac{3}{51} = \frac{12}{2,652}$$

This fraction, when divided by $\frac{12}{12}$, equals $\frac{1}{221}$.

Reading Comprehension

1. D: To define and describe instances of spinoff technology. This is an example of a purpose question—*why* did the author write this? The article contains facts, definitions, and other objective information without telling a story or arguing an opinion. In this case, the purpose of the article is to inform the reader. The only answer choice that is related to giving information is answer Choice *D:* to define and describe.

2. A: A general definition followed by more specific examples. This organization question asks readers to analyze the structure of the essay. The topic of the essay is about spinoff technology; the first paragraph gives a general definition of the concept, while the following two paragraphs offer more detailed examples to help illustrate this idea.

3. C: They were looking for ways to add health benefits to food. This reading comprehension question can be answered based on the second paragraph—scientists were concerned about astronauts' nutrition and began researching useful nutritional supplements. Choice *A* in particular is not true because it reverses the order of discovery (first NASA identified algae for astronaut use, and then it was further developed for use in baby food).

4. B: Even for readers who have never encountered the word "neurological" before, the passage does provide context clues. The sentence following the statement about neurological benefits says algae has "potential to boost brain health." From this context, readers should be able to infer that "neurological" is related to the brain.

5. D: To give an example of valuable space equipment. This purpose question requires readers to understand the relevance of the given detail. In this case, the author mentions "costly and crucial equipment" before mentioning space suit visors, which are given as an example of something that is very valuable. *A* is not correct because fashion is only related to sunglasses, not to NASA equipment. *B* can be eliminated because it is simply not mentioned in the passage. While *C* seems like it could be a true statement, it is also not relevant to what is being explained by the author.

6. C: It is difficult to make money from scientific research. The article gives several examples of how businesses have been able to capitalize on NASA research, so it is unlikely that the author would agree with this statement. Evidence for the other answer choices can be found in the article: In Choice *A*, the author mentions that "many consumers are unaware that products they are buying are based on NASA research." Choice *B* is a general definition of spinoff technology. Choice *D* is mentioned in the final paragraph.

7. D: To criticize a theory by presenting counterevidence. The author mentions anti-Stratfordian arguments in the first paragraph, but then goes on to debunk these theories with more facts about Shakespeare's life in the second and third paragraphs. *A* is not correct because, while the author does present arguments from both sides, the author is far from unbiased; in fact, the author clearly disagrees with anti-Stratfordians. *B* is also not correct because it is more closely aligned to the beliefs of anti-Stratfordians, whom the author disagrees with. *C* can be eliminated because, while it is true that the author gives historical background, the main purpose of the article is using that information to disprove a theory.

8. B: But in fact, there is not much substance to such speculation, and most anti-Stratfordian arguments can be refuted with a little background about Shakespeare's time and upbringing. The thesis is a statement that contains the author's topic and main idea. As seen in question 7, the main purpose of this article is to use historical evidence to provide counterarguments to anti-Stratfordians. *A* is simply a definition; *C* is a supporting detail, not a main idea; and *D* represents an idea of anti-Stratfordians, not the author's opinion.

9. B: By explaining grade school curriculum in Shakespeare's time. This question asks readers to refer to the organizational structure of the article and demonstrate understanding of how the author provides

487

details to support their argument. This particular detail can be found in the second paragraph: "even though he did not attend university, grade school education in Shakespeare's time was actually quite rigorous."

10. A: Busy. This is a vocabulary question that can be answered using context clues. Other sentences in the paragraph describe London as "the most populous city in England" filled with "crowds of people," giving an image of a busy city full of people. *B* is not correct because London was in Shakespeare's home country, not a foreign one. *C* is not mentioned in the passage. *D* is not a good answer choice because the passage describes how London was a popular and important city, probably not an undeveloped one.

11. D: In Shakespeare's time, glove-makers were not part of the upper class. Anti-Stratfordians doubt Shakespeare's ability because he was not from the upper class; his father was a glove-maker; therefore, in at least this instance, glove-makers were not included in the upper class (this is an example of inductive reasoning, or using two specific pieces of information to draw a more general conclusion).

12. C: It is an example of a play set outside of England. This detail comes from the third paragraph, where the author responds to skeptics who claim that Shakespeare wrote too much about places he never visited, so *Romeo and Juliet* is mentioned as a famous example of a play with a foreign setting. In order to answer this question, readers need to understand the author's main purpose in the third paragraph and how the author uses details to support this purpose. *A* and *D* are not mentioned in the passage, and *B* is clearly not true because the passage mentions more than once that Shakespeare never left England.

13. A: It is possible to learn things from reading rather than from firsthand experience. This inference can be made from the final paragraph, where the author refutes anti-Stratfordian skepticism by pointing out that books about life in Europe could easily circulate throughout London. From this statement, readers can conclude that the author believes it is possible that Shakespeare learned about European culture from books, rather than visiting the continent on his own. *B* is not true because the author believes that Shakespeare contributed to English literature without traveling extensively. Similarly, *C* is not a good answer because the author explains how Shakespeare got his education without university. *D* can also be eliminated because the author describes Shakespeare's genius and clearly Shakespeare is not from Italy.

14. B: A period of time. "Four score and seven years ago" is the equivalent of eighty-seven years, because the word "score" means "twenty." *A* and *C* are incorrect because the context for describing a unit of measurement or a literary movement is lacking. *D* is incorrect because although Lincoln's speech is a cornerstone in political rhetoric, the phrase "Four score and seven years ago" is better narrowed to a period of time.

15. D: Abraham Lincoln is the former president of the United States, so the correct answer is *D*, "The American Civil War." Though the U.S. was involved in World War I and II, *A* and *C* are incorrect because a civil war specifically means citizens fighting within the same country. *B* is incorrect, as "The War of Spanish Succession" involved Spain, Italy, Germany, and Holland, and not the United States.

16. A: The audience should perpetuate the ideals of freedom that the soldiers died fighting for. *B* is incorrect because, although they are there to "dedicate a portion of that field," there is no mention in the text of an annual memorial service. *C* is incorrect because there is no charged language in the text, only reverence for the dead. *D* is incorrect because "forget[ting] the lives that were lost" is the opposite of what Lincoln is suggesting.

17. A: Choice *A* is correct because Lincoln's intention was to memorialize the soldiers who had fallen as a result of war as well as celebrate those who had put their lives in danger for the sake of their country. Choices *B*, *C*, and *D* are incorrect because Lincoln's speech was supposed to foster a sense of pride among the members of the audience while connecting them to the soldiers' experiences, not to alienate or discourage them.

18. B: It scares children. The passage states that the Juggernaut causes the children to scream. Choices *A* and *D* don't apply because the text doesn't mention either of these instances specifically. Choice *C* is incorrect because there is nothing in the text that mentions space travel.

19. B: To constantly visit. The mention of *morning*, *noon*, and *night* make it clear that the word *haunt* refers to frequent appearances at various times. Choice *A* doesn't work because the text makes no mention of levitating. Choices *C* and *D* are not correct because the text makes mention of Mr. Utterson's anguish and disheartenment because of his failure to find Hyde but does not make mention of Mr. Utterson's feelings negatively affecting anyone else.

20. D: The speaker intends to continue to look for Hyde. Choices *A* and *B* are not possible answers because the text doesn't refer to any name changes or an identity crisis, despite Mr. Utterson's extreme obsession with finding Hyde. The text also makes no mention of a mistaken identity when referring to Hyde, so Choice *C* is also incorrect.

21. C: The author contrasts two different viewpoints, then builds a case showing preference for one over the other. Choice *A* is incorrect because the introduction does not contain an impartial definition, but rather, an opinion. Choice *B* is incorrect. There is no puzzling phenomenon given, as the author doesn't mention any peculiar cause or effect that is in question regarding poetry. Choice *D* does contain another's viewpoint at the beginning of the passage; however, to say that the author has no stake in this argument is incorrect; the author uses personal experiences to build their case.

22. B: Choice *B* accurately describes the author's argument in the text: that poetry is not irrelevant. While the author does praise, and even value, Buddy Wakefield as a poet, the author never heralds him as a genius. Eliminate Choice *A*, as it is an exaggeration. Not only is Choice *C* an exaggerated statement, but the author never mentions spoken word poetry in the text. Choice *D* is incorrect because this statement contradicts the writer's argument.

23. D: *Exiguously* means not occurring often, or occurring rarely, so Choice *D* would LEAST change the meaning of the sentence. Choice *A*, *indolently*, means unhurriedly, or slow, and does not fit the context of the sentence. Choice *B*, *inaudibly*, means quietly or silently. Choice *C*, *interminably*, means endlessly, or all the time, and is the opposite of the word *exiguously*.

24. D: A student's insistence that psychoanalysis is a subset of modern psychology is the most analogous option. The author of the passage tries to insist that performance poetry is a subset of modern poetry, and therefore, tries to prove that modern poetry is not "dying," but thriving on social media for the masses. Choice *A* is incorrect, as the author is not refusing any kind of validation. Choice *B* is incorrect; the author's insistence is that poetry will *not* lose popularity. Choice *C* mimics the topic but compares two different genres, while the author does no comparison in this passage.

489

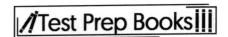
25. B: The author's purpose is to disprove Gioia's article claiming that poetry is a dying art form that only survives in academic settings. In order to prove his argument, the author educates the reader about new developments in poetry (Choice *A*) and describes the brilliance of a specific modern poet (Choice *C*), but these serve as examples of a growing poetry trend that counters Gioia's argument. Choice *D* is incorrect because it contradicts the author's argument.

26. C: The text mentions all of the listed properties of minerals except the instance of minerals being organically formed. Objects or substances must be naturally occurring, must be a homogeneous solid, and must have a definite chemical composition in order to be considered a mineral.

27. A: Choice *A* is the correct answer because geology is the study of earth related science. Choice *B* is incorrect because psychology is the study of the mind and behavior. Choice *C* is incorrect because biology is the study of life and living organisms. Choice *D* is incorrect because botany is the study of plants.

28. A: Choice *A* is the correct answer because the prefix "homo" means same. Choice *B* is incorrect because "differing in some areas" would be linked to the root word "hetero," meaning "different" or "other."

29: C: Choice *C* is the correct answer because *-logy* refers to the study of a particular subject matter.

30. D: A *rookery* is a colony of breeding birds. Although *rookery* could mean Choice *A,* houses in a slum area, it does not make sense in this context. Choices *B* and *C* are both incorrect, as this is not a place for hunters to trade tools or for wardens to trade stories.

31. B: An important bird colony. The previous sentence is describing "twenty colonies" of birds, so what follows should be a bird colony. Choice *A* may be true, but we have no evidence of this in the text. Choice *C* does touch on the tension between the hunters and wardens, but there is no official "Bird Island Battle" mentioned in the text. Choice *D* does not exist in the text.

32. D: To demonstrate the success of the protective work of the Audubon Association. The text mentions several different times how and why the association has been successful and gives examples to back this fact. Choice *A* is incorrect because although the article, in some instances, calls certain people to act, it is not the purpose of the entire passage. There is no way to tell if Choices *B* and *C* are correct, as they are not mentioned in the text.

33. C: To have a better opportunity to hunt the birds. Choice *A* might be true in a general sense, but it is not relevant to the context of the text. Choice *B* is incorrect because the hunters are not studying lines of flight to help wardens, but to hunt birds. Choice *D* is incorrect because nothing in the text mentions that hunters are trying to build homes underneath lines of flight of birds for good luck.

34. A: Not only does the article provide examples to disprove a myth, the title also suggests that the article is trying to disprove a myth. Further, the sentence, "But the 'fact' that the majority of your body heat is lost through your head is a lie," and then the subsequent "let me explain," demonstrates the author's intention in disproving a myth. *B* is incorrect because although the selection does compare elephants and anteaters, it does so in order to prove a point, and is not the primary reason that the selection was written. *C* is incorrect because even though the article mentions somebody wearing clothes in the winter, and that doing so could save your life, wearing clothes in the winter is not the

490

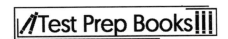

primary reason this article was written. *D* is incorrect because the article only mentions that people are gullible once, and makes no further comment on the matter, so this cannot be the primary purpose.

35. B: If the myth is that most of one's body heat is lost through their head, then the fact that heat loss is proportional to surface area exposed is the best evidence that disproves it, since one's head has a great deal less surface area than the rest of the body, making *B* the correct choice. "It is better to wear a shirt than a hat" does not provide evidence that disproves the fact that the head loses more heat than the rest of the body. Thus, *A* is incorrect. *C* is incorrect because gullibility is mentioned only once in this passage and the rest of the article ignores this statement, so clearly it is not the main idea. Finally, *D* is incorrect because though the article mentions that the human chest probably loses the most heat, it is to provide an example of the evidence that heat loss is proportional to surface area exposed, so this is not the main idea of the passage.

36. B: Choice *B* is correct because the author is trying to demonstrate the main idea, which is that heat loss is proportional to surface area, and so they compare two animals with different surface areas to clarify the main point. Choice *A* is incorrect because the author uses elephants and anteaters to prove a point, that heat loss is proportional to surface area, not to express an opinion. Choice *C* is incorrect because though the author does use them to show differences, they do so in order to give examples that prove the above points. Choice *D* is incorrect because there is no language to indicate favoritism between the two animals.

37. C: Since there is an opinion presented along with a fact, *C* is the correct answer. *A* is incorrect—"Not only would you look stupid," is an opinion because there is no way to prove that somebody would look stupid by not wearing a shirt in the cold, even if that may be a popular opinion. However, this opinion is sandwiched inside a factual statement. *B* is incorrect because again, this is a factual statement, but it has been editorialized by interjecting an opinion. Because of the presence of both a fact and an opinion, *D* is the opposite of the correct answer.

38. C: Because of the way the author addresses the reader and the colloquial language the author uses (i.e., "let me explain," "so," "well," didn't," "you would look stupid," etc.), Choice *C* is the best answer because it has a much more casual tone than the usual informative article. Choice *A* may be a tempting choice because the author says the "fact" that most of one's heat is lost through their head is a "lie" and that someone who does not wear a shirt in the cold looks stupid. However, this only happens twice within the passage, and the passage does not give an overall tone of harshness. Choice *B* is incorrect because again, while not necessarily nice, the language does not carry an angry charge. The author is clearly not indifferent to the subject because of the passionate language that they use, so Choice *D* is incorrect.

39. B: Choice *B* is correct. The primary purpose of the article is to provide evidence to disprove the myth that most of a person's heat is lost through their head. The fact that each part of the body loses heat in proportion to its surface area is the best evidence to disprove this myth. *A* is incorrect because again, gullibility is not a main contributor to this article, but it may be common to see questions on the test that give the same wrong answer in order to try and trick the test taker. Choice *C* only suggests what you should do with this information; it is not the primary evidence itself. Choice *D*, while tempting, is actually not evidence. It does not give any reason for why it is a lie; it simply states that it is. Evidence is factual information that supports a claim.

40. B: Choice *B* is correct because having very little drinking water on earth is a very good reason that one should limit their water usage so that the human population does not run out of drinking water and die out. People wasting water on superfluous things does not support the fact that we need to limit our water usage. It merely states that people are wasteful. Therefore, *A* is incorrect. Answer Choice *C* may be tempting, but it is not the correct one, as this article is not about reducing water usage in order to help those who don't have easy access to water, but about the fact that the planet is running out of drinking water. Choice *D* is incorrect because nowhere in the article does it state that only first world countries have access to drinking water.

41. C: The primary purpose is to present a problem (the planet is running out of water) with a solution (to reduce water waste), therefore the correct answer is *C*. Choice *A* is incorrect because the passage does not have a sequential timeline of events and is therefore not in chronological order. It may be tempting to think the author compares and contrasts people who do not have access to drinking water to those who do, but that does not fit with the primary purpose of the article, which is to convince people to reduce their water usage. Thus, Choice *B* is incorrect. Choice *D* is incorrect because descriptions are not the primary content of this article. Remember that a descriptive writing style describes people, settings, or situations in great detail with many adjectives. While a descriptive writing voice may be used alongside a persuasive writing style, it is generally not the primary voice when trying to convince a reader to take a certain stance.

42. A: If the assertion is that the earth does not have enough drinking water, then having abundant water stores that are not being reported would certainly challenge this assertion. Choice *B* is incorrect because even if much of the water we drink does come from rain, that means the human population would be dependent on rain in order to survive, which would more support the assertion than challenge it. Because the primary purpose of the passage is not to help those who cannot get water, then Choice *C* is not the correct answer. Even if Choice *D* were true, it does not dismiss the other ways in which people are wasteful with water, and is also not the point.

43. B: Choice *B* is correct because the article uses a lot of emotionally charged language and also suggests what needs to be done with the information provided. The article does not contain elements of a narrative, which include plot, setting, characters, and themes. Not only does the article lack these things, but it does not follow a timeline, which is a key element of a narrative voice. Thus, Choice *A* is incorrect. Choice *C* is incorrect because the article uses information in order to be persuasive, but the purpose is not solely to inform on the issue. Choice *D* is incorrect because the article is not written in primarily descriptive language.

44. C: Choice *C* is correct because people who waste water on lawns in the desert, or run a half-full dishwasher, or fill their personal pools are not taking into account how much water they are using because they get an unlimited supply, therefore they are taking it for granted. Choice *A* is incorrect because it is explicitly stated within the text: "running dishwashers that are only half full." Choice *B* is also explicitly stated: "meanwhile people in Africa are dying of thirst." While Choice *D* is implicitly stated within the whole article, it is not implicitly stated within the sentence.

45. B: Choice *B* is correct because the author uses this example in order to show people, through emotional appeal, that they take water for granted, because they get water freely from their faucets, while millions of people have to endure great hardships to get drinking water. Choice *A* does not pertain directly to the main idea of the article, nor does it pertain to the author's purpose. The main idea is that people should reduce their water usage, and the author's purpose is to persuade the reader to do so. A

492

person walking for miles in intense heat does not align with the main point. Choice *C* is incorrect because the selection never mentions that water is only available in first world countries. Choice *D* is the author's purpose for the entire passage, but not the purpose for mentioning the difficulty in getting water for some of the population.

46. C: To be mindful means to be aware, so *C* is the best answer. Choice *A* may be a tempting answer, because if people are interested in the water they are using, they may be more aware of it, but this is not the best answer of the choices. Being amused by water does not make sense in this context, so Choice *B* is incorrect. Being accepting of the amounts of water they use is the opposite of what the author is trying to get the reader to do. Thus, Choice *D* is incorrect.

47. A: The primary purpose and the main idea are essentially the same thing, and the main idea is that people should reduce their water usage because there is not a lot of available drinking water on Earth. Choice *B* is a *reason* that people should reduce their water usage, but it is not the main idea. Choice *C* is a demonstration of how people are not aware of the amount of water they use, but again, not the main idea. Choice *D* is a suggestion for reducing water usage, but still not the main idea.

48. D: The passage directly states that the larger sensor is the main difference between the two cameras. Choices *A* and *B* may be true, but these answers do not identify the major difference between the two cameras. Choice *C* states the opposite of what the paragraph suggests is the best option for amateur photographers, so it is incorrect.

49. D: An actuary assesses risks and sets insurance premiums. While an actuary does work in insurance, the passage does not suggest that actuaries have any affiliation with hospitalists or working in a hospital, so all other choices are incorrect.

50. A: The passage focuses mainly on the problems of hard water. Choice *B* is incorrect because calcium is not good for pipes and hard surfaces. The passage does not say anything about whether water softeners are easy to install, so Choice *C* is incorrect. Choice *D* is also incorrect because the passage does offer other solutions besides vinegar.

51. C: The main point of this paragraph is that parents need to change their poor behavior at their kids' sporting events. Choice *A* is incorrect because the coaches' behavior is not mentioned in the paragraph. Choice *B* suggests that sports are bad for kids, when the paragraph is about parents' behavior, so it is incorrect. While Choice *D* may be true, it offers a specific solution to the problem, which the paragraph does not discuss.

52. B: The main point of this passage is to show how a tornado forms. Choice *A* is off base because while the passage does mention that tornadoes are dangerous, it is not the main focus of the passage. While thunderstorms are mentioned, they are not compared to tornadoes, so Choice *C* is incorrect. Choice *D* is incorrect because the passage does not discuss what to do in the event of a tornado.

53. C: The purpose of this passage is to explain how the digestive system works. Choice *A* focuses only on the liver, which is a small part of the process and not the focus of the paragraph. Choice *B* is off-track because the passage does not mention healthy foods. Choice *D* only focuses on one part of the digestive system.

54. D: The main point of this passage is to define osteoporosis. Choice *A* is incorrect because the passage does not list ways that people contract osteoporosis. Choice *B* is incorrect because the passage does not mention any treatment options. While the passage does briefly mention prevention, it does not explain how, so Choice *C* is incorrect.

55. D: The passage compares Disney cruises with Disney parks. It does not discuss how to book a cruise, so Choice *A* is incorrect. Choice *B* is incorrect because though the passage does mention some of the park attractions, it is not the main point. The passage does not mention the cost of either option, so Choice *C* is incorrect.

Vocabulary

1. A: *Instigate* refers to initiating or bringing about an action. While instigating something can be overwhelming, *overwhelm* describes the action, not what the action is. None of these choices match this except for *begin*, which is synonymous with instigate.

2. D: The patient is displaying *displacement*, in which he is taking his negative feelings towards the doctor and expressing them towards the nurse aide, unfairly. *Reaction formation* is when the person feels negatively but reacts positively. *Intellectualization* is when a person focuses on minute details of the situation rather than coping with the negative emotions associated with it. *Undoing* is when the person has done something wrong and acts excessively in the opposite way to "redeem" themselves of their prior wrong-doing.

3. D: The other choices refer to *attitude*, a word spelled and pronounced similarly to altitude. Someone's attitude can reflect haughtiness, influence their outlook, and reflect their behavior. None of these terms describe *altitude*, which is the measure of height. *Height* is directly related to altitude.

4. A: The chest pain as described in this patient's situation most likely is cardiac in origin, so the patient could be experiencing a *myocardial infarction*, or heart attack. Chest pain associated with *gastroesophageal reflux* is more often described as a burning sensation, without the other symptoms described. *Pneumonia* and *pleuritis* may both cause the patient to have a different type of chest pain, in which a sharp, stabbing sensation is felt upon breathing.

5. A: *Reconnaissance* is a noun that means preliminary research or surveying. It is also used in a military context where a *reconnaissance* is the surveying or observation to obtain information for strategic planning or to locate an enemy.

6. C: Something *ineffable* cannot be described with words. It often is used in connection to something so impressive, emotional, or great. The heartwarming feelings of a family reuniting after a parent has been deployable may be said to be *ineffable.*

7. C: Someone that is described as *gregarious* is social and talkative. *Meek* is more of an antonym because it means quiet and submissive.

8. A: *Caustic* is an adjective that is often used in the chemical context to describe a substance that is corrosive or able to burn tissues. In this way, it is typically an acidic and abrasive chemical. However, it can also be used to describe a person's demeanor, which is bitterly sarcastic or scathing.

9. C: This type of seizure with muscle rigidity, convulsions, and unconsciousness is called a *grand mal* seizure. A *myoclonic* seizure only involves one part of the body making jerking movements. An *absence* seizure involves a brief loss of consciousness where the patient may stare off into space. A *tonic* seizure is characterized by rigidity and stiffness of the muscles.

10. D: The patient is most likely experiencing a stroke, as evidenced by the difficulty with speech and facial drooping. *Meningitis* is an inflammation of the meninges and does not fit the description of symptoms here. A *migraine* is a severe headache that can sometimes mimic stroke symptoms but is less severe. A stroke should be suspected until it is proven otherwise in order to get the patient timely and effective treatment. A *seizure* is characterized by muscle rigidity, convulsions, and loss of consciousness.

11. A: This patient is at risk for *hypoglycemia*, or a blood sugar less than 60mg/dL due to the missed meals and perhaps missed regular insulin and anti-diabetic medication dosages. A disruption in a diabetic patient's schedule can lead to hypoglycemia and the nurse aide should be vigilant in monitoring the patient's intake. *Diabetic ketoacidosis* is a result of too much blood sugar, or hyperglycemia. A *diabetic coma* is possible in both the cases of hyper- and hypoglycemia, but the patient is still conscious, so that rules that option out. *Hyperglycemia* is a blood sugar greater than 200mg/dL and is not likely, since this patient has not had any oral intake.

12. A: Someone that is *obtuse* is unintelligent or slow-witted. They might be described as ignorant or dense. In geometry, it refers to an angle greater than 90 degrees and less than 180 degrees, but this is a different usage of the word.

13. A: *Loquacious* reflects the tendency to talk a lot. While someone can be humorous and loquacious, *humorous* describes the kind of talk, not the fact that someone talks a lot. *Cranky* has nothing to do with the word, and *silent* is a clear opposite. This leaves *verbose*, meaning using an abundance of words; loquacious is a synonym.

14. B: The medical term for coughing up blood in the sputum is *hemoptysis*. *Hematopoiesis* is the process of creating new blood cells in the body. *Hematemesis* is when there is blood in the vomitus. *Hematochezia* refers to rectal bleeding.

15. C: *Sordid* means filthy, vile, or squalid. *Semantic* means referring to the meaning of words or language. *Surly* can mean either threatening in appearance or crabby (in terms of mood).

16. A: *Bereavement* may present as many different physical conditions and can be diagnosed by completing a thorough history. *Stroke* often presents as deficits on one side of the body. *Anorexia nervosa* presents with decreased appetite along with signs of malnutrition. *MI (myocardial infarction)* often presents with tingling or pain in the left arm or jaw and chest pressure or pain.

17. C: Alternative medications are often ordered in place of antispasmodics for treatment of urinary incontinence due to side effects of excessive thirst.

18. A: To *solicit* is to ask for something, often with the goal of obtaining something from someone else. *Solicitation* is the noun that is derived from the term; it refers to the act of asking for something. Sometimes, homes or businesses will post a notice that "no solicitation is allowed," meaning no one is to knock on the door trying to sell something, asking for signatures in support of a cause, etc.

19. C: *Venous* ulcers are commonly found between the knees and ankles. *Arterial* ulcers are located at the end of the toe on pressure points or in non-healing wounds. *Neuropathic* ulcers are found on the

495

toes and sides of the feet. *Staging* applies to all types of ulcers and is dependent upon size, tunneling, and other factors.

20. A: *Isometric* exercises are done against resistance without moving a joint. *Isotonic* exercise moves the joint, *isokinetic* exercise uses a machine, and *plyometric* exercise uses a combination of stretching followed by contraction.

21. A: *Plausible* means likely to be possible or accepted, the opposite of *skeptical*. *Diurnal* relates to daytime, so is unrelated. *Erudite* means clever or intelligent, but not necessarily possible or correct. *Conceivable* means that something is able to be thought of or able to be done. Conceivable is the best match for plausible.

22. C: *Discourse* refers to spoken and written communication, or debate. *Path* doesn't have anything to do with discourse, unless used figuratively. While discourse may consist of praise or disagreement, all discourse—written or verbal—is a form of speech. Therefore, *speech* is the best term that encompasses the same meaning as discourse.

23. A: The Latin root, *asper*, means rough. *Exasperate*, then, means to make relations with someone rough or to rub them the wrong way. *Disappointment* can be the result of an exasperating situation, but these are results of the term, not the same as exasperation itself. *Annoy* is a synonym, meaning to irritate and make someone slightly angry.

24. B: in a medical context, *genicular* or *geniculate* refer to something pertaining the knee. The term *geniculate* itself can be used in a more general context to refer to something bent sharply like the knee.

25. D: The prefix *trans* means across, beyond, over. Choices *A*, B, and C are incorrect because they are the meanings of other prefixes. Choice *A* is a meaning of the prefix *de*. Choice B is the meaning of the prefix *omni*. Choice C is one of the meanings of the prefix *pro*. The example words are helpful in determining the meaning of *trans*. All of the example words—*transfer, transact, translation, transport*—indicate something being *across, beyond,* or *over* something else. For example, *translation* refers to text going across languages. If no example words were given, you could think of words starting with *trans* and then compare their meanings to try to determine a common definition.

26. C: *Cubital,* in terms of body regions, refers to the elbow. For example, the inner elbow area where blood draws are often collected is called the antecubital space. The shoulder region is referred to as the *acromial* area.

27. A: *Mitigate* refers to easing tension or making less severe. *Focus, fiery,* and *conspire* do not relate. *Alleviate* is synonymous, meaning to make less severe. Note the ending -*ate*, which also indicates function. Both terms reflect the function of easing difficult circumstances.

28. A: *Keratin* is a structural protein, and it is the primary constituent of things like hair and nails. Choice *B* is incorrect; *antigens* are immune proteins that help fight disease. Choice *C* is incorrect because *channel proteins* are transport proteins that help move molecules into and out of a cell. Lastly, Choice *D* is incorrect because *actin*, like myosin, is a motor protein because it is involved in the process of muscle contraction.

29. B: Deep. The dermis is the deeper layer of skin under the more superficial epidermis.

30. C: A professional who draws blood. An x-ray technician takes x-rays, a prosthetist makes artificial limbs, and a psychologist, social worker, or therapist counsels patients.

31. C: Regress. *Rescind* means to revoke or repeal. It often is used in relation to an agreement or law. *Digress* means to temporarily deviate from the main topic when speaking or writing (for example, telling a story that is just somewhat related to the main point). *Diverge* is to fork or separate from the main path or road.

32. C: The shoulder. The acromion process is a bony protrusion on the scapula that extends laterally toward the shoulder joint. The acromioclavicular ligament connects the acromion process with the clavicle.

33. B: Expressionless. Glassy eyes, like a doll's, are shiny and empty; they are expressionless. Someone with glassy eyes may have a fixed stare. Different conditions, such as severe dehydration and cholera, can cause glassy eyes.

34. A: Flush. Though *flush* has several definitions, in the context of the provided sentence, it means to align in a smooth, consistent way, forming an unbroken surface. It's important for braces, for example AFOs (ankle foot orthoses), to be flush with the skin. Otherwise, friction will occur between the skin and the brace where it contacts a prominence and cause blistering or skin breakdown.

35. C: To supply nerves to. For example, the radial nerve innervates the extensors in the upper arm, such as the triceps.

36. A: Amputation. Gangrene is localized dead or necrotic tissue, which can be caused by insufficient blood flow. For example, a toe may be affected by gangrene in someone with poorly controlled, advanced diabetes.

37. C: Exigent. *Lenient* means permissive and easy-going, to *extoll* is to praise, and *lackadaisical* means apathetic or lazy.

38. D: Language impairment. *Aphasia* is a loss in the ability to express or understand speech, so it is language impairment. It is often caused by brain damage, whether due to a stroke, TBI, or other cause. An inability to recognize things is *agnosia*.

39. C: Nothing by mouth. NPO comes from the Latin *nil per os,* which means nothing by mouth. Do not resuscitate is abbreviated DNR.

40. A: Dull. Something that is *jejune* is simplistic, naïve, or unoriginal.

41. A: Deficit. *Diffident* means shy or lacking in confidence. *Dearth* means scarcity, so it might be an attractive choice, but *deficit* is a better word in the context of the sentence. *Diffident* means obstinate or uncooperative.

42. D: Contradiction. A paradox often seems self-contradictory; something that is true yet doesn't follow what's expected or logical.

43. A: Lithe. While Choice *B, ballerina,* may be described as agile and graceful, the correct choice is the adjective that describes the movement, *lithe.*

497

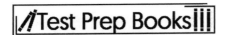

44. B: Cyanosis. Cyanosis often results from an occlusion or circulation impairment, which causes an insufficient amount of oxygen to perfuse the tissues.

45. A: Respect. Someone who is venerated is respected and revered.

46. B: Mycosis. The prefix *myco-* means something related to fungus.

47. C: Uremia. *Anuria* is no urine production, *nocturia* is nighttime urination, and *polyrurea* refers to abnormally large volumes of urine.

48. B: A sustained muscle contraction. A single nerve impulse initiates a muscle twitch, whereas when many impulses sum together, the muscle contraction is sustained in what is called tetanus. Tetanus occurs with repeated stimulation without a break for the muscle to relax.

49. A: Spatial awareness of the body. The body has sensory receptors, called proprioceptors, which help the body sense and respond to position and movement.

50. D: An *archetype* is an example of a person or thing, a recurrent symbol. An *ancestor* may be a good model of ideal behavior, but the term refers to someone who is related. Archetypes appear in literature, but these are different terms. *Policy* is unrelated. A *model* is a standard or representative, which is synonymous with archetype.

51. C: *Retort* is a verb that means "to answer back," usually in a sharp manner. This term embodies the idea of a response, emphasized by the "re-" prefix meaning "back, again." While a *retort* is used in conversations and even as a jest, neither term embodies the idea of addressing someone again. *Counter,* however, means to respond in opposition when used as a verb.

52. A: *Subliminal* and *subconscious* share the Latin prefix "sub-," meaning under or below, or more commonly used when talking about messages the sender doesn't want the receiver to consciously take note of. The word *subliminal* means beneath the consciousness. Thus, *subconscious* is the perfect match.

53. C: Although *incite* usually has negative connotations, leaders can incite their followers to benevolent actions as well. In both cases, people rally to support a cause.

54. B: *Sustain* is to revitalize, or to give strength. *Strength* would be a good choice, but strength alone does not describe the re-strengthening that sustain embodies. The best choice is *invigorate*, which is a verb like sustain, meaning to strengthen. This makes invigorate the better choice. *Expedite* is unrelated. While *embolden* means to give someone courage, which is a form of strength, invigorate and sustain speak more toward physical circumstances.

55. A: *Malevolent* literally means bad or evil-minded. The clue is also in the Latin root "mal-," which translates to bad.

Grammar

1. B: In Choice *B* the word *Uncle* should not be capitalized, because it is not functioning as a proper noun. If the word named a specific uncle, such as *Uncle Jerry*, then it would be considered a proper noun and should be capitalized. Choice *A* correctly capitalizes the proper noun *East Coast*, and does not capitalize *winter*, which functions as a common noun in the sentence. Choice *C* correctly capitalizes the name of a specific college course, which is considered a proper noun. Choice *D* correctly capitalizes the proper noun *Jersey Shore*.

2. C: In Choice *C, avid* is functioning as an adjective that modifies the word photographer. *Avid* describes the photographer Julia Robinson's style. The words *time* and *photographer* are functioning as nouns, and the word *capture* is functioning as a verb in the sentence. Other words functioning as adjectives in the sentence include, *local, business,* and *spare,* as they all describe the nouns they precede.

3. A: Choice *A* is correctly punctuated because it uses a semicolon to join two independent clauses that are related in meaning. Each of these clauses could function as an independent sentence. Choice *B* is incorrect because the conjunction is not preceded by a comma. A comma and conjunction should be used together to join independent clauses. Choice *C* is incorrect because a comma should only be used to join independent sentences when it also includes a coordinating conjunction such as *and* or *so.* Choice *D* does not use punctuation to join the independent clauses, so it is considered a fused (same as a run-on) sentence.

4. C: Choice *C* is a compound sentence because it joins two independent clauses with a comma and the coordinating conjunction *and.* The sentences in Choices *B* and *D* include one independent clause and one dependent clause, so they are complex sentences, not compound sentences. The sentence in Choice *A* has both a compound subject, *Alex and Shane,* and a compound verb, *spent and took,* but the entire sentence itself is one independent clause.

5. A: Choice *A* uses incorrect subject-verb agreement because the indefinite pronoun *neither* is singular and must use the singular verb form *is.* The pronoun *both* is plural and uses the plural verb form of *are.* The pronoun *any* can be either singular or plural. In this example, it is used as a plural, so the plural verb form *are* is used. The pronoun *each* is singular and uses the singular verb form *is.*

6. B: Choice *B* is correct because the pronouns *he* and *I* are in the subjective case. *He* and *I* are the subjects of the verb *like* in the independent clause of the sentence. Choices *A, C,* and *D* are incorrect because they all contain at least one objective pronoun (*me* and *him*). Objective pronouns should not be used as the subject of the sentence, but rather, they should come as an object of a verb. To test for correct pronoun usage, try reading the pronouns as if they were the only pronoun in the sentence. For example, *he* and *me* may appear to be the correct answer choices, but try reading them as the only pronoun.

He like[s] to go fishing...

Me like to go fishing...

When looked at that way, *me* is an obviously incorrect choice.

7. B: Answer Choice *A* uses the plural form of the verb, when the subject is the pronoun *none,* which needs a singular verb. *C* also uses the wrong verb form and uses the word *all* in place of *none,* which doesn't make sense in the context of the sentence. *D* uses *all* again, and is missing the comma, which is necessary to set the dependent clause off from the independent clause.

8. C: In this answer, the article and subject agree, and the subject and predicate agree. Answer Choice *A* is incorrect because the article *an* and *issues* do not agree in number. *B* is incorrect because an article is needed before *important issue. D* is incorrect because the plural subject *issues* does not agree with the singular verb *is.*

9. D: Choices *A* and *C* use additional words and phrases that aren't necessary. *B* is more concise, but uses the present tense of *is.* This does not agree with the rest of the sentence, which uses past tense. The best choice is *D,* which uses the most concise sentence structure and is grammatically correct.

10. C: Choice *A* is missing the word *that,* which is necessary for the sentence to make sense. Choice *B* pluralizes *trains* and uses the singular form of the word *include,* so it does not agree with the word *set.* Choice *D* changes the verb to *were,* which is in plural form and does not agree with the singular subject.

11. A: Choices *B* and *D* both use the expression *attributed to the fact* incorrectly. It can only be attributed *to* the fact, not *with* or *in* the fact. Choice *C* incorrectly uses a gerund, *saying,* when it should use the present tense of the verb *say.*

12. B: Choice *B* is correct because it uses correct parallel structure of plural nouns. Choice *A* is incorrect because the word *accessory* is in singular form. Choice *C* is incorrect because it pluralizes *makeup,* which is already in plural form. Choice *D* is incorrect because it again uses the singular *accessory,* and it uses the singular *shoe.*

13. D: In a cause/effect relationship, it is correct to use the word because in the clausal part of the sentence. This can eliminate both Choices *A and* C which don't clearly show the cause/effect relationship. Choice *B* is incorrect because it uses the present tense, when the first part of the sentence is in the past tense. It makes grammatical sense for both parts of the sentence to be in present tense.

14. A: In answer Choice *B,* the present tense form of the verb *consider* creates an independent clause joined to another independent clause with only a comma, which is a comma splice and grammatically incorrect. Choices *C* and *D* use the possessive form of *its,* when it should be the contraction *it's* for *it is.* Choice *D* also includes incorrect comma placement.

15. B: Choice *B* is an imperative sentence because it issues a command. In addition, it ends with a period, and an imperative sentence must end in a period or exclamation mark. Choice *A* is a declarative sentence that states a fact and ends with a period. Choice *C* is an exclamatory sentence that shows strong emotion and ends with an exclamation point. Choice *D* is an interrogative sentence that asks a question and ends with a question mark.

16. C: Choice *C* is a compound sentence because it joins two independent clauses—*The baby was sick* and *I decided to stay home from work*—with a comma and the coordinating conjunction *so.* Choices *A,* B, and D, are all simple sentences, each containing one independent clause with a complete subject and predicate. Choices *A* and *D* each contain a compound subject, or more than one subject, but they are still simple sentences that only contain one independent clause. Choice *B* contains a compound verb (more than one verb), but it's still a simple sentence.

17. C: The simple subject of this sentence, the word *lots,* is plural. It agrees with the plural verb form *were.* Choice *A* is incorrect, because the simple subject *there,* referring to the two constellations, is considered plural. It does not agree with the singular verb form *is.* In Choice *B,* the plural subject *four,* does not agree with the singular verb form *needs.* In Choice *D* the singular subject *everyone* does not agree with the third person plural verb form *have.*

500

18. B: *Excellent* and *walking* are adjectives modifying the noun *tours*. *Rich* is an adjective modifying the noun *history*, and *brotherly* is an adjective modifying the noun *love*. Choice *A* is incorrect because all of these words are functioning as nouns in the sentence. Choice *C* is incorrect because all of these words are functioning as verbs in the sentence. Choice *D* is incorrect because all of these words are considered prepositions, not adjectives.

19. D: The object pronouns *her* and *me* act as the indirect objects of the sentence. If *me* is in a series of object pronouns, it should always come last in the series. Choice *A* is incorrect because it uses subject pronouns *she* and *I*. Choice *B* is incorrect because it uses the subject pronoun *she*. Choice *C* uses the correct object pronouns, but they are in the wrong order.

20. A: In this example, a colon is correctly used to introduce a series of items. Choice *B* places an unnecessary comma before the word *because*. A comma is not needed before the word *because* when it introduces a dependent clause at the end of a sentence and provides necessary information to understand the sentence. Choice *C* is incorrect because it uses a semi-colon instead of a comma to join a dependent clause and an independent clause. Choice *D* is incorrect because it uses a colon in place of a comma and coordinating conjunction to join two independent clauses.

21. B: Choice *B* correctly uses the contraction for *you are* as the subject of the sentence, and it correctly uses the possessive pronoun *your* to indicate ownership of the jacket. It also correctly uses the adverb *there*, indicating place. Choice *A* is incorrect because it reverses the possessive pronoun *your* and the contraction for *you are*. It also uses the possessive pronoun *their* instead of the adverb *there*. Choice *C* is incorrect because it reverses *your* and *you're* and uses the contraction for *they are* in place of the adverb *there*. Choice *D* incorrectly uses the possessive pronoun *their* instead of the adverb *there*.

22. A: Slang refers to non-standard expressions that are not used in elevated speech and writing. Slang tends to be specific to one group or time period and is commonly used within groups of young people during their conversations with each other. Jargon refers to the language used in a specialized field. The vernacular is the native language of a local area, and a dialect is one form of a language in a certain region. Thus, *B*, *C*, and *D* are incorrect.

23. D: Colloquial language is that which is used conversationally or informally, in contrast to professional or academic language. While *ain't* is common in conversational English, it is a non-standard expression in academic writing. For college-bound students, high school should introduce them to the expectations of a college classroom, so *B* is not the best answer. Teachers should also avoid placing moral or social value on certain patterns of speech. Rather than teaching students that their familiar speech patterns are bad, teachers should help students learn when and how to use appropriate forms of expression, so *C* is wrong. *Ain't* is in the dictionary, so *A* is incorrect, both in the reason for counseling and in the factual sense.

24. C: A complex sentence joins an independent or main clause with a dependent or subordinate clause. In this case, the main clause is "The restaurant is unconventional." This is a clause with one subject-verb combination that can stand alone as a grammatically-complete sentence. The dependent clause is "because it serves both Chicago style pizza and New York style pizza." This clause begins with the subordinating conjunction *because* and also consists of only one subject-verb combination. *A* is incorrect because a simple sentence consists of only one verb-subject combination—one independent clause. *B* is incorrect because a compound sentence contains two independent clauses connected by a conjunction.

D is incorrect because a complex-compound sentence consists of two or more independent clauses and one or more dependent clauses.

25. A: Parallelism refers to consistent use of sentence structure or word form. In this case, the list within the sentence does not utilize parallelism; three of the verbs appear in their base form—*travel, take,* and *eat*—but one appears as a gerund—*going*. A parallel version of this sentence would be "This summer, I'm planning to travel to Italy, take a Mediterranean cruise, go to Pompeii, and eat a lot of Italian food." *B* is incorrect because this description is a complete sentence. *C* is incorrect as a misplaced modifier is a modifier that is not located appropriately in relation to the word or words they modify. *D* is incorrect because subject-verb agreement refers to the appropriate conjugation of a verb in relation to its subject.

26. C: In this sentence, the modifier is the phrase "Forgetting that he was supposed to meet his girlfriend for dinner." This phrase offers information about Fred's actions, but the noun that immediately follows it is Anita, creating some confusion about the "do-er" of the phrase. A more appropriate sentence arrangement would be "Forgetting that he was supposed to meet his girlfriend for dinner, Fred made Anita mad when he showed up late." *A* is incorrect as parallelism refers to the consistent use of sentence structure and verb tense, and this sentence is appropriately consistent. *B* is incorrect as a run-on sentence does not contain appropriate punctuation for the number of independent clauses presented, which is not true of this description. *D* is incorrect because subject-verb agreement refers to the appropriate conjugation of a verb relative to the subject, and all verbs have been properly conjugated.

27. B: A comma splice occurs when a comma is used to join two independent clauses together without the additional use of an appropriate conjunction. One way to remedy this problem is to replace the comma with a semicolon. Another solution is to add a conjunction: "Some workers use all their sick leave, but other workers cash out their leave." *A* is incorrect as parallelism refers to the consistent use of sentence structure and verb tense; all tenses and structures in this sentence are consistent. *C* is incorrect because a sentence fragment is a phrase or clause that cannot stand alone—this sentence contains two independent clauses. *D* is incorrect because subject-verb agreement refers to the proper conjugation of a verb relative to the subject, and all verbs have been properly conjugated.

28. D: The problem in the original passage is that the second sentence is a dependent clause that cannot stand alone as a sentence; it must be attached to the main clause found in the first sentence. Because the main clause comes first, it does not need to be separated by a comma. However, if the dependent clause came first, then a comma would be necessary, which is why Choice *C* is incorrect. *A* and *B* also insert unnecessary commas into the sentence.

29. A: A noun refers to a person, place, thing, or idea. Although the word *approach* can also be used as a verb, in the sentence it functions as a noun within the noun phrase "a fresh approach," so *B* is incorrect. An adverb is a word or phrase that provides additional information of the verb, but because the verb is *need* and not *approach*, then *C* is false. An adjective is a word that describes a noun, used here as the word *fresh*, but it is not the noun itself. Thus, *D* is also incorrect.

30. D: An adjective modifies a noun, answering the question "Which one?" or "What kind?" In this sentence, the word *exhaustive* is an adjective that modifies the noun *investigation*. Another clue that this word is an adjective is the suffix *–ive*, which means "having the quality of." The nouns in this sentence are *investigators, inquiry, accusations,* and *corruption*; therefore, *A* is incorrect. The verb in this sentence is *conducted* because this was the action taken by the subject *the investigators*; therefore, *B* is incorrect. *C* is incorrect because an adverb is a word or phrase that provides additional information about the verb, expressing how, when, where, or in what manner.

31. B: In this case, the phrase functions as an adverb modifying the verb *report*, so *B* is the correct answer. "To the student center" does not consist of a subject-verb combination, so it is not a clause; thus, Choices *A* and *C* can be eliminated. This group of words is a phrase. Phrases are classified by either the controlling word in the phrase or its function in the sentence. *D* is incorrect because a noun phrase is a series of words that describe or modify a noun.

32. D: In this sentence, the first answer choice requires a noun meaning *impact* or *influence*, so *effect* is the correct answer. For the second answer choice, the sentence is drawing a comparison. *Than* shows a comparative relationship whereas *then* shows sequence or consequence. *A* and *C* can be eliminated because they contain the choice *then*. *B* is incorrect because *affect* is a verb while this sentence requires a noun.

33. D: Since the sentence contains two independent clauses and a dependent clause, the sentence is categorized as compound-complex:

Independent clause: *I accepted the change of seasons*

Independent clause: *I started to appreciate the fall*

Dependent clause: *Although I wished it were summer*

34. D: Students can use context clues to make a careful guess about the meaning of unfamiliar words. Although all of the words in a sentence can help contribute to the overall sentence, in this case, the adjective that pairs with *ubiquitous* gives the most important hint to the student—cars were first *rare*, but now they are *ubiquitous*. The inversion of *rare* is what gives meaning to the rest of the sentence and *ubiquitous* means "existing everywhere" or "not rare." *A* is incorrect because *ago* only indicates a time frame. *B* is incorrect because *cars* does not indicate a contrasting relationship to the word *ubiquitous* to provide a good context clue. *C* is incorrect because it also only indicates a time frame, but used together with *rare*, it provides the contrasting relationship needed to identify the meaning of the unknown word.

35. B: Proper nouns are specific. *Statue of Liberty* is a proper noun and specifies exactly which statue is being discussed. Choice *A* is incorrect because the word *people* is a common noun and it is only capitalized because it is at the beginning of the sentence. Choice *C* is incorrect. The word *awesome* is an adjective describing the sight. Choice *D* is incorrect. The word *sight* is a common noun. A clue to eliminate answer Choices *C* and *D* is that they were not capitalized. Proper nouns are always capitalized.

36. D: The word *kittens* is plural, meaning more than one kitten. Choice *A* is incorrect. The word *kitten* is singular. Choice *B* is incorrect. The word *girl's* is a singular possessive form. The girl is making the choice. There is only one girl involved. Choice *C* is incorrect. The word *choice* is a singular noun. The girl has only one choice to make. The word *litter* in this sentence is a collective plural noun meaning a group of kittens.

37. C: The word *who* in the sentence is a subjective interrogative pronoun and the sentence needed a subject that begins a question. Choice *A* is incorrect. The word *whose* is a possessive pronoun and it is not being asked who owns the flowers. Choice *B* is incorrect. The word *whom* is always an objective

503

pronoun—never a subjective one; a subjective pronoun is needed in this sentence. Choice *D* is incorrect. The word *who've* is a contraction of the words *who* and *have*. We would not say, *"Who have ordered the flowers?"*

38. D: The word *its* in the sentence is the singular possessive form of the pronoun that stands in place for the word *giraffe's*. There is one baby that belongs to one giraffe. Choice *A* is incorrect. It is a contraction of the words *it* and *is*. You would not say, *"The giraffe nudged it is baby."* Choice *B* is incorrect. We do not know the gender of the giraffe and if it was female the proper word would be *her* baby not *hers* baby. Choice *C* is incorrect. The word *their* is a plural possessive pronoun and we need a singular possessive pronoun because there is only one giraffe doing the nudging.

39. B: The word *several* stands in for a plural noun at the beginning of the sentence, such as the noun *people*. It is also an indefinite pronoun because the number of people, for example, is not defined. Choice *A* is incorrect. The pronoun is plural not singular. It indicates more than one person. We can tell because the sentence works with the plural word *are* for the verb; substituting the singular word *is* would not make sense. We wouldn't say, *"Several is laughing loudly on the bus."* Choice *C* is incorrect. *Several* is the subject of the sentence. Therefore, it is a subjective pronoun not an objective one. Choice *D* is incorrect. The word *several* does not modify a noun in the sentence. If the sentence said, *"Several people are laughing loudly on the bus,"* then the word *several* would be an indefinite adjective modifying the word *people*.

40. A: The word *delectable* is an adjective modifying the noun *meal* in the sentence. It answers the question: *"What kind of meal?"* Choice *B* is incorrect. The word *connoisseur* is a noun that is the subject of the sentence. Choice *C* is incorrect. The word *slowly* is an adverb telling how the subject enjoyed the meal. Choice *D* is incorrect. The word *enjoyed* is the past-tense verb in the sentence telling us what action the subject had taken.

41. B: The word *by* is a positional preposition telling where we are in relation to the water. The word *near* is also a positional preposition telling where *we* are in relation to the lake. The word *before* is a time preposition telling when in relation to the time of day, dawn. Choice *A* is incorrect because *went* and *to see* are both verbs and *pretty* is an adjective modifying the word *sunrise*. Choice *C* is incorrect because *water, lake, dawn,* and *sunrise* are all nouns in the sentence. Choice *D* is incorrect because the word *we* is a pronoun, the word *down* is an adverb modifying the verb *went*, the word *the* is an article, and the word *pretty* is an adjective modifying *sunrise*.

42. B: The word *well* at the beginning of the sentence is set apart from the rest of the sentence with a comma and is a mild interjection. Choice *A* is incorrect. The word *goodness* at the end of the sentence is a noun. It is the idea/state of being for the cookie. Choice *C* is incorrect. It is an interrogative sentence and all of the words in the sentence can be identified as other parts of speech. *Can't* is a contraction of the word cannot and it works with the word *see* as the verb in the sentence. The word *you* is a pronoun; the word *that* is an adjective modifying the word *cookie*; *cookie* is a noun; *is* is another verb; and *broken* is an adjective modifying the word *cookie*. Choice *D* is incorrect because the exclamation mark at the end of the sentence is not there to set apart an interjection. Rather, it is there to punctuate the exclamatory sentence.

43. C: The simple subject is *bike* and its modifiers *the heaviest* and *green* are included to form the complete subject. Choice *A* is incorrect because *bike* is the simple subject. Choice *B* is incorrect because it includes only one of the modifiers (*green*) of the word *bike*. Choice *D* is incorrect because *is mine* is the predicate of the sentence, not the subject.

44. D: The subject of the sentence is *my house;* therefore, the rest of the sentence is the predicate. Choice *A* is incorrect because *my house* is the subject, not the predicate. Choice *B* is incorrect because *is the yellow one* is only part of the predicate, but the sentence does not end there. Choice *C* is incorrect because *at the end of the street* is only a portion of the predicate.

45. B: The *kitten* is a singular subject and so the singular verb *pounces* should be used instead of *pounce*. Choice *A* is incorrect because the plural subject *kittens* agrees with the plural verb *show*. Choice *C* is incorrect because the singular subject *kitten* agrees with the singular verb *eats*. Choice *D* is incorrect because the singular subject *kitten* agrees with the singular verb *snuggles*.

46. C: *Her mother* is to whom Calysta brought the lamp. Choice *A* is incorrect because *stained-glass lamp* is the direct object of the sentence. Choice *B* is incorrect because *brought* is the verb. Choice *D* is incorrect because *beautiful* is an adjective modifying the noun *lamp*.

47. C: *They're* (they are) on *their* (possessive) way to New Jersey but *they're* (they are) not *there* (location) yet. This sentence makes sense. Choice *A* is incorrect because after the word *but* should be the word *they're* (they are). Choice *B* is incorrect because the sentence should begin with *they're* (they are) instead of *their* (possessive). Choice *D* is incorrect because after the word *not* should be *there* (location) instead of *their* (possessive).

48. D: *For the longest time* is an introductory prepositional phrase beginning with the preposition *for* and all the modifiers for the word *time*. Choice *A* is incorrect because it includes the past-tense verb *have wanted* creating a clause. Choice *B* is incorrect because it includes the verb *wanted* and the infinitive *to learn*. Choice *C* is incorrect because it includes the verb *learn* and the infinitive *to skate*.

49. B: *The weight of the world was on his shoulders* and *he took a long walk* are both independent clauses connected with a comma and a coordinating conjunction. Choice *A* is incorrect because there are two independent clauses and a simple sentence has only one independent clause. Choice *C* is incorrect because the sentence has no dependent clauses and a complex sentence needs at least one dependent clause. Choice *D* is incorrect because, although there are two independent clauses, there are no dependent clauses and a compound-complex sentence will have at least two independent clauses and at least one dependent clause.

50. A: *The last thing she wanted to do was see the Eiffel Tower before the flight* has only one independent clause and no dependent clauses therefore it is a simple sentence. Choice *B* is incorrect because the sentence has only one independent clause. *The last thing she wanted to do* is a gerund phrase serving as the noun subject of the sentence, therefore it is not an independent clause. Choice *C* is incorrect because the sentence has no dependent clauses therefore it cannot be a complex sentence. Choice *D* is incorrect because the sentence has only one independent clause and no dependent clauses. A compound-complex sentence needs at least two independent clauses and at least one dependent clause.

51. C: Choice *C* correctly adds a comma after *style*, successfully joining the dependent and the independent clauses as a single sentence. Choice *A* is incorrect because the dependent and independent clauses remain unsuccessfully combined without the comma. Choices *B* and *D* do nothing to fix this.

52. A: Choice *A* is correct, as *not only* and *but also* are correlative pairs. In this sentence, *but* successfully transitions the first part into the second half, making punctuation unnecessary. Additionally, the use of *to* indicates that an idea or challenge is being presented to the reader. Choice *B*'s *with*, *C*'s *for*, and *D*'s *there before* are not as active, meaning these revisions weaken the sentence.

53. B: Choice *B* correctly joins the two independent clauses with a comma before *but*. Choice *A* is incorrect because, without the comma, it is a run-on sentence. Choice *C* also lacks punctuation and uses *however*, which should be reserved for starting a new sentence or perhaps after a semicolon. Choice *D* is incorrect because the semicolon throws off the sentence structure and is incorrectly used; the correct revision would have also removed *but*.

54. A: Choice *A* is correct because the sentence does not require modification. Choice *B* is incorrect because it uses the faulty subject/verb agreement, "Physical proof are." Choice *C* is incorrect because a comma would need to follow *exists*. Choice *D* is incorrect because the comma after *science* is unnecessary.

55. A: Choice *A* is the best answer for several reasons. To begin, the section is grammatically correct in using a semicolon to connect the two independent clauses. This allows the different two ideas to be connected without separating them. In this context, the semicolon makes more sense for the overall sentence structure and passage as a whole. Choice *B* is incorrect because it forms a run-on. Choice *C* applies a comma in inc.

Biology

1. C: A hypothesis is a statement that makes a prediction between two variables. The two variables here are the amount of poison and how quickly the rat dies. Choice *C* states that the more poison a rat is given, the more quickly it will die, which is a prediction. Choice *A* is incorrect because it's simply an observation. Choice *B* is incorrect because it's a question posed by the observation but makes no predictions. Choice *D* is incorrect because it's simply a fact.

2. D: Water's unique properties are due to intermolecular hydrogen bonding. These forces make water molecules "stick" to one another, which explains why water has unusually high cohesion and adhesion (sticking to each other and sticking to other surfaces). Cohesion can be seen in beads of dew. Adhesion can be seen when water sticks to the sides of a graduated cylinder to form a meniscus. The stickiness to neighboring molecules also increases surface tension, providing a very thin film that light things cannot penetrate, which is observed when leaves float in swimming pools. Water has a low freezing point, not a high freezing point, due to the fact that molecules have to have a very low kinetic energy to arrange themselves in the lattice-like structure found in ice, its solid form.

3. A: Catabolic reactions release energy and are exothermic. Catabolism breaks down complex molecules into simpler molecules. Anabolic reactions are just the opposite—they absorb energy in order to form complex molecules from simpler ones. Proteins, carbohydrates (polysaccharides), lipids, and nucleic acids are complex organic molecules synthesized by anabolic metabolism. The monomers of these organic compounds are amino acids, monosaccharides, triglycerides, and nucleotides.

4. C: Metabolic reactions utilize enzymes to decrease their activation energy. Enzymes that drive these reactions are protein catalysts. Their mechanism is sometimes referred to as the "lock-and-key" model. "Lock and key" references the fact that enzymes have exact specificity with their substrate (reactant)

506

like a lock does to a key. The substrate binds to the enzyme snugly, the enzyme facilitates the reaction, and then product is formed while the enzyme is unchanged and ready to be reused.

5. B: The structure exclusively found in eukaryotic cells is the nucleus. Animal, plant, fungi, and protist cells are all eukaryotic. DNA is contained within the nucleus of eukaryotic cells, and they also have membrane-bound organelles that perform complex intracellular metabolic activities. Prokaryotic cells (archae and bacteria) do not have a nucleus or other membrane-bound organelles and are less complex than eukaryotic cells.

6. A: The Golgi complex, also known as the Golgi apparatus, is not found in the nucleus. Chromosomes, the nucleolus, and chromatin are all found within the nucleus of the cell. The Golgi apparatus is found in the cytoplasm and is responsible for protein maturation, the process of proteins folding into their secondary, tertiary, and quaternary configurations. The structure appears folded in membranous layers and is easily visible with microscopy. The Golgi apparatus packages proteins in vesicles for export out of the cell or to their cellular destination.

7. B: The cell structure responsible for cellular storage, digestion, and waste removal is the lysosome. Lysosomes are like recycle bins. They are filled with digestive enzymes that facilitate catabolic reactions to regenerate monomers.

8. B: The mitochondria are cellular energy generators and the "powerhouses" of the cell. They provide cellular energy in the form of adenosine triphosphate (ATP). This process, called aerobic respiration, uses oxygen plus sugars, proteins, and fats to produce ATP, carbon dioxide, and water. Mitochondria contain their own DNA and ribosomes, which is significant because according to endosymbiotic theory, these structures provide evidence that they used to be independently-functioning prokaryotes.

9. B: Plastids are the photosynthesizing organelles of plants that are not found in animal cells. Plants have the ability to generate their own sugars through photosynthesis, a process where they use pigments to capture the sun's light energy. Chloroplasts are the most prevalent plastid, and chlorophyll is the light-absorbing pigment that absorbs all energy carried in photons except that of green light. This explains why the photosynthesizing parts of plants, predominantly leaves, appear green.

10. B: During telophase, two nuclei form at each end of the cell and nuclear envelopes begin to form around each nucleus. The nucleoli reappear, and the chromosomes become less compact. The microtubules are broken down by the cell, and mitosis is complete. The process begins with prophase as the mitotic spindles begin to form from centrosomes. Prometaphase follows, with the breakdown of the nuclear envelope and the further condensing of the chromosomes. Next, metaphase occurs when the microtubules are stretched across the cell and the chromosomes align at the metaphase plate. Finally, in the last step before telophase, anaphase occurs as the sister chromatids break apart and form chromosomes.

11. B: Phenotypes are observable traits, such as eye color, hair color, blood type, etc. They can also be biochemical or have physiological or behavioral traits. A genotype is the collective gene representation of an individual, whether the genes are expressed or not. Alleles are different forms of the same gene that code for specific traits, like blue eyes or brown eyes. In simple genetics, there are two forms of a gene: dominant and recessive. More complex genetics involves co-dominance, multiple alleles and sex-linked genes. The other answer choices are incorrect because gender is determined by the presence of an entire chromosome, the Y chromosome, and a karyotype is an image of all of an individual's chromosomes.

12. D: Reproductive cells are referred to as gametes: egg (female) and sperm (male). These cells have only 1 set of 23 chromosomes and are haploid so that when they combine during fertilization, the zygote has the correct diploid number, 46. Reproductive cell division is called meiosis, which is different from mitosis, the type of division process for body (somatic) cells.

13. A: The process of cell division in somatic is mitosis. In interphase, which precedes mitosis, cells prepare for division by copying their DNA. Once mitotic machinery has been assembled in interphase, mitosis occurs, which has five distinct phases: prophase, prometaphase, metaphase, anaphase, and telophase, followed by cytokinesis, which is the final splitting of the cytoplasm. The two diploid daughter cells are genetically identical to the parent cell.

14. D: Equal sharing of electrons is correct. In water, the electronegative oxygen sucks in the electrons of the two hydrogen atoms, making the oxygen slightly negatively-charged and the hydrogen atoms slightly positively-charged. This unequal sharing is called "polarity." This polarity is responsible for the slightly-positive hydrogen atoms from one molecule being attracted to a slightly-negative oxygen in a different molecule, creating a weak intermolecular force called a hydrogen bond, so *A* and *B* are true. *C* is also true, because this unique hydrogen bonding creates intermolecular forces that literally hold molecules with low enough kinetic energy (at low temperatures) to be held apart at "arm's length" (really, the length of the hydrogen bonds). This makes ice less dense than liquid, which explains why ice floats, a very unique property of water. *D* is the only statement that is false, so it is the correct answer.

15. A: All the other answer choices are functions of lipids. Choice *B* is true because steroid hormones are lipid based. Long-term energy is one of the most important functions of lipids, so *C* is true. *D* is also true because the cell membrane is not only composed of a lipid bilayer, but it also has cholesterol (another lipid) embedded within it to regulate membrane fluidity.

16. A: An alteration in the normal gene sequence is called a DNA point mutation. Mutations can be harmful, neutral, or even beneficial. Sometimes, as seen in natural selection, a genetic mutation can improve fitness, providing an adaptation that will aid in survival. DNA mutations can happen as a result of environmental damage, for example, from radiation or chemicals. Mutations can also happen during cell replication, as a result of incorrect pairing of complementary nucleotides by DNA polymerase. There are also chromosomal mutations as well, where entire segments of chromosomes can be deleted, inverted, duplicated, or sent or received from a different chromosome.

17. B: 50%. According to the Punnett square, the child has a 2 out of 4 chance of having A-type blood, since the dominant allele I^A is present in two of the four possible offspring. The O-type blood allele is masked by the A-type blood allele since it is recessive.

I^A i	ii
I^A i	ii

18. D: The building blocks of DNA are nucleotides. A nucleotide is a five-carbon sugar with a phosphate group and a nitrogenous base (Adenine, Guanine, Cytosine, and Thymine). DNA is a double helix and looks like a spiral ladder. Each side has a sugar/phosphate backbone, and the rungs of the ladder that connect the sides are the nitrogenous bases. Adenine always pairs with thymine via two hydrogen bonds, and cytosine always pairs with guanine via three hydrogen bonds. The weak hydrogen bonds are important because they allow DNA to easily be opened for replication and transcription.

19. C: DNA contains chemical bases that form chemical bonds with each other. The four bases in DNA are adenine, cytosine, thymine, and guanine. Uracil is a chemical base found in RNA, not DNA, so Choice *C* is the correct answer.

20. C: Endergonic reactions absorb free energy from its surroundings. Answer Choices *A*, B, and D are all qualities of exergonic reactions.

21. D: Cellular respiration is the term used for the set of metabolic reactions that convert chemical bonds to energy in the form of ATP. All respiration starts with glycolysis in the cytoplasm, and in the presence of oxygen, the process will continue to the mitochondria. In a series of oxidation/reduction reactions, primarily glucose will be broken down so that the energy contained within its bonds can be transferred to the smaller ATP molecules. It's like having a $100 bill (glucose) as opposed to having one hundred $1 bills. This is beneficial to the organism because it allows energy to be distributed throughout the cell very easily in smaller packets of energy.

When glucose is broken down, its electrons and hydrogen atoms are involved in oxidative phosphorylation in order to make ATP, while its carbon and oxygen atoms are released as carbon dioxide. Anaerobic respiration does not occur frequently in humans, but during rigorous exercise, lack of available oxygen in the muscles can lead to anaerobic ATP production in a process called lactic acid fermentation. Alcohol fermentation is another type of anaerobic respiration that occurs in yeast. Anaerobic respiration is extremely less efficient than aerobic respiration, as it has a net yield of 2ATP, while aerobic respiration's net yield exceeds 30 ATP.

22. C: The secondary structure of a protein refers to the folds and coils that are formed by hydrogen bonding between the slightly charged atoms of the polypeptide backbone. The primary structure is the sequence of amino acids, similar to the letters in a long word. The tertiary structure is the overall shape of the molecule that results from the interactions between the side chains that are linked to the polypeptide backbone. The quaternary structure is the complete protein structure that occurs when a protein is made up of two or more polypeptide chains.

23. C: In the Linnaean system, organisms are classified as follows, moving from comprehensive and specific similarities to fewer and more general similarities: domain, kingdom, phylum, class, order, family, genus, and species. A popular mnemonic device to remember the Linnaean system is "Dear King Philip came over for good soup."

24. A: All the other answer choices are functions of lipids. *B* is true because steroid hormones are lipid based. Long-term energy is one of the most important functions of lipids, so *C* is true. *D* is also true because the cell membrane is not only composed of a lipid bilayer, but it also has cholesterol (another lipid) embedded within it to regulate membrane fluidity.

25. D: Ribosomes are the structures responsible for protein synthesis using amino acids delivered by tRNA molecules. They are numerous within the cell and can take up as much as 25% of the cell.

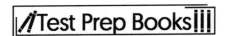
Ribosomes are found free-floating in the cytoplasm and also attached to the rough endoplasmic reticulum, which resides alongside the nucleus. Ribosomes translate messenger RNA into chains of amino acids that become proteins. Ribosomes themselves are made of protein as well as rRNA. Choice *B* might be an attractive choice, since the Golgi is the site of protein maturation; however, it is not where proteins are synthesized. Choice *A* might be an attractive choice as well because DNA provides the instructions for proteins to be made, but DNA does not make the protein itself.

26. D: The color reagent is attached to the secondary antibody. It is released only when the secondary antibody attaches to the activated primary antibody. The antigen, primary antibody, and capture antibody, Choices *A, B,* and *C*, do not have any color reagent attached to them, so only the secondary antibody can cause the color reaction.

27. B: The color reagent is attached to the secondary antibody. If more antigen is present, more primary and secondary antibody will be attached to it and more color reagent will be released. Row 1 has the darkest green color of all the samples tested in the plate in Figure 2.

28. C: Looking at the graph in Figure 3, the highest amount of IL-1β is found in the spleen. IL-1β is a marker of inflammation and indicates that the spleen had the most inflammation of the areas tested. Serum, Choice *A,* had no IL-1β in the sample. Plasma, Choice *B,* had the second highest amount of IL-1β in the sample, and bone marrow, Choice *D,* had the second lowest amount of IL-1β.

29. B: Looking at the diagram in Figure 1, the antigen is located between the capture antibody and the primary antibody. The capture antibody keeps the antigen attached to the surface of the plate. The primary antibody recognizes the specific antigen. The secondary antibody generally recognizes the primary antibody is not specific to the antigen.

30. A: ELISAs are used to analyze specific substances within a larger sample. The antibodies used in an ELISA are designed specifically for a particular antigen. Sandwich ELISAs are generally used to quantify one antigen and not all substances in a larger sample, making Choice *B* incorrect. When used to quantify an antigen, the antibodies need to already be developed and able to detect the antigen, making Choice *D* incorrect.

Chemistry

1. A: Review the following conversion:

$$°F = \frac{9}{5}(°C) + 32$$

$$°F = \frac{9}{5}(45) + 32$$

$$°F = 113 \ °F$$

Choices *B, C,* and *D* all incorporate a mistake in the order of operations necessary for this calculation to convert degrees Celsius to degrees Fahrenheit: divide by 5, multiply by 9, and then add 32.

2. A: The neutrons and protons make up the nucleus of the atom. The nucleus is positively charged due to the presence of the protons. The negatively charged electrons are attracted to the positively charged nucleus by the electrostatic or Coulomb force; however, the electrons are not contained in the nucleus.

The positively charged protons create the positive charge in the nucleus, and the neutrons are electrically neutral, so they have no effect. Radioactivity does not directly have a bearing on the charge of the nucleus.

3. B: The conversion from Celsius to Fahrenheit is:

$$°F = \frac{9}{5}(°C) + 32$$

Substituting the value for °C gives $°F = \frac{9}{5}(35) + 32$ which yields 95°F. The other choices do not apply the formula correctly and completely.

4. B: Choices A and D both suggest a different number of protons, which would make a different element. It would no longer be a sodium atom if the proton number or atomic number were different, so those are both incorrect. An atom that has a different number of electrons is called an ion, so Choice C is incorrect as well.

5. B: They form covalent bonds. If nonmetals form ionic bonds, they will fill their electron orbital (and become an anion) rather than lose electrons (and become a cation), due to their smaller atomic radius and higher electronegativity than metals. A is, therefore, incorrect. There are some nonmetals that are diatomic (hydrogen, oxygen, nitrogen, and halogens), but that is not true for all of them; thus, D is incorrect. Organic compounds are carbon-based due to carbon's ability to form four covalent bonds. In addition to carbon, organic compounds are also rich in hydrogen, phosphorus, nitrogen, oxygen, and sulfur, so C is incorrect as well.

6. B: The basic unit of matter is the atom. Each element is identified by a letter symbol for that element and an atomic number, which indicates the number of protons in that element. Atoms are the building block of each element and are comprised of a nucleus that contains protons (positive charge) and neutrons (no charge). Orbiting around the nucleus at varying distances are negatively-charged electrons. An electrically-neutral atom contains equal numbers of protons and electrons. Atomic mass is the combined mass of protons and neutrons in the nucleus. Electrons have such negligible mass that they are not considered in the atomic mass. Although the nucleus is compact, the electrons orbit in energy levels at great relative distances to it, making an atom mostly empty space.

7. A: Nuclear reactions involve the nucleus, and chemical reactions involve electron behavior alone. If electrons are transferred between atoms, they form ionic bonds. If they are shared between atoms, they form covalent bonds. Unequal sharing within a covalent bond results in intermolecular attractions, including hydrogen bonding. Metallic bonding involves a "sea of electrons," where they float around non-specifically, resulting in metal ductility and malleability, due to their glue-like effect of sticking neighboring atoms together. Their metallic bonding also contributes to electrical conductivity and low specific heats, due to electrons' quick response to charge and heat, given to their mobility. Their floating also results in metals' property of luster as light reflects off the mobile electrons. Electron movement in any type of bond is enhanced by photon and heat energy investments, increasing their likelihood to jump energy levels. Valence electron status is the ultimate contributor to electron behavior as it determines their likelihood to be transferred or shared.

8. A: Electrons give atoms their negative charge. Electron behavior determines their bonding, and bonding can either be covalent (electrons are shared) or ionic (electrons are transferred). The charge of an atom is determined by the electrons in its orbitals. Electrons give atoms their chemical and electromagnetic properties. Unequal numbers of protons and electrons lend either a positive or negative charge to the atom. Ions are atoms with a charge, either positive or negative.

9. B: On the periodic table, the elements are grouped in columns according to the configuration of electrons in their outer orbitals. The groupings on the periodic table give a broad view of trends in chemical properties for the elements. The outer electron shell (or orbital) is most important in determining the chemical properties of the element. The electrons in this orbital determine charge and bonding compatibility. The number of electron shells increases by row from top to bottom. The periodic table is organized with elements that have similar chemical behavior in the columns (groups or families).

10. B: In chemical equations, the reactants are on the left side of the arrow. The direction of the reaction is in the direction of the arrow, although sometimes reactions will be shown with arrows in both directions, meaning the reaction is reversible. The reactants are on the left, and the products of the reaction are on the right side of the arrow. Chemical equations indicate atomic and molecular bond formations, rearrangements, and dissolutions. The numbers in front of the elements are called coefficients, and they designate the number of moles of that element accounted for in the reaction. The subscript numbers tell how many atoms of that element are in the molecule, with the number "1" being understood. In H_2O, for example, there are two atoms of hydrogen bound to one atom of oxygen. The ionic charge of the element is shown in superscripts and can be either positive or negative.

11. B: The law of conservation of mass states that matter cannot be created or destroyed, but that it can change forms. This is important in balancing chemical equations on both sides of the arrow. Unbalanced equations will have an unequal number of atoms of each element on either side of the equation and violate the law.

12. D: Solids all increase solubility with Choices *A–C*. Powdered hot chocolate is an example to consider. Heating (*A*) and stirring (*B*) make it dissolve faster. Regarding Choice *C*, powder is in chunks that collectively result in a very large surface area, as opposed to a chocolate bar that has a very small relative surface area. The small surface area to volume ratio dramatically increases solubility. Decreasing the solvent (most of the time, water) will decrease solubility.

13. A: The quantity of a solute in a solution can be calculated by multiplying the molarity of the solution by the volume. The equivalence point is the point at which an unknown solute has completely reacted with a known solute concentration. The limiting reactant is the reactant completely consumed by a reaction. The theoretical yield is the quantity of product produced by a reaction.

14. A: When salt is added to water, it increases its boiling point. This is an example of a colligative property, which is any property that changes the physical property of a substance. This particular colligative property of boiling point elevation occurs because the extra solute dissolved in water reduces the surface area of the water, impeding it from vaporizing. If heat is applied, though, it gives water particles enough kinetic energy to vaporize. This additional heat results in an increased boiling point. Other colligative properties of solutions include the following: their melting points decrease with the addition of solute, and their osmotic pressure increases (because it creates a concentration gradient that was otherwise not there).

15. C: Pressure has little effect on the solubility of a liquid solution because liquid is not easily compressible; therefore, increased pressure won't result in increased kinetic energy. Pressure increases solubility in gaseous solutions, since it causes them to move faster.

16. B: Nonpolar molecules have hydrophobic regions that do not dissolve in water. Oils are nonpolar molecules that repel water. Polar molecules combine readily with water, which is, itself, a polar solvent. Polar molecules are hydrophilic or "water-loving" because their polar regions have intermolecular bonding with water via hydrogen bonds. Some structures and molecules are both polar and nonpolar, like the phospholipid bilayer. The phospholipid bilayer has polar heads that are the external "water-loving portions" and hydrophobic tails that are immiscible in water. Polar solvents dissolve polar solutes, and nonpolar solvents dissolve nonpolar solutes. One way to remember these is "Like dissolves like."

17. A: A catalyst increases the rate of a chemical reaction by lowering the activation energy. Enzymes are biological protein catalysts that are utilized by organisms to facilitate anabolic and catabolic reactions. They speed up the rate of reaction by making the reaction easier (perhaps by orienting a molecule more favorably upon induced fit, for example). Catalysts are not used up by the reaction and can be used over and over again.

18. C: Proteins are made up of chains of amino acids. Lipids are usually nonpolar, hydrophobic molecules. Nucleic acids are made of nucleotides. Carbohydrates are ring-like molecules built using carbon, oxygen, and hydrogen.

19. C: 2:9:10:4. These are the coefficients that follow the law of conservation of matter. The coefficient times the subscript of each element should be the same on both sides of the equation.

20. A: Ionic bonding is the result of electrons transferred between atoms. When an atom loses one or more electrons, a cation, or positively-charged ion, is formed. An anion, or negatively-charged ion, is formed when an atom gains one or more electrons. Ionic bonds are formed from the attraction between a positively-charged cation and a negatively-charged anion. The bond between sodium and chlorine in table salt, or sodium chloride ($NaCl$), is an example of an ionic bond.

21. A: Oxidation is when a substance loses electrons in a chemical reaction, and reduction is when a substance gains electrons. Any element by itself has a charge of 0, as iron and oxygen do on the reactant side. In the ionic compound formed, iron has a +3 charge, and oxygen has a -2 charge. Because iron had a zero charge that then changed to +3, it means that it lost three electrons and was oxidized. Oxygen that gained two electrons was reduced.

22. C: Fission occurs when heavy nuclei are split and is currently the energy source that fuels power plants. Fusion, on the other hand, is the combining of small nuclei and produces far more energy, and it is the nuclear reaction that powers stars like the sun. Harnessing the extreme energy released by fusion has proven impossible so far, which is unfortunate since its waste products are not radioactive, while waste produced by fission typically is.

23. A: Alpha decay involves a helium particle emission (with two neutrons). Beta decay involves emission of an electron or positron, and gamma is just high-energy light emissions.

24. B: Choice *A* is false because it is possible to have a very strong acid with a pH between 0 and 1. *C* is false because the pH scale is from 0 to 14, and -2 is outside the boundaries. *D* is false because a solution with a pH of 2 has ten times fewer hydronium ions than a pH of 1 solution.

25. C: Gamma is the lightest radioactive decay with the most energy, and this high energy is toxic to cells. Due to its weightlessness, gamma rays are extremely penetrating. Alpha particles are heavy and can be easily shielded by skin. Beta particles are electrons and can penetrate more than an alpha particle because they are lighter. Beta particles can be shielded by plastic.

26. D: The equivalence point occurs when just enough of the unknown solution is added to completely neutralize the known solution. In Figure 1, at the halfway point of the curve, the equivalence point is when 25 volumes of NaOH have been added to the solution. The pH is 7 at this point also, which is a neutralization of the HCl, strong acid.

27. C: The acid dissociation constant is the pK_a of the solution. It is found at the halfway point between the beginning of the curve and the equivalence point, where the solution would have a pH of 7 and be completely neutralized. In Figure 3, it is marked as 4.76.

28. A: Looking at Figure 3, the vertical axis on the left side has information about the pH of the solution. The horizontal axis at the bottom has information about how much basic solution containing OH^- is being added to the acetic acid. When the OH^- is at 0, and none has been added yet, the pH of the acetic acid is marked as 2.

29. B: Looking at the chemical equation in Figure 2, the reactants are on the left side and the products are on the right side. HCl and NaOH, Choices *A* and *C*, are the reactants of the equation. NaCl is the salt that is formed as one of the products of the reaction. The chloride ion, Choice *D*, is not formed in this reaction.

30. A: The equivalence point occurs in all titration reactions when the solution is neutralized. If an acid and base are being titrated, the solution is no longer acidic or basic, Choices *B* and *C*. It reaches a pH of 7 and is considered neutral.

Anatomy and Physiology

1. D: Veins have valves, but arteries do not. Valves in veins are designed to prevent backflow, since they are the furthest blood vessels from the pumping action of the heart and steadily increase in volume (which decreases the available pressure). Capillaries diffuse nutrients properly because of their thin walls and high surface area and are not particularly dependent on positive pressure.

2. D: Mechanical digestion is physical digestion of food and tearing it into smaller pieces using force. This occurs in the stomach and mouth. Chemical digestion involves chemically changing the food and breaking it down into small organic compounds that can be utilized by the cell to build molecules. The salivary glands in the mouth secrete amylase that breaks down starch, which begins chemical digestion. The stomach contains enzymes such as pepsinogen/pepsin and gastric lipase, which chemically digest protein and fats, respectively. The small intestine continues to digest protein using the enzymes trypsin and chymotrypsin. It also digests fats with the help of bile from the liver and lipase from the pancreas. These organs act as exocrine glands because they secrete substances through a duct. Carbohydrates are digested in the small intestine with the help of pancreatic amylase, gut bacterial flora and fauna, and brush border enzymes like lactose. Brush border enzymes are contained in the towel-like microvilli in the small intestine that soak up nutrients.

514

3. D: The urinary system has many functions, the primary of which is removing waste products and balancing water and electrolyte concentrations in the blood. It also plays a key role in regulating ion concentrations, such as sodium, potassium, chloride, and calcium, in the filtrate. The urinary system helps maintain blood pH by reabsorbing or secreting hydrogen ions and bicarbonate as necessary. Certain kidney cells can detect reductions in blood volume and pressure and then can secrete renin to activate a hormone that causes increased reabsorption of sodium ions and water. This serves to raise blood volume and pressure. Kidney cells secrete erythropoietin under hypoxic conditions to stimulate red blood cell production. They also synthesize calcitriol, a hormone derivative of vitamin D3, which aids in calcium ion absorption by the intestinal epithelium.

4. C: The blood leaves the right ventricle through a semi-lunar valve and goes through the pulmonary artery to the lungs. Any increase in pressure in the artery will eventually affect the contractibility of the right ventricle. Blood enters the right atrium from the superior and inferior venae cava veins, and blood leaves the right atrium through the tricuspid valve to the right ventricle. Blood enters the left atrium from the pulmonary veins carrying oxygenated blood from the lungs. Blood flows from the left atrium to the left ventricle through the mitral valve and leaves the left ventricle through a semi-lunar valve to enter the aorta.

5. D: Sodium bicarbonate, a very effective base, has the chief function to increase the pH of the chyme. Chyme leaving the stomach has a very low pH, due to the high amounts of acid that are used to digest and break down food. If this is not neutralized, the walls of the small intestine will be damaged and may form ulcers. Sodium bicarbonate is produced by the pancreas and released in response to pyloric stimulation so that it can neutralize the acid. It has little to no digestive effect.

6. D: A reflex arc is a simple nerve pathway involving a stimulus, a synapse, and a response that is controlled by the spinal cord—not the brain. The knee-jerk reflex is an example of a reflex arc. The stimulus is the hammer touching the tendon, reaching the synapse in the spinal cord by an afferent pathway. The response is the resulting muscle contraction reaching the muscle by an efferent pathway. None of the remaining processes is a simple reflex. Memories are processed and stored in the hippocampus in the limbic system. The visual center is located in the occipital lobe, while auditory processing occurs in the temporal lobe. The sympathetic and parasympathetic divisions of the autonomic nervous system control heart and blood pressure.

7. B: Ligaments connect bone to bone. Tendons connect muscle to bone. Both are made of dense, fibrous connective tissue (primary Type 1 collagen) to give strength. However, tendons are more organized, especially in the long axis direction like muscle fibers themselves, and they have more collagen. This arrangement makes more sense because muscles have specific orientations of their fibers, so they contract in somewhat predictable directions. Ligaments are less organized and more of a woven pattern because bone connections are not as organized as bundles of muscle fibers, so ligaments must have strength in multiple directions to protect against injury.

8. A: The three primary body planes are coronal, sagittal, and transverse. The coronal or frontal plane, named for the plane in which a corona or halo might appear in old paintings, divides the body vertically into front and back sections. The sagittal plane, named for the path an arrow might take when shot at the body, divides the body vertically into right and left sections. The transverse plane divides the body horizontally into upper or superior and lower or inferior sections. There is no medial plane, per se. The anatomical direction medial simply references a location close or closer to the center of the body than another location.

9. C: Although the lungs may provide some cushioning for the heart when the body is violently struck, this is not a major function of the respiratory system. Its most notable function is that of gas exchange for oxygen and carbon dioxide, but it also plays a vital role in the regulation of blood pH. The aqueous form of carbon dioxide, carbonic acid, is a major pH buffer of the blood, and the respiratory system directly controls how much carbon dioxide stays and is released from the blood through respiration. The respiratory system also enables vocalization and forms the basis for the mode of speech and language used by most humans.

10. A: The forebrain contains the cerebrum, the thalamus, the hypothalamus, and the limbic system. The limbic system is chiefly responsible for the perception of emotions through the amygdala, while the cerebrum interprets sensory input and generates movement. Specifically, the occipital lobe receives visual input, and the primary motor cortex in the frontal lobe is the controller of voluntary movement. The hindbrain, specifically the medulla oblongata and brain stem, control and regulate blood pressure and heart rate.

11. C: Nephrons are responsible for filtering blood. When functioning properly they allow blood cells and nutrients to go back into the bloodstream while sending waste to the bladder. However, nephrons can fail at doing this, particularly when blood flood to the kidneys is limited. The medulla (also called the renal medulla) (*A*) and the renal cortex (*D*) are both parts of the kidney but are not specifically responsible for filtering blood. The medulla is in the inner part of the kidney and contains the nephrons. The renal cortex is the outer part of the kidney. The heart (*B*) is responsible for pumping blood throughout the body rather than filtering it.

12. B: Ossification is the process by which cartilage, a soft, flexible substance is replaced by bone throughout the body. All humans regardless of age have cartilage, but cartilage in some areas goes away to make way for bones.

13. D: The seminiferous tubules are responsible for sperm production. Had *testicles* been an answer choice, it would also have been correct since it houses the seminiferous tubules. The prostate gland (*A*) secretes enzymes that help nourish sperm after creation. The seminal vesicles (*B*) secrete some of the components of semen. The scrotum (*C*) is the pouch holding the testicles.

14. C: The parasympathetic nervous system is related to calm, peaceful times without stress that require no immediate decisions. It relaxes the fight-or-flight response, slows heart rate to a comfortable pace, and decreases bronchiole dilation to a normal size. The sympathetic nervous system, on the other hand, is in charge of the fight-or-flight response and works to increase blood pressure and oxygen absorption.

15. C: The parathryroid gland impacts calcium levels by secreting parathyroid hormone (PTH). Osteotoid gland is not a real gland. The pineal gland regulates sleep by secreting melatonin, and the thymus gland focuses on immunity. *Thyroid* would also be a correct answer choice as it influences the levels of circulating calcium.

16. D: Bony matrix is an intricate lattice of collagen fibers and mineral salts, particularly calcium and phosphorus. The mineral salts are strong but brittle, and the collagen fibers are weak but flexible, so the combination of the two makes bone resistant to shattering and able to withstand the normal forces applied to it.

17. D: Arteries carry oxygen-rich blood from the heart to the other tissues of the body. Veins carry oxygen-poor blood back to the heart. Intestines carry digested food through the body. Bronchioles are passageways that carry air from the nose and mouth to the lungs.

18. C: The somatic nervous system is the voluntary nervous system, responsible for voluntary movement. It includes nerves that transmit signals from the brain to the muscles of the body. Breathing is controlled by the autonomic nervous system. Thought and fear are complex processes that occur in the brain, which is part of the central nervous system.

19. A: Platelets are the blood components responsible for clotting. There are between 150,000 and 450,000 platelets in healthy blood. When a clot forms, platelets adhere to the injured area of the vessel and promote a molecular cascade that results in adherence of more platelets. Ultimately, the platelet aggregation results in recruitment of a protein called fibrin, which adds structure to the clot. Too many platelets can cause clotting disorders. Not enough leads to bleeding disorders.

20. C: The sinuses function to warm, filter, and humidify air that is inhaled. Choice *A* is incorrect because mucus traps airborne pathogens. Choice *B* is incorrect because the epiglottis is the structure in the pharynx that covers the trachea during swallowing to prevent food from entering it. Lastly, Choice *D,* sweeping away pathogens and directing them toward the top of the trachea, is the function of cilia. Respiratory structures, such as the nasal passages and trachea, are lined with mucus and cilia.

21. D: In mechanical processing the teeth tear up large chunks of food into smaller pieces. In secretion, Choice *A,* buffers, enzymes, and acids are secreted to help break complex molecules into simpler ones. In absorption, Choice *B,* nutrients are absorbed through the digestive epithelium. In excretion, Choice *C,* waste products are removed from the body.

22. C: A cluster of capillaries that functions as the main filter of the blood entering the kidney is known as the glomerulus, so Choice *C* is correct. The Bowman's capsule surrounds the glomerulus and receives fluid and solutes from it; therefore, Choice *A* is incorrect. The loop of Henle is a part of the kidney tubule where water and nutrients are reabsorbed, so *B* is false. The nephron is the unit containing all of these anatomical features, making Choice *D* incorrect as well.

23. C: The alveoli are small sac-shaped structures at the end of the bronchioles where gas exchange takes place. The bronchioles are tubes through which air travels. The kidneys and medulla oblongata do not directly affect oxygen and carbon dioxide exchange.

24. C: The uterus and ovaries aren't part of the birth canal, so Choices *A* and *D* are false. The cervix is the uppermost portion of the birth canal, so Choice *B* is incorrect, making Choice *C* the correct answer, as the vagina is the muscular tube on the lowermost portion of the birth canal that connects the exterior environment to the cervix.

25. C: The pancreas functions as an exocrine gland because it secretes enzymes that break down food components. It also functions as an endocrine gland because it secretes hormones that regulate blood sugar levels. The kidney isn't a gland; it is an organ located directly below the adrenal glands. The stomach is an exocrine gland because it secretes hydrochloric acid. Like the kidney, the spleen is an organ, not a gland. Therefore, the only correct answer is *C.*

26. D: In the secondary immune response, suppressor T lymphocytes are activated to negate the potential risk of damage to healthy cells, brought on by an unchecked, overactive immune response.

Choice *A* is incorrect because the activity is characteristic of the primary response, not the secondary response. Choice *B* is incorrect because humeral immunity is mediated by antibodies produced by B, not T, lymphocytes. Choice *C* is wrong because the secondary response is faster than the primary response because the primary response entails the time-consuming process of macrophage activation.

27. D: Massive urine production, or polyuria, is the result of a hyperglycemic state in the body and a hallmark sign of any diabetic condition. Urine is not concentrated, but rather diluted. Sodium, potassium, and other electrolyte imbalances may occur as a result of polyuria but are not a direct effect of hyperglycemia.

28. B: Basophils are the white blood cells that secrete histamine, the substance that causes itching in allergic reactions. Lymphocytes are responsible for antibody creation. Neutrophils take out bacterial and fungal organisms and are quite numerous. Monocytes assist in breaking down bacterial organisms.

29. B: The ventricles of the brain are responsible for the production of cerebrospinal fluid. The pons is located at the end of the brain stem and is responsible for regulating breathing. The thalamus acts as a message exchange center for the cerebrum and limbic system, and is located just above the brain stem. The corpus callosum is the fibrous tissue of white matter that connects the left and right brain.

30. A: Since electrolytes need to be suspended in a certain amount of liquid to move optimally and carry out their intended function, fluid level in the body is important. As fluid levels increase beyond a state of fluid-electrolyte balance, electrolyte levels will decrease, since there is too much fluid present. If fluid levels are too low, such as in a state of dehydration, there will be too many electrolytes per unit of fluid, which also prevents the electrolytes from carrying out their intended function.

Physics

1. A: Velocity is a measure of speed with direction. To calculate velocity, find the distance covered and the time it took to cover that distance; change in position over the change in time. A standard measurement for velocity is in meters per second (m/s). The change in velocity over change in time is acceleration, while acceleration with direction has no specific name.

2. B: Acceleration is the rate of change in velocity. Speed is the rate at which an object moves, velocity is speed in a given direction, and momentum is the velocity of an object multiplied by its mass.

3. B: While this is an important brainchild of Einstein's general relativity, it is not one of Newton's original three laws of motion. Newton's three laws describe how a force is defined as how much a mass is accelerated, how an object resists changes in inertia, and how all forces act with an equal and opposite reaction.

4. C: This is the actual force recognized in a rotational situation. The reactive force acting opposite of the centripetal force is named the centrifugal force, but it is not an actual force on its own. A common mistake is to interchange the two terms. The real force acting in a rotational situation is pulling in toward the axis of rotation and is called the centripetal force. Gravity technically only acts between all mass, so it is not specific enough for the question.

5. B: Kinetic energy is energy an object has while moving; potential energy is energy an object has based on its position or height. Electric and electromagnetic energies are other descriptions of generally potential energy contained in waves or fields, but neither has anything directly to do with movement.

518

6. B: Waves are periodic disturbances in a gas, liquid, or solid as energy is transmitted. Waves don't carry or slow down matter, but instead transfer energy.

7. A: The definition of refraction is when a wave bends (such as when the medium it is traveling through changes). Diffraction is when a wave bends around an object (such as when the medium it is traveling through runs into a barrier), so is too specific an answer for the question. Reflection is when a wave bounces off a surface without losing energy or becoming distorted, and convection is the thermal energy transferred through gases and liquids by convection currents.

8. A: Protons and neutrons are both found in the atomic nucleus, while electrons move freely in the electron cloud of an atom. Ions are a different name for entire atoms with unequal numbers of protons and electrons; since this includes electrons, it cannot describe things solely found in the nucleus (unless you were visualizing a hydrogen ion, which is a particular case and is arguably not general enough for the question).

9. C: Electricity moves from objects with greater potential energy to objects with less potential energy. Similar to how warm air spreads towards colder environments or how gasses and liquids move from areas of high concentration to areas of low concentration, electric currents are generated by the electric field moving electrons from areas of high voltage potential to areas of low voltage potential.

10. A: The recurring theme in electricity and magnetism is that like, similar, or identical charges repel one another (whether it is two negative charges or two positive charges) while unlike, dissimilar, or different charges attract one another. This is exemplified by Coulomb's law, which states that charges of the same sign produce a positive force (which repels the particles) and that charges of opposite signs produce a negative force (which attracts the particles).

11. B: The answer is 735.75 N. This is a simple calculation:

$$\frac{9.81 \text{ m}}{s^2} \times 150 \text{ kg} \times 1.5 \text{ m} = 3 \text{ m} \times F$$

$$F = \frac{2{,}207.25 \text{ N} \cdot \text{m}}{3 \text{ m}} = 735.75 \text{ N}$$

12. D: The answer is 40 N. Use the equation $F = L \times r/R$. Note that for an axle with a given, set radius, the larger the radius of the wheel, the greater the mechanical advantage:

$$F = 600 \text{ N} \times \frac{20 \text{ mm}}{300 \text{ mm}} = 40 \text{ N}$$

13. D: The answer is counterclockwise at 30 RPM. The driver gear is turning clockwise, and the gear meshed with it turns counter to it. Because of the 2:1 gear ratio, every revolution of the driver gear causes half a revolution of the follower.

14. B: The answer is 30 RPM, counterclockwise (B). While meshed gears rotate in different directions, wheels linked by a belt turn in the same direction. This is true unless the belt is twisted, in which case they rotate in opposite directions. So, the twisted link between the upper two wheels causes the right-hand wheel to turn counterclockwise, and the bigger wheel at the bottom also rotates counterclockwise. Since it's twice as large as the upper wheel, it rotates with half the RPMs.

15. C: The answer is $F_1 = 1000$ N; $F_2 = 500$ N. In case (a), the fixed wheels only serve to change direction. They offer no mechanical advantage because the lever arm on each side of the axle is the same. In case (b), the lower moveable block provides a 2:1 mechanical advantage. A quick method for calculating the mechanical advantage is to count the number of lines supporting the moving block (there are two in this question). Note that there are no moving blocks in case (a).

16. C: In any system, the total mechanical energy is the sum of the potential energy and the kinetic energy. Either value could be zero but it still must be included in the total. Choices A and B only give the total potential or kinetic energy, respectively.

17. D: The decibel scale is used to measure the intensity of sound waves. The decibel scale is a ratio of a particular sound's intensity to a standard value. Since it is a logarithmic scale, it is measured by a factor of 10. Choice A is the name of the effect experienced by an observer of a moving wave; Choice B is a particle in an atom; Choice C is a unit for measuring power.

18. D: Polarization changes the oscillations of a wave and can alter the appearance in light waves. For example, polarized sunglasses remove the "glare" from sunlight by altering the oscillation pattern observed by the wearer. Choice A, reflection, is the bouncing back of a wave, such as in a mirror; Choice B is the bending of a wave as it travels from one medium to another, such as going from air to water; and Choice C, dispersion, is the spreading of a wave through a barrier or a prism.

19. A: In an elastic collision, the objects collide and then travel in different directions; in an inelastic collision, the objects collide and then stick together in their final direction of travel. Both types of collisions adhere to the principle of the conservation of linear momentum. As such, the total momentum for the objects in either an elastic or inelastic collision will be the same before and after a collision.

20. D: The *mechanical advantage* is calculated by comparing the force input by the user to the simple machine with the force output from the use of the machine. This calculation is performed through a ratio:

$$Mechanical\ Advantage = \frac{output\ force}{input\ force}$$

$$MA = \frac{F_{out}}{F_{in}}$$

Choice A, the force input divided by the force output, is the reciprocal of the mechanical advantage. Choice B is an incorrect equation and would result in a force, not a ratio. Choice C is not used for any calculation.

Index

Muscle, 111, 146, 148, 151, 152, 164

Mutations, 116

Myofibrils, 151

Narrative Writing, 51

Nephrons, 168

Nerve Cell Body, 153

Nervous, 74, 146, 150, 152, 153, 154, 155, 156, 157, 165

Neuroglia, 153

Neurons, 146, 152, 153, 157

Neurotransmitters, 138, 146, 153

Neutral, 52, 54, 94, 124, 133, 134, 184

Neutral Tone, 52

Neutrons, 124, 135, 184

Neutrophils, 160

Newtons, 176

Nonmetals, 126

Nuclear Chemistry, 135

Nuclear Envelope, 106, 107, 114

Nucleic Acids, 102, 104, 136, 139

Nucleoid, 106

Nucleolus, 106, 113

Nucleotides, 104, 139

Nucleus, 100, 106, 113, 114, 124, 135, 152, 184

Numerator, 19, 20, 21, 25, 26, 27, 28, 29, 32, 34, 35

Object of the Preposition, 77, 93

Objective Pronouns, 74

Observation, 100

Occipital Lobe, 155

Odd Numbers, 11

Ohms, 185

Okazaki Fragments, 117

Orbitals, 124

Order of Operations, 37, 40

Organ Systems, 142, 146

Organelles, 106, 107, 108

Organs, 54, 74, 142, 146, 147, 149, 157, 159, 165, 168, 170

Ossification, 150

Osteoblasts, 150

Osteoclasts, 150

Osteocytes, 150

Ovaries, 170

Ovum, 170

Oxidation Numbers, 133

Oxidation-Reduction (or Redox) Reactions, 132

Oxidative Phosphorylation, 109, 110, 111

Pancreas, 159, 165, 167

Parallel Circuits, 186

Parallel Structure, 85

Parallelism, 85, 86

Parasympathetic, 156

Parathyroid Glands, 158

Parentheses, 12, 16, 37, 38, 89, 90, 129

Parietal Lobe, 155

Participial Phrases, 76

Participles, 76

Particles, 76, 108, 124, 129, 135, 148, 181

Past, 61, 76

Past Participle, 76

Pelvic Cavity, 142

Peptide Bonds, 104, 138

Percent Concentration, 131

Percent Yield, 132

Percentage, 30, 32, 33, 34, 35, 94

Perineal Structures, 170

Periodic Table, 124, 125, 126, 128

Periods, 47, 80, 126

Periosteum, 150

Peripheral Nervous System (PNS), 156

Peristalsis, 165

Peroxisome, 107

Personal Pronouns, 73

Persuasive Writing, 52

pH, 123, 134, 165, 166, 167, 168

Phagocytosis, 108

Phenotype, 115

Phosphate Group, 103, 104, 105, 106, 109, 113, 138, 139

Phospholipids, 103, 104, 138

Phrase, 48, 54, 74, 75, 76, 77, 78, 82, 84, 86, 89, 91

Physiology, 142

Pineal Gland, 158

Pituitary Gland, 142, 158

Place Value, 21, 29

Plane, 114, 142, 176

Plasma Membrane, 106, 108

Plasmodesmata, 107

Platelets, 149, 160

Polarity, 101

Polymers, 102, 104

Polynucleotides, 104

Dear HESI Admission Assessment Test Taker,

We would like to start by thanking you for purchasing this study guide for your HESI exam. We hope that we exceeded your expectations.

Our goal in creating this study guide was to cover all of the topics that you will see on the test. We also strove to make our practice questions as similar as possible to what you will encounter on test day. With that being said, if you found something that you feel was not up to your standards, please send us an email and let us know.

We would also like to let you know about other books in our catalog that may interest you.

ATI TEAS 7

This can be found on Amazon: amazon.com/dp/1637759886

NCLEX-RN

amazon.com/dp/1637753292

We have study guides in a wide variety of fields. If the one you are looking for isn't listed above, then try searching for it on Amazon or send us an email.

Thanks Again and Happy Testing!
Product Development Team
info@studyguideteam.com

FREE Test Taking Tips Video/DVD Offer

To better serve you, we created videos covering test taking tips that we want to give you for FREE. **These videos cover world-class tips that will help you succeed on your test.**

We just ask that you send us feedback about this product. Please let us know what you thought about it—whether good, bad, or indifferent.

To get your **FREE videos**, you can use the QR code below or email freevideos@studyguideteam.com with "Free Videos" in the subject line and the following information in the body of the email:

    a. The title of your product

    b. Your product rating on a scale of 1-5, with 5 being the highest

    c. Your feedback about the product

If you have any questions or concerns, please don't hesitate to contact us at info@studyguideteam.com.

Thank you!